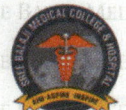

SREE BALAJI MEDICAL COLLEGE & HOSPITAL

A constituent college of

BHARATH INSTITUTE OF HIGHER EDUCATION AND RESEARCH

(Declared as Deemed to be University under section 3 of UGC Act, 1956)

(Vide Notification No.F.9-5/2000-U.3,Ministry of Humand Resource Development, Govt. of India, dated 4ᵗʰ July, 2002)

Phone: 044-42911000, Telefax:044-22415051

Website: www.sbmch.ac.in

7, Works Road, Chromepet,

Chennai 600 044,Tamil Nadu

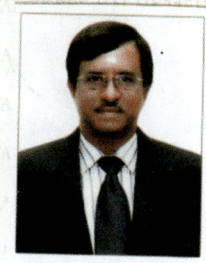

FOREWORD

I am just recollecting the release of the first edition of this book earlier and am delighted with the success of the first edition. I have great pleasure to write the foreword for the 2nd edition of this book titled TEST BOOK OF MODERN PHARMACOLOGY authored by Dr. M. Muniappan, Ph.D, Dr. R. Sivaraj, M.D., and Dr. Somasundaram, M.D., and edited by Dr. N.S. Muthiah, MD., all senior faculty of Pharmacology of repute.

This book will be useful for the undergraduates as well as Post Graduate students in order to learn the latest and modern Pharmacology to prescribe the needy patients. Medical knowledge and practice change constantly. This book is designed to provide accurate, authoritative information about the subject matter. This book is a valuable addition to the already existing books of Pharmacology.

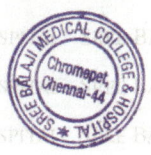

Dr. P. SAIKUMAR, M.D., Ph.D.,

DEAN - SBMCH

Dr. G. M. Yahya, M.B.B.S., M.sc.
Professor of Pharmacology
Dean, Thanjavur Medical College & Hospital (Retd.)

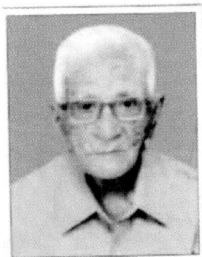

"Amir Mahal"
257 Bharathi Salai
Royapettah
Chennai - 600 014
Ph: 044-4215 8463

Date: 17-07-2018

FOREWORD

It gives me immense pleasure to write the foreword for this book in pharmacology, authored by Dr. M. Muniappan and edited by Dr. N.S. Muthiah.

It is the short, concise book of pharmacology concentrating more on commonly used approved drugs in the treatment of common clinical conditions. It is more like clinically oriented without much detail about pharmacokinetics, chemistry etc., of the drugs.

In a short book of this nature, there may be some deficiencies. The students may refer to the standard books for more information. The author has taken lot of pains to write this text to make the subject of pharmacology more interesting by illustrations, designs and diagrams.

I have no doubt that this book will help the medical students and general practitioners to read, understand, apply the knowledge of pharmacology in the treatment of sick patients to cure and reduce their sufferings.

The science of pharmacology has progressed, tremendously in all directions over half a century. So, my sincere advice to the medical students and the young medical practitioners is to be in touch in clinical pharmacology and recent advances to be a successful clinician which will be useful to them.

The country in general and Chennai, Tamil Nadu in particular is on the world medical map because of the hard dedicated work of some of the physicians and surgeons. Follow them as example and reach their standard.

DR. G. M. YAHYA, M.B.B.S., M Sc.,
PROFESSOR OF PHARMACOLOGY
Dean, Thanjavur Medical College & Hospitals
(RETD.)
Amir Mahal, Pycrofts Road,
Royapettah: Chennai - 600 014

Third Edition

Textbook of
Modern
Pharmacology
for MBBS Students

Pharmacology Made Easier

As per the latest syllabus prescribed by MCI

M Muniappan PhD (Pharmacology)
Ex-Professor
Department of Pharmacology
Sree Balaji Medical College and Hospital
(BIHER, Deemed to be University)
Chennai

G Somasundaram MD
Professor and Head
Department of Pharmacology
SLIMS, Puducherry
(BIHER, Deemed to be University)

R Sivaraj MD, DIH
Professor and Head
Department of Pharmacology
Arupadai Veedu Medical College and Hospital
Kirumampakkam, Puducherry
Vinayaka Mission's Research Foundation
(Deemed to be University under Section 3 of the UGC Act, 1956)

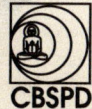

CBSPD

CBS Publishers & Distributors Pvt Ltd

New Delhi • Bengaluru • Chennai • Kochi • Kolkata • Lucknow • Mumbai
Hyderabad • Jharkhand • Nagpur • Patna • Pune • Uttarakhand

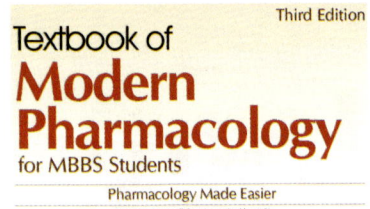

ISBN: 978-93-89688-01-6

Third Edition: 2021
Reprint: 2024
First Edition: 2018
Second Edition: 2019

Published by Satish Kumar Jain and produced by Varun Jain for

CBS Publishers & Distributors Pvt Ltd

4819/XI Prahlad Street, 24 Ansari Road, Daryaganj, New Delhi 110 002, India.
Ph: 23289259, 23266861   Website: www.cbspd.com

e-mail: delhi@cbspd.com

Corporate Office: 204 FIE, Industrial Area, Patparganj, Delhi 110 092
Ph: 011-4934 4934   Fax: 011-4934 4935 e-mail: publishing@cbspd.com

Branches

- **Bengaluru:** Seema House 2975, 17th Cross, K.R. Road, Banasankari 2nd Stage, Bengaluru 560 070, Karnataka, India
  Ph: +91-80-26771678/79   Fax: +91-80-26771680   e-mail: bangalore@cbspd.com
- **Chennai:** 7, Subbaraya Street, Shenoy Nagar, Chennai 600 030, Tamil Nadu, India
  Ph: +91-44-26680620, 26681266   Fax: +91-44-42032115   e-mail: chennai@cbspd.com
- **Kochi:** 42/1325, 1326, Power House Road, Opp KSEB, Ernakulam 682 018, Kochi, Kerala, India
  Ph: +91-484-4059061-67   Fax: +91-484-4059065   e-mail: kochi@cbspd.com
- **Kolkata:** 147, Hind Ceramics Compound, 1st Floor, Nilgunj Road, Belghoria, Kolkata 700 056, West Bengal, India
  Ph: +91-33-25633055/56   e-mail: kolkata@cbspd.com
- **Lucknow:** Basement, Khushnuma Complex, 7-Meerabai Marg (Behind Jawahar Bhawan), Lucknow 226 001, UP, India
  Ph: +0552-4000032   e-mail:tiwari.lucknowi@cbspd.com
- **Mumbai:** PWD Shed. Gala no. 25/26, Ramchandra Bhatt Marg, Next to JJ Hospital Gate no. 2, Opp. Union Bank of India, Noorbaug, Mumbai 400 009, Maharashtra, India
  Ph: 022-66661880/89   e-mail: mumbai@cbspd.com

Representatives

• Hyderabad	0-9885175004	• Jharkhand	0-9811541605	• Nagpur	0-8692091830
• Patna	0-9334159340	• Pune	0-9664372571	• Uttarakhand	0-9716462459

Printed at : Goyal Offset Works Pvt. Ltd. Haryana (INDIA)

CONTRIBUTORS

The following professors have contributed some topics and also given good suggestions to improve the standard of this book:

▷ **Dr. N.Venkatadri,** M.D., Professor & Head, Department of Pharmacology, Sathyasai Medical College, Chennai

▷ **Dr A. Ruckmani,** M.D., Professor & Head, Department of Pharmacology, Chettinad Institute of medical Sciences & Research, Chennai.

▷ **Dr. P. Durairajan,** M.D., Professor and Head, Department of Pharmacology, Muthukumaran Medical College, Mangadu, Chennai.

▷ **Dr. S. Priestly Vivek kumar,** M.D., Professor and Head, Department of Pharmacology, Tagore Medical College & Hospital, Chennai.

▷ **Dr. Thirunavukkarasu,** M.D., Professor and Head, Department of Pharmacology, Saveetha Medical College and Hospital, Thandalam, Chennai.

PREFACE

Pharmacology is the dynamic medical subject. So many new chapters are added in this edition as per MCI. All the diagrams are imposed and computerized. The headings are given in different colours to make easy capture for the students.

Learning objectives are given in the beginning of every chapter, so as the students should concentrate more on those points. Unnecessary details are excluded. All the diagrams are made simple and colourful so as the students can easily understand the subject.

Every care has been taken to make the book free from the errors, but absolute perfection may not be there. Hence, error if any, may please be communicated to us.

We are thankful to Dr. Nagesh Simhadri, Assistant Professor, Tagore Medical College and Hospital, Chennai, for nice, simple computerized pictures.

M.Muniappan
mmuniappan@yahoo.com

R.Sivaraj
sivaraj.rangaraj@avmc.edu.in

CONTENTS

Chapters   Pages

SECTION-III PERIPHERAL NERVOUS SYSTEM

SECTION- IV AUTACOIDS

SECTION-V   CARDIO VASCULAR SYSTEM INCLUDING DIURETICS

SECTION–VI RESPIRATORY SYSTEM

SECTION-VII   CENTRAL NERVOUS SYSTEM

SECTION–VIII   BLOOD AND BLOOD FORMING ORGANS

SECTION-IX GASTROINTESTINAL SYSTEM

SECTION–X HORMONES

SECTION–XI   CHEMOTHERAPY

SECTION-XII MISCELLANEOUS

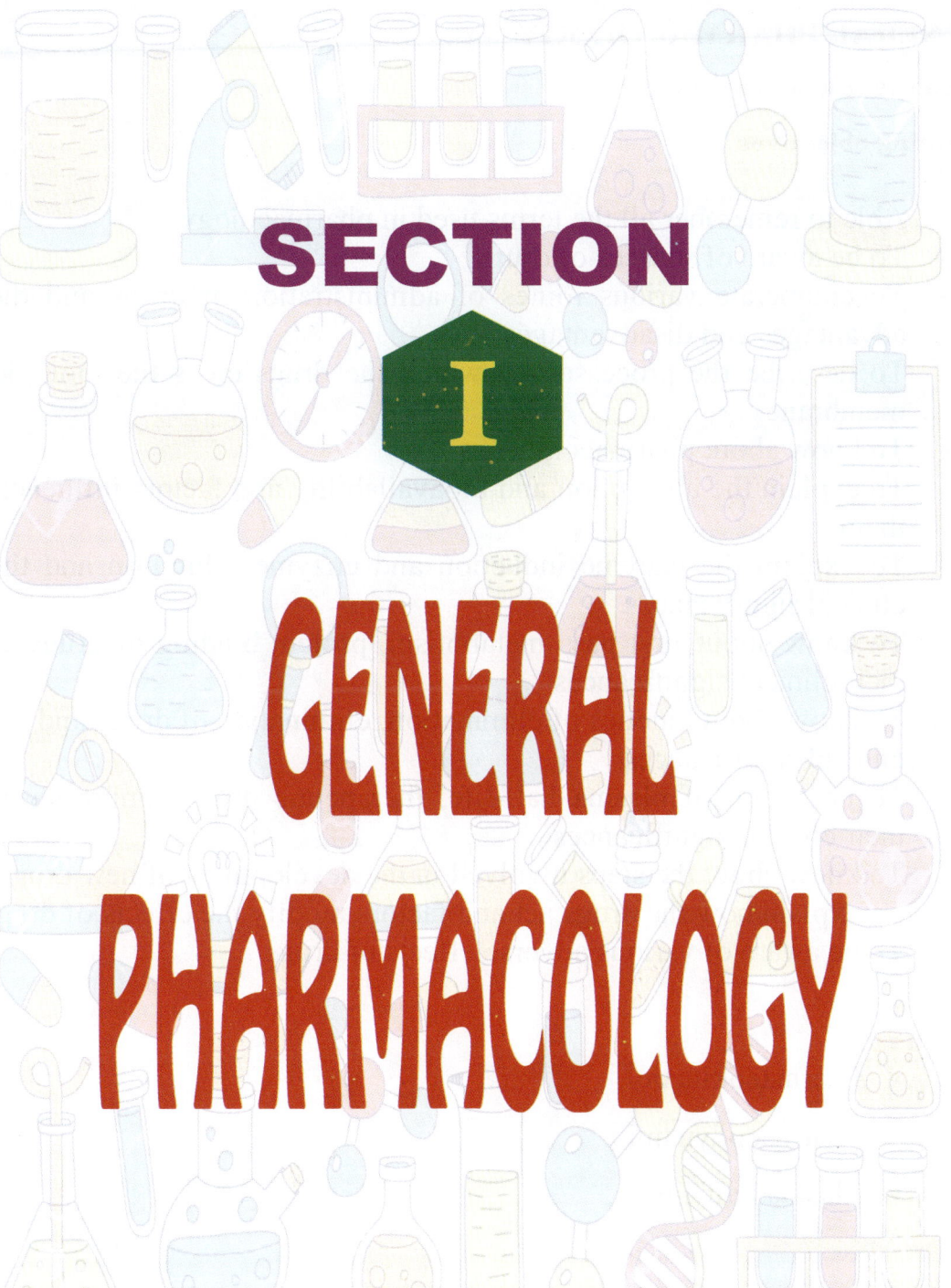

SECTION

I

GENERAL
PHARMACOLOGY

GENERAL PHARMACOLOGY

General considerations

Learning objectives

- Able to remember all the terms used in pharmacology
- To be aware of sources of drugs
- To enumerate various routes of administration of drugs and their advantages and disadvantages
- To describe the processes by which the drugs cross the biological membrane
- To know about pharmacokinetics
- To explain the absorption and bioavailability and factors influencing them
- To explain the enzyme induction and enzyme inhibition and their clinical significances
- To know about first pass metabolism, protein binding of drugs and their clinical significances
- To know about kinetics of elimination, elimination of drugs and their clinical significances
- To be aware of plasma half-life, therapeutic drug monitoring and their clinical significances
- To know about the steps involved in the development of new drug
- To explain how the drugs act and factors modify the effects of drugs
- To be aware of various adverse effects of drugs

Key terms

- ✓ Pharmacokinetic
- ✓ Pharmacodynamic
- ✓ Plasma half-life

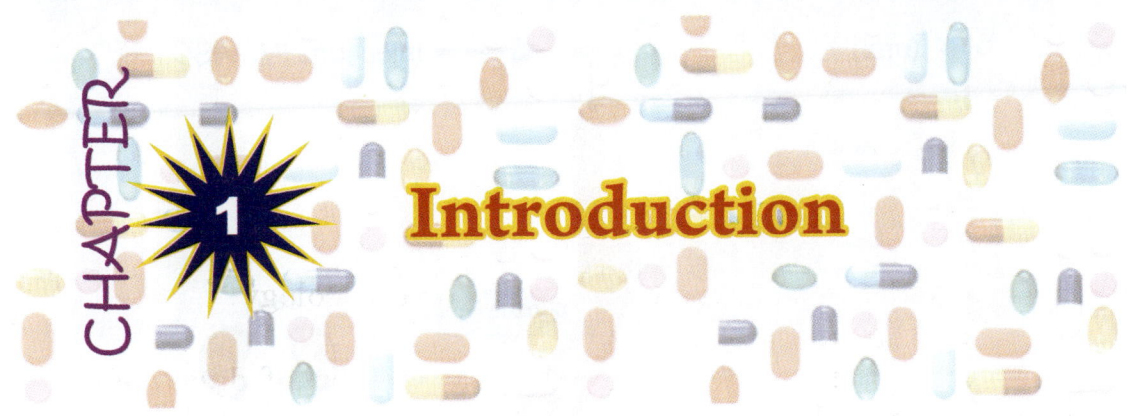

Introduction

CHAPTER 1

It is better to know some terms commonly used in pharmacology before going to general pharmacology.

PHARMACOLOGY is derived from Greek word, 'Pharmakon'=drug and 'logos'='science' or 'study'. In short, Pharmacology means, 'study of drugs' (i.e., everything about the drugs).

The term DRUG is derived from French word 'Drough' means, 'herb'. Since in the earlier days, most of the agents used in the treatment of diseases are derived from 'herbs'.

Earlier the term Drug is defined as a chemical agent that is used to prevent, diagnose and cure or treat the diseases. But the oral contraceptive is used to prevent pregnancy, which is not a disease. It is physiological process and also general anaesthetic does not fit in the above definition. The general anaesthetic does not cure / prevent disease.

As per WHO, the definition of a drug is "any chemical agent used either to modify or explore pathological states or physiological system to the benefit of the recipients".

PHARMACOKINETIC: (Fig.1) Kinetic means, movement. It deals with the study of the movement of drug in and out of the body. That is to study what happens to the drug from the entry till it comes out of the body.

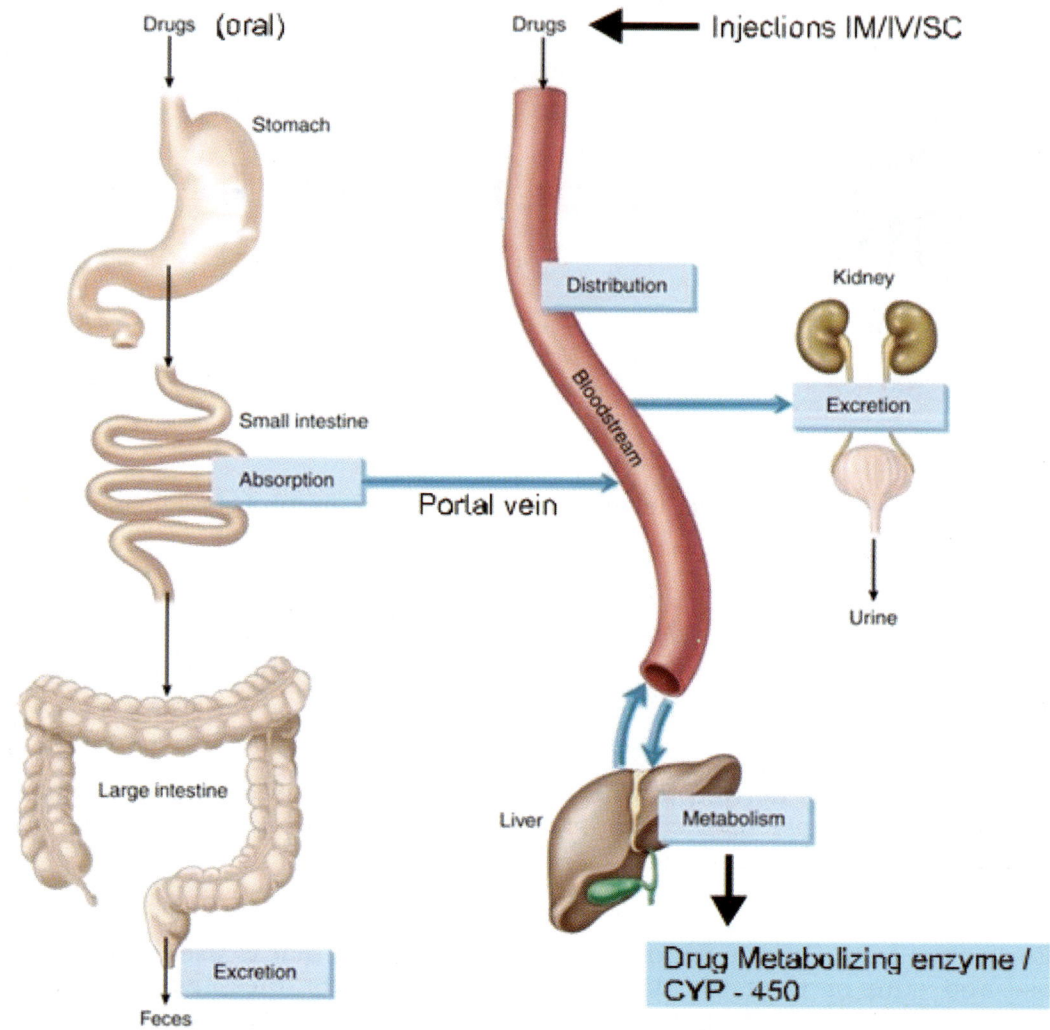

Fig. 01 : Pharmacokinetic

This includes absorption, metabolism, distribution and excretion of drugs and their CLINICAL SIGNIFICANCES. In short we can also refer this process as "what body does to the drug".

PHARMACODYNAMIC: (Fig. 02) Dynamic means, power. It deals with the power of the drug i.e., to produce pharmacological actions and how it produces that actions? (Mechanism of action of drugs). In short it deals with the study of the pharmacological actions and mechanism of actions of drugs.

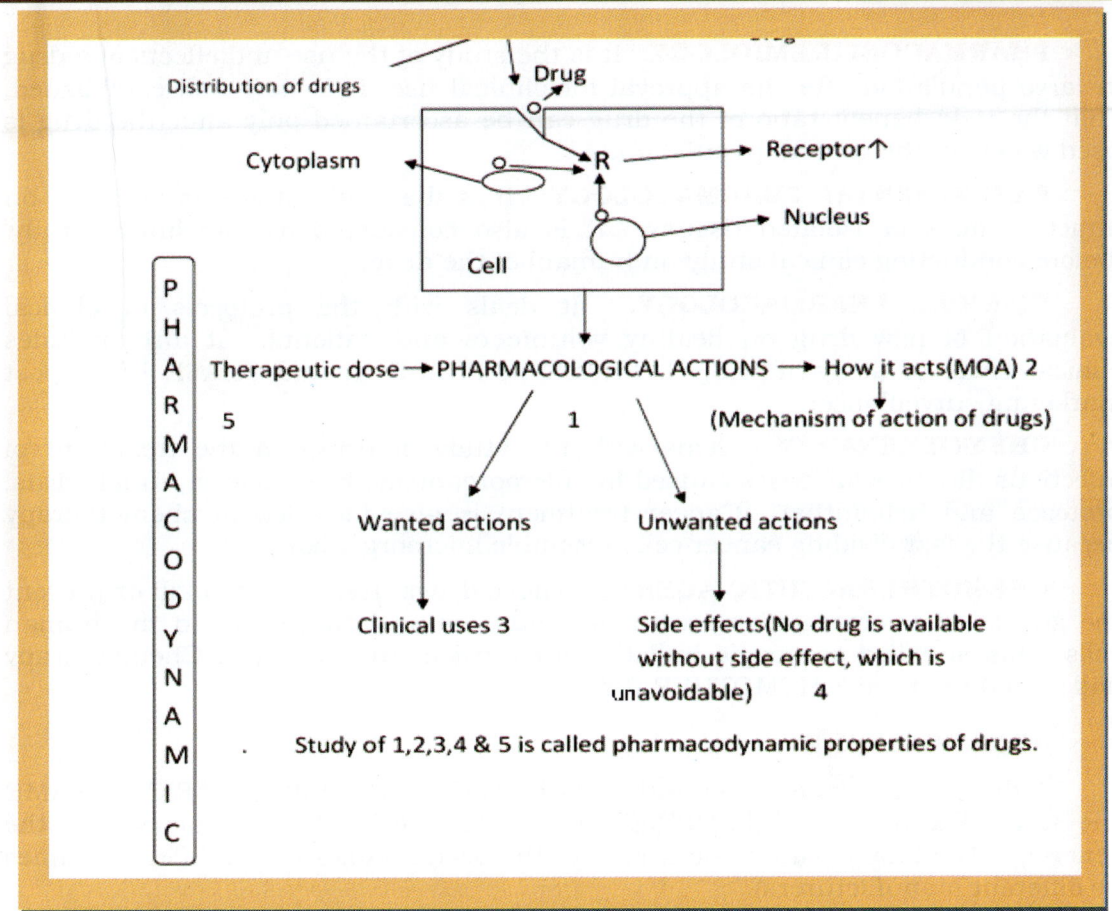

Fig. 02 : Pharmacodynamic

PHARMACOTHERAPHY: is the application of pharmacological actions in therapy (treatment).

PHARMACOVIGILANCE: Many rare adverse effects have been found out during the post marketing surveillance of the drugs. So, pharmacovigilance means continuous monitoring for unwanted effects of marketed drugs. It is the science related to the Detection, Assessment, Understanding and Prevention (DAUP) of adverse effects or any other drug related problems.

PHARMACOGENETIC: To study the genetic variation in drug metabolism or drug response (example: Haemolysis is common in the individual who is showing deficiency of Glucose 6 Phosphate Dehydrogenase (G6PDH). Example : Primaquine inhibit the enzyme G6PDH and cause haemolysis in the above said individual.

PHARMACOGENOMIC: Treatment of diseases by genetic material according to the gene mapping of the individual.

PHARMACOEPIDEMIOLOGY: It is the study of the use and effects of a drug in large population after its approval for clinical use. It is now well established. That the risk: benefit ratio of the drug can be ascertained only after the drug is used widely in the general population.

EXPERIMENTAL PHARMACOLOGY: It is the study of effects of drugs on intact animals or isolated tissues. It is also considered as 'preclinical study' (before conducting clinical study on human) of the drug.

CLINICAL PHARMACOLOGY: It deals with the protocols of clinical evaluation of new drug on healthy volunteers and patients. It also includes clinical trials of drugs (PHASE I, PHASE II, PHASE III and PHASE IV or post marketing surveillance).

CHEMOTHERAPHY: deals with the study of drugs in the treatment of infectious diseases (diseases caused by microorganisms like bacteria, fungi, virus, protozoa and helminths). Cancer treatment is also included in chemotherapy because the fast dividing cancer cells resemble microorganisms.

CHEMOTHERAPEUTIC AGENTS: Those drugs used either to kill or prevent the growth of microorganisms with minimum or no lethal effect to the human cells. This is called as 'magic bullet'. Paul Ehrlich, the Father of Chemotherapy has coined the term 'CHEMOTHERAPY'.

NOMENCLATURE:

A drug may be prescribed either by its GENERIC NAME / OFFICIAL NAME OR BY ITS BRAND NAME (PROPRIETARY NAME). But in Pharmacology, only the generic/ official name should be used, not the brand names (given different names by different manufacturers).

Official name / Generic name	Proprietary name / Trade name
(1) Paracetamol	Crocin, dolo-650
(2) Diazepam	Valium, Calmpose
(3) Zolpidem	Zolfresh
(4) Metronidazole	Flagyl
(5) Clotrimazole	Candid

COMPLIANCE: If a patient follows fully the doctor's prescription, then the patient compliance is good. If the patients do not follow strictly as per doctor's prescription or advice is called patient's poor compliance due to many reasons.

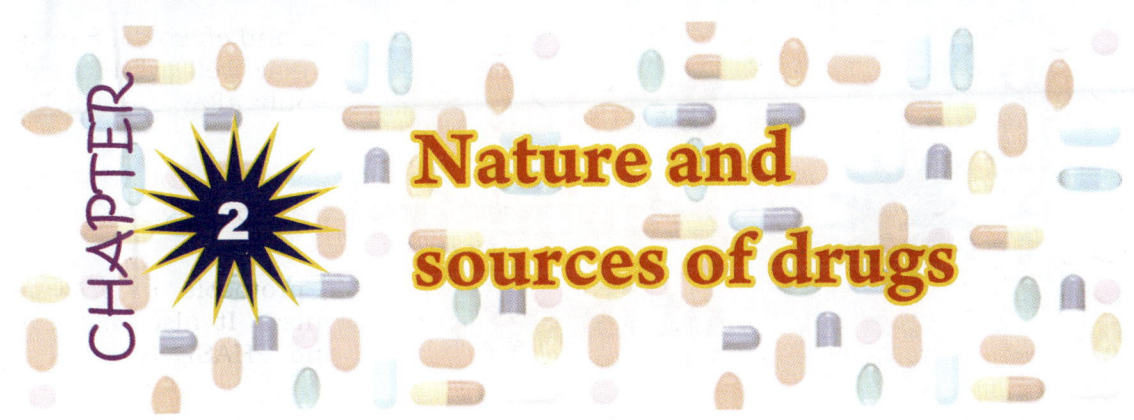

CHAPTER

2

Nature and sources of drugs

This will be also dealt at the time of explaining the individual drugs. It is briefly explained here.

Sources of drugs mean, from where the drugs have been obtained. Nature means, the chemical nature of the drug.

1. From Plants: Alkaloids (Atropine, Morphine), Glycosides (cardiac glycoside like digoxin)

2. From Animals: Pig (Insulin), Horse serum (Anti Serum), Human urine (Pregnant)-Gonadotropic Hormones.

3. From Microbes: (ANTIBIOTICS) Antibiotic is a drug that derived from the microorganisms and used either to kill or prevent the growth of **other** microorganisms Example: Ampicillin, Amoxicillin, Cephalosporins, Gentamicin etc.,

4. Synthetic: More than 90% of the drugs are synthetic in nature (manufactured in the drug industry)

5. DNA Recombinant technology: It is also one type of synthesizing the drugs. Large amount can be synthesized. Example : Humulin (very closely resemble human Insulin). A note about DNA recombinant technology: They are genetically engineered drugs. A desired gene is inserted into a very fast multiplying non-pathogenic strain of some bacteria e.g., E.coli-K12 by this method. This host cell will now produce large amount of the gene-directed proteins (DRUGS), which are required. E.coli, otherwise, does not synthesize these proteins. e.g., Humulin (a human Insulin synthesized by inserting proinsulin gene). Humulin is very closely resembles human Insulin.

6. Mineral Source: Ferrous sulphate (used in anaemia), Aluminium hydroxide (antacid).

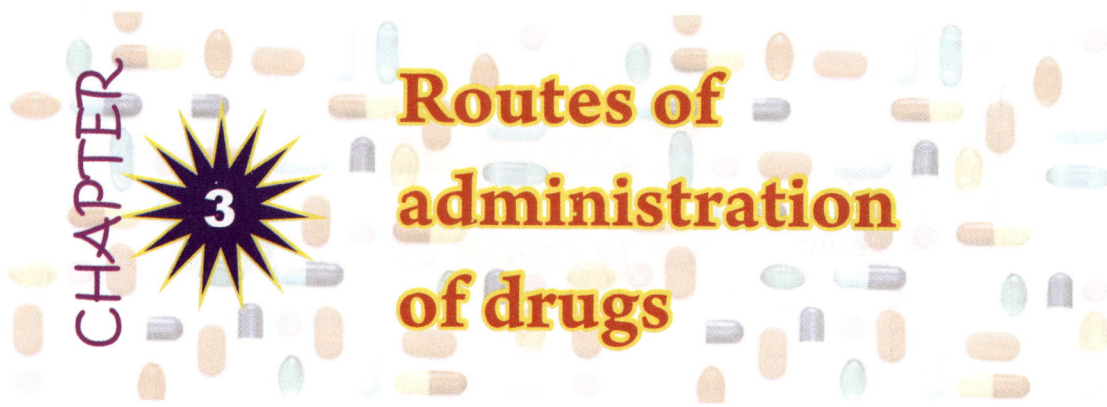

Routes of administration of drugs

CHAPTER 3

Routes of administration of drugs is the method by which the drug is introduced into the body.

CLASSIFICATION OF ROUTES OF ADMINISTRATION OF DRUGS. (Fig.3)

Enteral	Parenteral (par=away, enteral = GIT, away from GIT)	Topical
1.Oral 2.Sublingual 3.Rectal 4.Buccal	1.Injections i)subcutaneous ii)intramuscular iii)intravenous iv)intradermal v)interathecal/epidural vi)intraarticular vii)intraarterial 2.Inhalational administration 3.Transdermal administration	1.Drops i)nasal, eye and ear drops) 2.Vaginal, urethral tablets 3.Dermal – gel, ointment

For local action: The drug need not be absorbed. But for systemic action, the drug should be absorbed (absorption means, entry of the drug into the blood stream from the site of administration)

ORAL ROUTE: The drugs are administered by swallowing from the mouth. This route is meant for both local and systemic actions.

Dosage forms: tablet, capsule, powder, liquid preparations.

ORAL   SUB-LINGUAL   RECTAL - SUPPOSITORIES

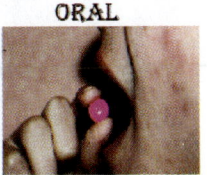 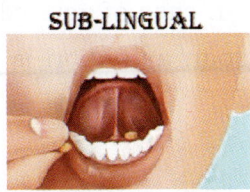 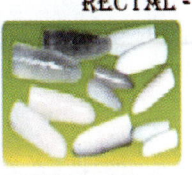 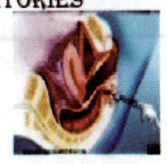

Fig. 03   ROUTES OF DRUG ADMINISTRATION

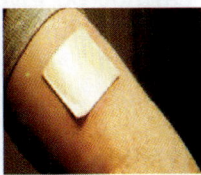 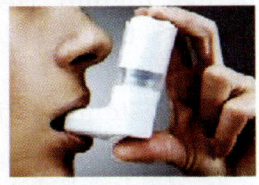 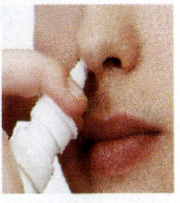 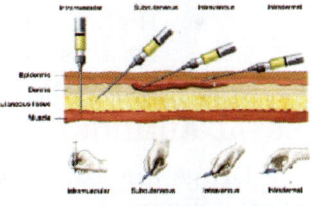

TRANSDERMAL PATCH   INHALATIONAL   NASAL   PARENTERAL

Advantages/merits of oral administration:

- Most common method.
- Very safe
- Self administration is possible.
- Non invasive
- Painless
- Economical, since sterilization and other procedure are not needed.

Disadvantages/demerits:

- Slow onset of action. Not suitable in emergency condition.
- Many drugs being polar are not absorbed (Gentamicin).
- The drugs which are destroyed by the gastric juice cannot be given by this route.
- The drugs which are having high first pass metabolism cannot be given by this route. (Example : GTN (Glyceryl Tri Nitrate)
- This route is not suitable in unconscious, noncooperative patients or in patients having severe vomiting.
- Unpalatable substances cannot be given by this route.

SUBLINGUAL ADMINISTRATION:

The drug is kept under the tongue mainly for systemic action. Example : Glyceryl Tri Nitrate (GTN)

Merits:

- This route is suitable for those drugs which have got high first pass metabolism, since this route bypasses liver (portal circulation) for the first time. The drug directly goes to the systemic circulation.

- Quick onset of action.

- Self administration is possible in case of emergency.
- The drug can be spit out as soon as action is over in order to avoid the side effects.

Demerits:

- Distasteful, irritant drugs cannot be given by this route.
- Higher molecular weight drugs like Insulin, Heparin cannot be given by this route, (otherwise it will be the best route for Insulin and Heparin).

RECTAL ADMINISTRATION for both local and systemic actions.

Drugs are administered through rectum. Dosage forms: suppository (conical shape) - Example : Dulcolax – (purgative in children). Liquids are administered with high pressure (enema). Example: Evacuant enema (soap water) is used to clear the GIT in case of emergency evacuation of bowel.

Merits:

- Useful in patients having severe nausea and vomiting.
- This route may be convenient in noncooperative children, (Diazepam suppository in febrile convulsion in children)
- It is alternate route for gastric irritant drugs.

Demerits:

- Inconvenient and embrassing to the patients.
- The drugs soil the clothes.
- Rectal inflammation is possible.
- Absorption is unreliable.

PARENTERAL ROUTES:

- Drugs are administered away from GIT (par= away, enteral=GIT) usually by injections or by inhalation.
- Injection → It is given by using needle and puncturing the skin. This route is preferred mainly for systemic action.
- Inhalation → The drug is administered through nose and mouth to the respiratory tract for local or systemic action.

INTRAMUSCULAR INJECTION:

Drugs are injected deep into the skeletal muscles.

Sites: Deltoid muscle, gluteal muscle of buttock (preferred for depot or long acting preparations of drugs).

Merits:

- Injections are suitable for those drugs which cannot be given by oral route. Injections are preferred, when quick action is required.
- Bioavailability is high (90 to 100%) after injection.
- Depot or long acting preparations are given by this route.

Demerits:

- Painful at the site of injection.
- Self administration is difficult.
- Expensive.
- Perfect aseptic conditions are required.
- Chances of abscesses or nerve damage at the site of injection is possible.
- Large volume cannot be given through this route.

SUBCUTANEOUS INJECTION:

The drugs are injected into the subcutaneous tissues of forearm, abdomen and thigh.

Merits:

- Self administration is possible.
- This is the best route for administering highly potent drug (among injections). Because of less blood supply, there will be slow absorption and hence less toxic. (Morphine, Insulin, Low molecular weight Heparin).
- Also depot preparation for prolonged action is given by this route (Example: Progesterone implant into the subcutaneous tissues for prolonged action as contraceptive).

Demerits:

- Only small volume can be given (maximum of 1 ml).
- Irritant drugs produce necrosis.
- Not suitable in shock as reduced blood circulation decreases the rate of absorption.

DERMOJET:

Subcutaneous administration of drugs with pressure (without needle). Useful for mass inoculation. No need for repeated sterilization.

INTRAVENOUS INJECTION (I.V.): (Slow administration of drugs into the vein is called as infusion)

Site: The drugs are injected into antecubital vein.

Merits:

- I.V. Injection is suitable for those drugs which cannot be given by oral route. I.V. injections preferred, when quick action is required.
- Bioavailability is 100%
- It is the best route in emergency.
- Large volume can be given (Example : IV infusion of Dextrose, Saline, Blood).
- For controlled dosage administration; (IV infusion of Oxytocin and IV General Anaesthetics).

Demerits:

- Painful at the site of injection.
- Self administration is difficult.
- Expensive.
- Perfect aseptic conditions are required.
- Chances of abscesses or nerve damage at the site of injection is possible.
- Necrosis and thrombophlebitis are common.
- Care should be taken that air should not enter into the vein (air embolism is fatal).
- Drugs of oily or suspension in nature (used for long action) cannot be given by this route.

INHALATIONAL ADMINISTRATION OF DRUGS:

The drugs are administered by inhalation through mouth and nose (through respiratory tract).

Example: Volatile general anaesthetics, Salbutamol in bronchial asthma, steroid (Beclomethasone) in bronchial asthma.

The drugs are administered and excreted through the same route.

Absorption is through alveoli (plenty of blood supply and also vast surface area). So the absorption is quick and there will be quick onset of action.

General anaesthetic dose is accurately monitored. (Fig.12)

TOPICAL ROUTES: Mainly for local action.

Example: Eye drops, Ear drops, Nasal drops, vaginal tablet, foam etc., Diclofenac sodium spray on skin is for systemic action (analgesic and anti-inflammatory actions).

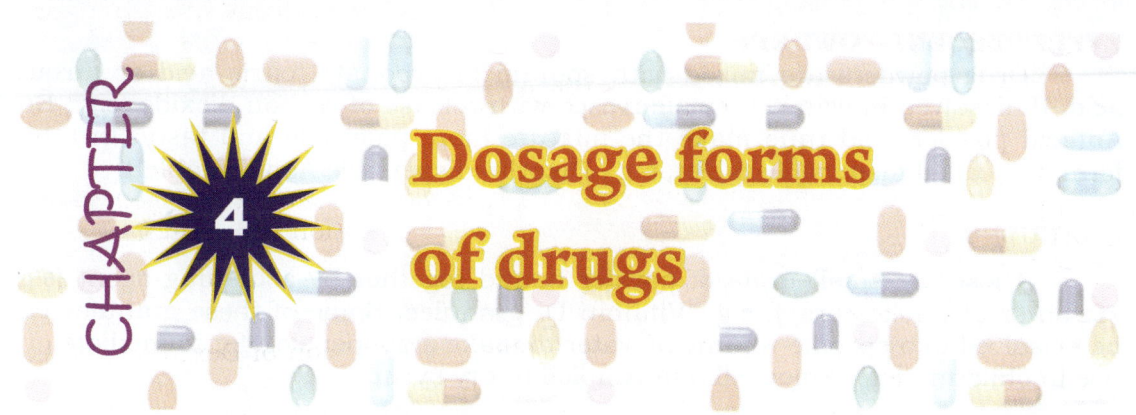

CHAPTER

4

Dosage forms of drugs

In the modern days, the pharmacist is no longer required to prepare or to dispense the drugs for doctors' prescription. Drugs are now prepared and well packed by the pharmaceutical companies and supplied in various dosage forms and formulations for dispensing to the patients. The drugs are not administered as formulated Syrups, capsules, tablets or injections.

FORMULATION OF DRUGS

It is a recipe of drug preparation. It consists of active ingredients (the drug) and other substances like excipients, vehicles, flavouring agents and preservatives, with the quantity of each components.

DOSAGE FORM

It is the form (e.g., as tablet or capsule or injection or oral liquid) in which the above formulation of the drug can be administered to a patient.

EXCIPIENTS

Pharmacologically inert substances which are added to the pharmaceutical preparation either to add bulk of the tablet (active drug is extremely small in quantity) or to mask (or reduce) the unpalatable taste e.g., lactose, calcium lactate, starch etc.,

VEHICLES

These are the substances which are used to dissolve or suspend the drugs, in a pharmaceutical preparation, to make them suitable into usage form (as in ointments) or more palatable (as in liquids), e.g., sugar syrups, cherry syrup, gum acacia and petroleum jelly etc.,

CLASSIFICATION OF DOSAGE FORMS :

SOLID DOSAGE FORMS

POWDERS

These may be one drug or combination of drugs in a dried and finely powdered form intended for external use (e.g., dusting powders, boric acid) or for oral use (e.g., Aspirin powder).

EFFERVESCENT POWDERS

Drug powders are mixed with sodium bicarbonate, citric acid or tartaric acid. If dissolved in water, they effervesce with release of carbon dioxide (e.g., Eno Antacid powder) and thus make the mixture more palatable and tasty. In tablet form it is called dispersible tablet, e.g., Disprin (dispersible Aspirin tablet).

GRANULES

These are small units of powder bound together by a binding agent (e.g., starch or alcoholic spray), e.g., Vitamin D_3 granules. Some of these granules can be dissolved in a specific volume of water to make a suspension for immediate oral use in children, e.g., Amoxicillin or Ampicillin dry syrup.

TABLETS

Drugs which are powdered or granulated form are compressed under heavy pressure into a round or oval shaped making them suitable for swallowing.

i) **Ordinary Tablets**
   These are uncoated compressed tablets, e.g., Paracetamol tablets.

ii) **Sugar-coated Tablets**
   These tablets are coated with sugar to avoid bitter taste of ingredients, e.g., tab, Chloroquine, tab. Metronidazole.

iii) **Film-coated Tablets**
   A transparent film coating is done by gelatin or cellulose derivatives just to mask the unpleasant taste. But the tablet size or weight remains the same. E.g., Cefuroxime film coated tablet, Diltiazem film coated tablet etc.,

iv) **Enteric-coated Tablets**
   Coating of the tablet is made by cellulose acid phthalate, shellac or keratin which are resistant to gastric acid but dissolve at intestinal alkaline pH. The active drug is protected from destruction by acidic pH. Gastric irritation is reduced, e.g., Diclofenac enteric coated tab Enteric coated enzyme preparation), Enteric coated Aspirin tablets.

v) **Long acting tablets (retard tablets-R, sustained release tablets-SR)**
   Each unit of drug particles have individual coating with different types of inert resins so that each type of coating dissolves at different time intervals. Such tablets provide a steady and sustained release of the drug over a period of 10-12 hr and hence have a lesser side effects, e.g., Pot.chloride retard tabs, Diclofenac sod.sustained release tablet. Nifedipine retard tab. Controlled release drugs are most suitable for drugs of short $t_{1/2}$. Therapeutic failure can occur for life saving drugs such as Nitro glycerine controlled release capsules.

vi) **Pellets**

Drugs which are in sterile spheres prepared by compression of drug powders such as hormonal preparations. Used for subcutaneous depot implantation of the drugs which will be slowly released for a long duration . e.g., Testosterone pellets.

vii) **Lozenges**

It is a tablet form of drug prepared with sugar and resin, and is meant for chewing to provide local effects in mouth or throat e.g., various cough lozenges, throat smoothening agents.

Capsules

These are inert gelatin coated shells of suitable size, incorporating powdered drug and excipients meant for swallowing, e.g., Doxycycline cap., Amoxicillin cap., etc., Thick gelatin capsules are used to incorporate powder form of drug (e.g., Amoxicillin) while soft, thin gelatin capsules are used to incorporate oily drug (e.g., Vit E). The gelatin coating quickly dissolves in gastric juice and release the drug in the GIT.

a) Spansules

These are longer acting capsules, similar to long acting tablets., e.g., Iron formulations, Isosorbide dinitrate Spansules, Nitroglycerine Spansules. These are visible coloured drug granules inside a transparent capsule. These beads are impregnated with various resins which will dissolve at different time intervals.

LIQUID DOSAGE FORMS OF DRUGS

AQUEOUS SOLUTIONS

These are subdivided into the following forms:

i) **Syrups**

Drug(s) present in concentrated solution. Sugar or Sugar free liquids plus flavouring agents and permitted colours, e.g., Commonly used cough syrups, vitamin syrups.

ii) **Solutions (Liquor)**

These are aqueous solutions of therapeutic agents e.g., hydrogen peroxide solution, liquor ammonia and iodine solution.

iii) **Linctus**

Viscous syrupy liquid formulations consist of the drug and demulcents, like menthol. Linctus provides soothing effect in sore throat, e.g., cough linctus.

iv)   **Injections**

These are sterile solutions or suspensions of the drug in appropriate solvent and preservatives which are meant for parenteral use, e.g., Injection Diclofenac, Injection Lignocaine. Some drugs are supplied as dry powders which should be dissolved in aqueous vehicles like water for injection e.g. Cephalosporins, Amoxycillin etc.,

a) **Depot injection**

It is a longer acting injectable preparation similar to long acting Tablets or Spansules, but in injection form. The drug is suspended in sterile oily base from which it is slowly released for a prolonged duration, e.g., Testosterone depot inj. Fluphenazine depot inj.

AQUEOUS SUSPENSION

i)   **Mixtures**

Solid drugs dispersed homogeneously in water by suitable suspending agent (agar agar), e.g.,Milk of magnesia etc.,

ii)   **Emulsions**

They are prepared by mixing two or more immiscible liquid medicaments by means of a suitable suspending agent (Gum acacia). One liquid serves as continuous phase in which the other liquid is dispersed uniformly in fine droplet form, e.g., cod liver oil emulsion, liquid paraffin emulsion. This preparation helps for better absorption of the drugs.

ALCOHOLIC SOLUTIONS

i)   **Spirits**

These are 10% v/v solution of volatile essential oils plus alcohol and are used as flavouring agents, masking agents and to some extent as preservatives, e.g., spirit chloroform, spirit ammonia aromaticus,

ii)   **Elixirs**

These are pleasantly flavoured solutions of a drug in sugar syrup or glycerol along with higher proportions of alcohol,e.g., vitamin B – complex elixirs, cough elixirs; but these preparations are now on the decline. Alcohol is used in elixir as a solvent for drugs that are not suitable for water alone.

iii)   **Tinctures**

These are alcoholic extracts of plant drugs (10-20 w/v), e.g., tinct. belladonna . Many tinctures are used as flavouring agents, e.g., tinct.cardamom . and tinct. Zingibaris (in such cases drug contents many range from 20% to 50%). Hydroalcoholic solutions of inorganic substances known as tinctures, e.g., Tinct.iodine which is used as an antiseptic.

Drops

Used mainly in paediatrics. These formulations contain small quantity of concentrated solutions of drug (s), e.g., vitamin drops and enzyme drops. Eye/ear drops are also included in this category. These are sterile, isotonic buffered solutions of the drug. These are usually supplied in a vial with a dropper, e.g., Ciprofloxacin eye/ear drops, gentamicin eye/ear drops etc.,

Enema

Medicated liquid preparations for rectal route of administration with high pressure and are used for emergency evacuvation of bowel e.g., soap and water enema

DOSAGE FORMS FOR EXTERNAL USE

Liniments

Liquid medicaments to be rubbed on skin with friction. It contains drug (s) in a liniment vehicle (fixed oil or soap) and water or alcohol. One ingredient is usually incorporated with another medium (Capsaicin, camphor which serve as counterirritant). These are mainly used as pain relievers or as rubefacient (making skin red), e.g., liniment capsaicin, and liniment turpentine.

Lotions

Liquid medicaments used for local application but without rubbing. They are generally used as antiseptics, soothing agents, astringents and antipruritic agents, e.g., Permethrin lotion, zinc calamine lotion, povidone iodine scrub lotion.

Ointments

These are soft, semi-solid substances containing the drug in a greasy base (paraffin or wool fat), e.g., Povidine Iodine skin ointment and Silver sulfadiazine ointment. Some ointments are in a water miscible base (vehicle). Ophthalmic ointments are sterile medicated ointments for eye ailments, e.g., Ciprofloxacin eye ointment, Atropine eye ointment.

Paste

It is like an ointment with some adhesive material (like starch) or a foaming agent (like carboxymethyl cellulose),e.g., zinc oxide paste, etc.,

Plaster

It consists of a drug mixed in a resinous base spread over a muslin cloth. Some plasters are coated with water repellent film also. The preparation remains hard at room temperature but becomes sticky at body temperature. These are used for protective, analgesic and antiseptic action, e.g., Flurbiprofen plaster, belladonna plaster and Band-Aid.

Gels/ Colloidal aqueous Suspensions

The drug is dissolved in a liquid and then dispersed in soft gelatin. These are usually transparent preparations, e.g., contraceptive gels. The colloidal aqueous suspensions of hydrated inorganic substances used as antacids, e.g., aluminium hydroxide gel.

Inhalants

Liquid preparations of a drug which is meant to be inhaled as vapour. e.g., Eucalyptol, Menthol, tincture benzoin inhalation. The contents may be poured into a jug of boiling water and inhaled to relieve nasal or chest congestion. Solid powdered inhalants, e.g., Salbutamol, Budesonide are inhaled with the use of rotahaler, turbo spin inhaler.

Aerosols

The drug is dissolved in a liquid form is kept inside a cylindrical container (canister) and is then filled with a propellant gas (air or oxygen) under pressure. A compression at the valve releases the microfine drug through a tiny nozzle in the form of mist which is inhaled. If one compression releases a measured dose of drug ,then these are called as "metered aerosols", e.g., Salbutamol metered aerosol, Budesonide metered aerosol.

Suppositories (rectal), Pessaries (vaginal) and Bougies (urethral)

The drug is mixed with any one of the incredients e.g., glycerine, gelatine, soap, paraffin, cocoa butter. These remain solid at room temperature but become soft and melt at body temperature. Suppositories are bullet shaped, pessaries are conical, while bougies (for both male and female urethra) are pencil shaped. For example: Bisacodyl suppositories and Clotrimazole vaginal pessaries.

Transdermal drug delivery system - Transdermal patch

These are adhesive patches, the drug is incorporated into a polymer (usually polyisobutylene) which in turn is bonded to an adhesive plaster. The drug is delivered at the skin surface by diffusion, by percutaneous absorption it enters into circulation. These preparations are designed to provide steady and smooth plasma concentration of the drug for a period ranging from 1-3 days from the site of their application (usually chest, abdomen, upper arm or mastoid region). Examples are transdermal patches of Nitroglycerin patch, Nicotine patch and Estradiol patch.

TARGETED DRUG DELIVERY SYSTEMS

To improve the drug delivery at the site of action and to reduce the systemic adverse drug reactions special drug delivery systems have been developed recently which have an added advantage of reduced dosage with prolonged drug action. Examples of targeted drug delivery systems are:

Ocuserts
These are thin elliptical microunits of drug in a reservoir from which the drug is slowly released through a semipermeable membrane by diffusion at a steady rate. e.g., Pilocarpine ocusert used in glaucoma, which is placed under the lower eyelid to deliver pilocarpine for a period of 7 days, thus avoiding cumbersome frequent administration of eye drops every day.

Progestaserts
Intrauterine contraceptive device to deliver progesterone into uterus. It is inserted into uterus which delivers progesterone uniformily at a specified rate for a period of one year.

Liposomal drug encapsulation for Intravenous Infusion
Liposomes are minute spherical vesicles of phospholipids containing an aqueous suspension . They can be artificially filled with soluble drug particles, which may be delivered to target tissues. Amphotericin (an antifungal drug used to treat systemic mycoses) is available in a liposomal formulation for intravenous infusion; the preparation is less nephrotoxic and better tolerated. The cost is high due to the manufacturing.

Prodrugs
This is a form of inactive drug which will be converted in the body to an active drug. These are used to overcome the pharmacokinetic disadvantage of bioavailability of the therapeutically very useful drug. For example: Dopamine is very useful in treating parkinsonism, but it does not cross blood-brain barrier (Fig.56). Levodopa, its prodrug, can cross BBB, which is then converted to dopamine in the CNS. Prodrug may also be used to provide longer duration of drug action, e.g., esters of penicillins get slowly hydrolysed in the body to provide slow and sustained release of penicillins (e.g., Procaine Penicillin – G and Benzathine Penicillin –G).

Computerised Miniature Pumps (Fig.06)
These are Computer programmed pumps to release drugs at a definite rate, either continuously as in the case of insulin pumps or intermittently in pulses as in the case of GnRH (gonadotrophin-releasing hormone) pumps. These pumps may also be synchronized with glucose sensor devices which release the desired dose of insulin as per the blood glucose level.

Monocclonal Antibodies (MAbs) as Drug Carriers

These are   antibodies which are produced by a single antigenic determinant (epitope) and directed against that particular antigen are called "monoclonal antibodies".

Large scale production of monoclonal antibodies against any specific antigen is now done by using "hybridoma technology". Hybridomas are somatic cell hybrids, obtained by fusing a specific B-lymphocyte (forming antibody against a specific antigen) with a mouse myeloma (tumour) cell. The resultant hybridoma, therefore, retains the antibody forming capacity of the B-lymphocyte with an ability of the myeloma tumour cell to proliferate endlessly.

To generate these antibodies, the mouse myeloma cells are first grown in a culture deficient in hypoxanthine phosphoribosyl transferase (HPRT) enzyme so as to inactivate antigen and to prevent the subsequent formation of immunoglobulins (because a tumour cell itself has a specific antigen on its surface). These myeloma cells are then fused with B-lymphocytes, obtained from the spleen of mouse immunised with the desired antigen, in polyethylene glycol. The fused cells (hybridomas) are then placed in HAT medium and cloned.In HAT medium, only the hybridomas can be maintained endlessly in this culture and can continue to produce monoclonal antibodies (MAbs) which can be eluted and purified for clinical use.

However, totally humanised MAbs are the least antigenic. These are obtained either by recombinant DNA technology (by replacing a part of mouse gene sequence with human gene sequence) or by grafting of "complimentarity determining regions (CDRs)" of murine MAbs on human immunoglobulins framework.

The name of any monoclonal antibody ends with a suffix "mab". The letter before "mab" indicates the source of the antibody e.g., "o" for murine (omab), "xi" for chimeric (ximab) and "zu" for human (zumab). The letters appearing before these words denote their therapeutic use, e.g., "tu" for tumour, "vi" for virus and "ci" for circulation. If there is no prefix then such a "Mab" is generally an immunomodulatory.

For example, muromonab – CD3 is a murine anti – CD3 monoclonal antibody which is used to prevent transplant rejections. Rituximab is a chimeric monoclonal antibody used to treat non Hodgkin's lymphoma (tumour). Palivizumab is a Mab that binds to fusion protein of respiratory syncytical virus (RSV) and thus prevents RS-viral infections in airways. Abciximab is a chimeric Mab which binds to GP IIb/IIIa receptors present on activated platelets to prevent their aggregations and very useful in preventing platelet aggregation in coronary angioplasty.

Mechanism of action of monoclonal antibodies: MAbs bind with specific antigens (virus, grafted tissues and neutralize (kills virus, prevent graft rejection) and also neutralize the specific antigens like non-self antigen and prevent the destruction of non-self tissues), prevent antigen antibody reaction on mast cell and prevent the release of chemical mediators from mast cells.

Clinical uses of monoclonal antibodies:

1. As antiviral : Palavizumab- it neutralizes RSV (Respiratory Syncytial Virus) and inhibits its fusion with human cell membrane. It is used to prevent lower respiratory tract infections due to RSV.
2. As anticancer: i) Rituximab : Used in B-cell lymphoma, chronic lymphocytic leukaemia. ii) Epratuzumab (humanized): Used in Non-Hodgkin's lymphoma. iii) Alemtuzumab- Used in B- cell chronic lymphoid leukaemia and T- cell lymphoma.
3. As antiasthmatic: Omalizumab: Used in allergic type of asthma. It inhibits the binding of IgE with mast cells and suppressses IgE mediated release of bronchoconstrictor chemical mediators (Histamine/LTs)
4. As immunosuppressive agents: Muromonab-CD-3 (anti CD3). It depletes cytotoxic T-cell (CD8+Tc) Hence it is useful to prevent graft rejection in organ transplantation. It is also useful in autoimmune diseases, since it inhibits the antigen and antibody reaction, which prevent the destruction of non-self tissues.

Fig.05 Insulin Delivery Devices

- Insulin syringes
- External Insulin Pumps
- Implantable Insulin Pumps
- Insulin Pens
- Insulin Injection Aids
- Insulin Jet Injectors
- Insulin Inhalers

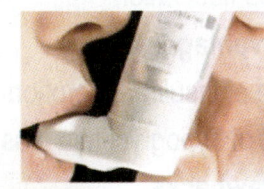
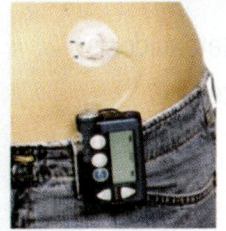
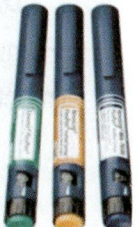

(Fig.06)

Continuous subcutaneous insulin infusion (CSII) through pumps

Most physiological method of insulin delivery

Preferred in patients uncontrolled on multiple injections
& those needing excellent control(pregnancy)

Specially suitable for patients with risk of hypoglycemia,
uncertain lifestyles,meal times.

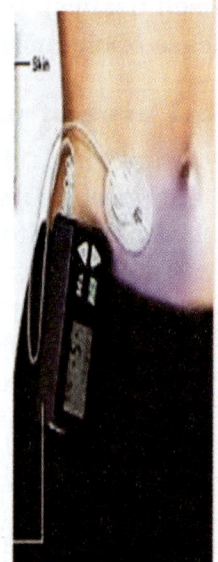

□Consists of insulin reservoir, program chip, keypad&
screen. Insulin infused through plastic tubings connected
to s/c inserted infusion set .

INSULIN DELIVERY – short acting insulin analogues like Aspart(lispro) used.

o Provides constant basal infusion of insulin & patient can activate pre-meal boluses.

o Pumps can be discontinued for short periods for activities like exercise

o Pump can be pre-programmed to compensate for nocturnal & early morning glucose fluctuation.

Advantages

- Rate of insulin absorption more predictable than multiple injections
- Risk of hypoglycemia less

Drawbacks

Pump failure -→ketoacidosis

Injection site abscess

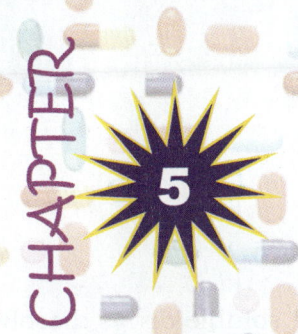

Biological membrane and the mechanism by which the drugs cross (transported) the membrane

CHAPTER 5

Before going to the pharmacokinetic properties of the drugs, it is better to know how the drugs cross the biological membrane or are transported across the membrane.

The drugs are carried all over the body mainly through blood stream. The drugs enter into blood stream and leave the blood to reach the site of action on the cell membrane or into the cell. Two membranes are involved for the drugs to cross and reach the site of action. One is capillary endothelium and another one is cell membrane. Biological membrane is present in all those places.

Structure of biological membrane (Fig.07)

It is made up of lipid bilayers. On the surface of the membrane, water filled pores are present. There are also carrier proteins present on the cell membrane. On the cell membranes, some specialised cells are also present to transport the big molecular sized drugs by engulfing.

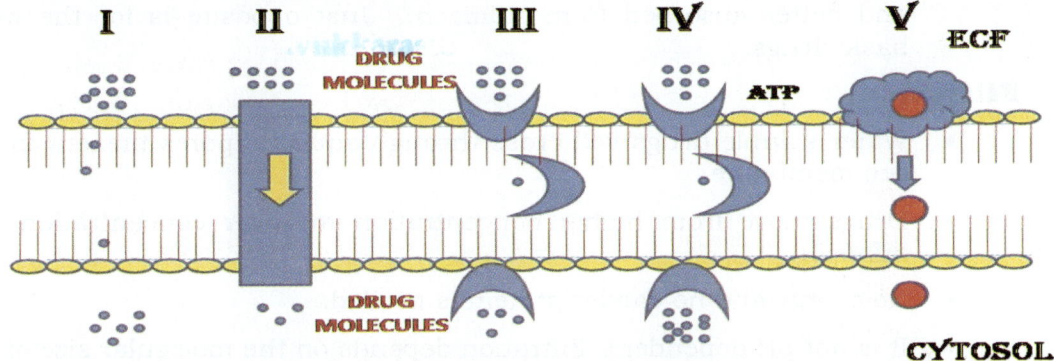

I – PASSIVE DIFUSSION (LIPID SOLUBLE)
II – AQUEOUS PORE – FILTERATION (WATER SOLUBLE)
III - FACILITATED DIFFUSION
IV – ACTIVE TRANSPORT
V - PINOCYTOSIS

Fig.07 - STRUCTURE OF BIOLOGICAL MEMBRANE AND MECHANISM OF DRUG TRANSPORT

Mechanims of drug transport: (Fig.07)

1. Passive diffusion

2. Filtration

3. Carrier protein mediated transport:

   i) Facilitated diffusion

   ii) Active transport

4. Pinocytosis

1. Passive diffusion: It is the process by which the lipid soluble drugs dissolve in lipid layer of biological membrane and cross (move) from one end (from higher concentration of drugs) to the other end (lower concentration of drug) of the membrane till the concentration of the drug becomes equal on both sides. So in this process, the drugs move from higher concentration to lower concentration (along the concentration gradient).

- Only the lipid soluble drugs will cross by this process.

- No carrier protein or energy is needed for this transport

- Lipid soluble drugs are better absorbed, better penetrating BBB (Blood Brain Barrier) and better crossing all the cell membranes.

- This transport process depends on pH of the medium. i.e., pH dependent.

- All the drugs are either weak acids or weak bases

- Weak acidic drug in acidic medium→ unionized→ lipid soluble→ better diffusion→better absorbed/crossed. Example: Aspirin is a weak acidic drug and in the acidic medium of the stomach, it is unionized and better absorbed from stomach. Just opposite is for the weak basic drugs.

2. Filtration:

- Water soluble drugs will cross through aqueous pores present in the cell membrane.

- Drugs move from higher concentration to lower concentration like diffusion.

- No energy and no carrier protein is needed.

- It is not pH dependent. Filtration depends on the molecular size of the drug. If the molecular size of the drug is bigger than that of the pore, then the drugs will not cross. Only smaller molecular sized drugs are allowed to cross by filtration.

- The pore size of the capillary endothelium is 40 A^0. The pore size of renal capillary endothelium is the biggest. Hence, most of the drugs and metabolites except protein/protein bound drugs are filtered and excreted.

BBB (Blood Brain Barrier) and its CLINICAL SIGNIFICANCES: There is no pore in the endothelium of capillaries entering into CNS. So water soluble drugs will not cross BBB and reach CNS. Only lipid soluble drugs will cross BBB.

3. Carrier protein mediated transport

i) Facilitated Diffusion:

- Carrier protein is needed for the transport of drugs (the carrier protein combines with the drug and carries to the other end and leaves it there, comes back and takes another molecule of the drug and the process is repeated (ferry like transfer).
- Drugs move from higher concentration towards lower concentration like that of passive diffusion.
- Energy is not required.

ii) Active Transport:

- Carrier protein is needed for the transport of drugs.
- Drugs can also move from lower concentration to higher concentration (against concentration gradient).
- Energy is needed (obtained from ATP).

Example: Glucose transport to the peripheral tissues, Gentamicin enters into g^{-ve} bacteria by active transport only, α methyl dopa etc.,

4. Pinocytosis:

- Pino=I drink. Bigger molecules are engulfed.
- Cell engulfs bigger molecule in solution and transfers across the membrane. (Example :Insulin, which is a bigger molecular size is transported through BBB).

COMPARATIVE STATEMENTS OF EACH TRANSPORT:

Passive diffusion	Active transport
1. Drugs move from higher concentration to lower concentration (along concentration gradient, till the concentration become equal at both ends)	1. Drugs also move from lower concentration to higher concentration (against concentration gradient)
2. Energy is not required	2. Energy is required
3. Carrier protein is not required	3. Carrier protein is required
4. Lipid soluble drugs and all drugs acting on CNS will cross by this mechanism	4. Non lipid soluble and bigger water soluble drugs will cross by this mechanism
5. pH dependent	5. Not pH dependent

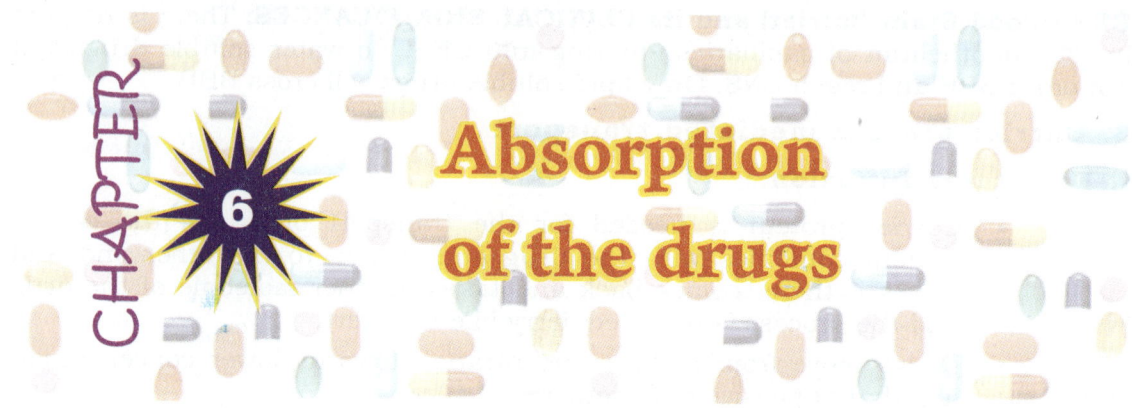

CHAPTER 6

Absorption of the drugs

Absorption of drugs means the entry of drugs into blood stream from the site of administration of drugs. It is possible by the drugs only after crossing the capillary endothelium. All the drugs cross the capillary endothelium and enter into venules (absorbed) and taken into the systemic circulation→to the heart→ reach all the body tissues through arterioles while cardiac out put. Remember, the capillaries (arterioles and venules) are important for absorption of drugs (through venules) and distribution of drugs (through arterioles) (Fig.08 and 09)

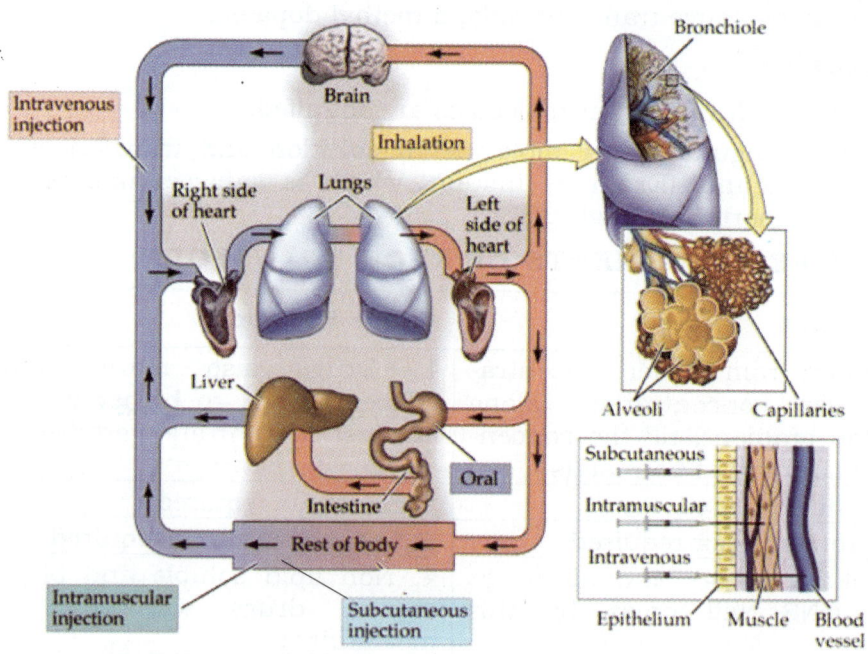

Fig. 08 Absorption of Drugs

Fig. 09 Absorption through capillary

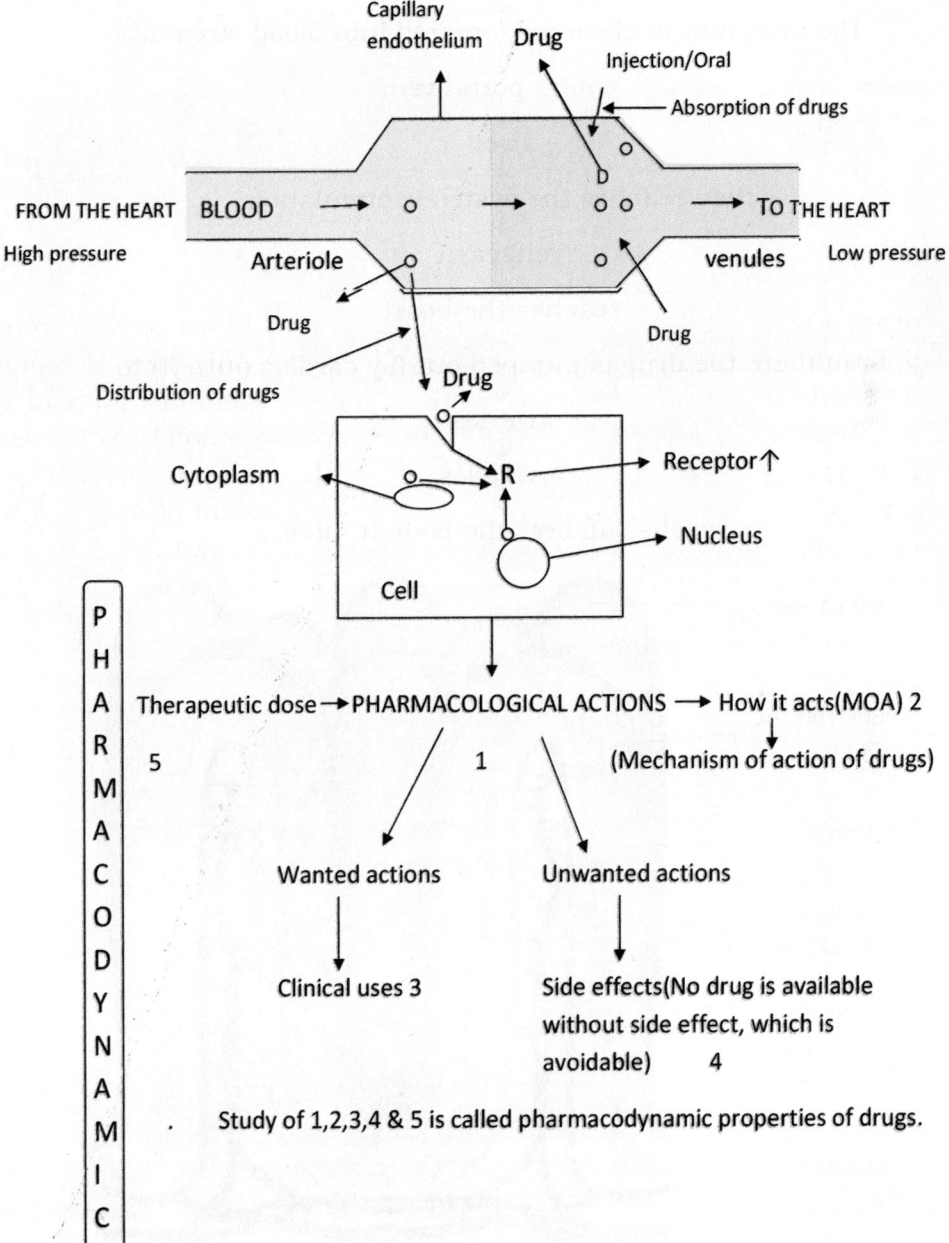

Therapeutic dose → PHARMACOLOGICAL ACTIONS → How it acts(MOA) 2

5   1   (Mechanism of action of drugs)

Wanted actions   Unwanted actions

Clinical uses 3   Side effects(No drug is available without side effect, which is avoidable)   4

Study of 1,2,3,4 & 5 is called pharmacodynamic properties of drugs.

PHARMACODYNAMIC

Absorption after oral administration: (Fig.10)

First the drug has to cross intestinal epithelium

↓

and then it has to cross capillary endothelium (capillaries supplying the villi)

↓

the drug now is absorbed (entered into blood stream)

↓

enters portal vein

↓

liver

↓

then reaches the systemic circulation

↓

venacava

↓

reaches the heart

↓

from there the drug is pumped out (by cardiac output) to

↓

arteries

↓

arterioles

↓

reaches all over the body tissues.

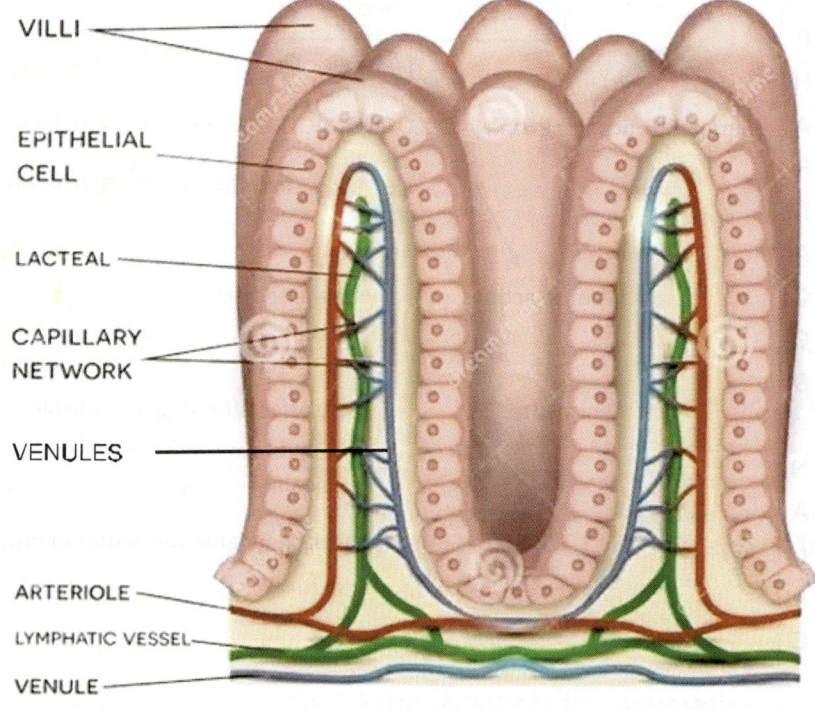

VILLI

EPITHELIAL CELL

LACTEAL

CAPILLARY NETWORK

VENULES

ARTERIOLE

LYMPHATIC VESSEL

VENULE

Fig. 10 Absorption of drugs after oral administration

The drugs are not absorbed or poorly absorbed after oral administration due to the following reasons:

1. If the drugs are in ionized form in the intestinal pH medium will become less lipid soluble and less or not capable of crossing the intestinal epithelium (villi) before reaching the capillaries, from where the drugs get absorbed and hence the drugs are poorly absorbed or not absorbed. (e.g., Gentamicin)
2. Certain drugs are degraded by gastric acid (Peniccilin - G) or by peptidase (Insulin), so they could not reach the intestine in sufficient concentration for absorption.
3. Some drugs form complexes and become bigger molecular size and not absorbed or poorly absorbed. Tetracyclines form complex with Ca++ (milk products) or antacids. Both the drugs are given two hours apart to prevent from forming complexes.
4. Certain drugs back diffuse into the intestinal lumen and hence poor absorption (Digoxin, Cyclosporine)

Absorption of drugs from sublingual

buccal mucosa
↓
buccal vein
↓
absorbed
↓
systemic circulation
↓
heart
↓
to all over body tissues through arterioles

parenteral injection
↓
cross the capillary endothelium
↓
absorbed
↓
systemic circulation
↓
heart
↓
to all over the body tissues through arterioles.

Absorption of drugs after injections:

The drugs which are not absorbed orally given by parenteral route for quick onset of action. The drug is injected (SC/IM) directly into the vicinity of capillaries. There is no need of crossing any other membrane except capillary endothelium, so there is quick onset of action. The drugs are also injected directly into the vein, hence there is no question of absorption and the onset of action is immediate.

Absorption after inhalation (via lungs): (Fig.11)

The lipid soluble drugs are administered in vaporized form (general anaesthetics), Salbutamol (aqueous solution spray) are absorbed (reach the blood stream) by crossing two membrane, first cross pulmonary epithelium/mucous membrane of trachea and lungs by simple diffusion and then capillary endothelium (now the drug enters into blood stream and hence absorbed). The absorption is rapid due to two reasons, 1. Vast surface area for absorption is available and 2. High vascularity for better absorption. As soon as the administration of the drug is discontinued, the drug back diffuses and is rapidly eliminated in the expired air. The control of the dose of general anesthetics accurately is possible.

Absorption of drugs after inhalation: (fig: 11A)

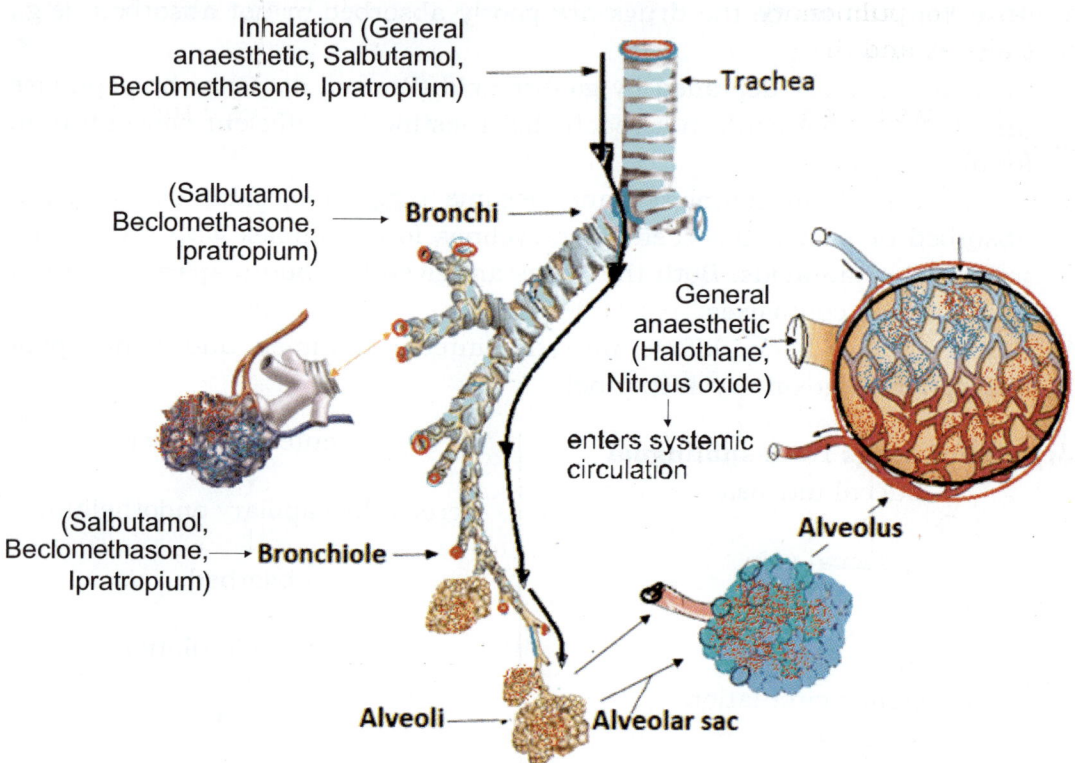

The drugs are administered through nose, mouth, respiratory tract. The drugs travel trachea→ bronchus → bronchioles→ alveoli→ capillaries → absorbed →systemic circulation.

For local action: (Fig.11A) Inhalation of Solbutamol, Iprotropium and Beclomethasone (all the drugs are used in bronchial asthma)→ reach the site of action directly only by crossing pulmonary epithelium (no need of absorption through capillaries). The action is quick.(hence systemic side effects are minimum). The inhalational Salbutamol produces less or no tremor, when compare to oral administration.

For systemic action: (Fig.11-B) The volatile General anaesthetics like Halothane will reach the alveoli quickly, crosses quickly and absorbed quickly through capillaries, which are plenty surrounding the alveoli, reach the site of action (CNS) through the systemic circulation quickly and produce the anaesthetic action quickly.

As soon as the drug administration is discontinued, the drug back diffuses from blood to pulmonary epithelium and crosses pulmonary epithelium and reaches airway and then exhaled (Rapidly eliminated in expired air).

The drugs are administered through inhaled air and excreted through exhaled air.

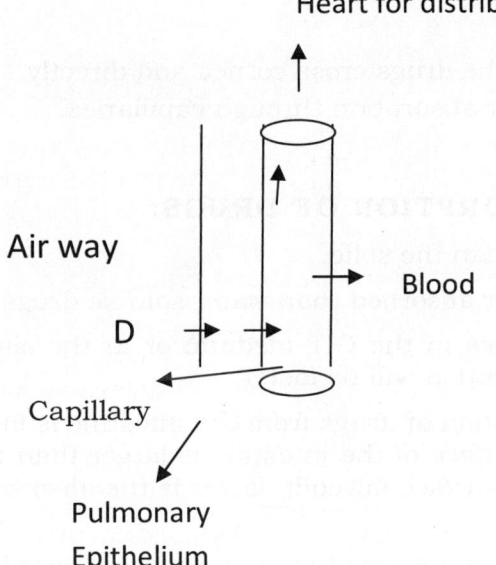

After Discontinuation:

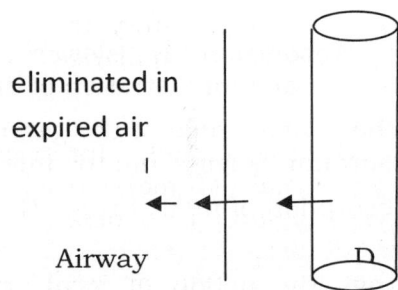

Fig. 11-B Absorption and elimination of drugs after inhalation

Note: The drug is absorbed through venules and distributed through arterioles.

Clinical significances of absorption of drugs:

- The drug has to be absorbed for systemic effect.
- Absorption of drugs from oral administration is through intestinal epithelium of villi and then capillary endothelium.
- If the absorption is faster, the action of drug will be faster (oral absorption-50-60%, IM, SC absorption is 90-95%. IV -100% absorption (where the drug directly comes to the blood circulation) and hence bioavailability.
- Absorption from SC inj. is slow when compared to IM inj. Hence the highly potent drugs like Morphine, Insulin, Low molecular weight Heparin are given by SC route. (Refer below)

Absorption of drugs from eye:

- After applying the eye drops, the drugs cross cornea and directly reach the site of action or after absorption through capillaries.

FACTORS INFLUENCING THE ABSORPTION OF DRUGS:

1. Liquid preparation is better absorbed than the solid.

2. Solubility; Lipid soluble drugs are better absorbed than water soluble drugs.

3. **Dissolution time:** If any drug dissolves in the GIT medium or at the site of parenteral administration faster, the absorption will be faster.

4. **Area of absorbing surface:** The absorption of drugs from the intestine is faster than from the stomach (the absorption surface of the intestine is larger than that of stomach). Larger the area of absorbing surface (alveoli), faster is the absorbtion of drug.

5. **Blood supply to the absorbing area:** more blood supply→ more absorption. Blood supply to the SC tissue is less than that of skeletal muscle. So less absorption from SC inj. than from IM inj. So potent drugs like Morphine, Insulin are given by SC route.

6. **Route of administration of drug:** Absorption is slower after oral administration. Absorption is faster after parenteral administration of drugs.

7. **GIT motility:** If GIT motility is faster, the contact time of the gastric content (which contains the drug) is less and the absorption is less from the intestine.

8. Presence of food will interfere with the absorption of many drugs. Drugs will be absorbed faster in empty stomach.

9. Vasoconstrictor like Adrenaline prolongs the action of local anaesthetic, Lignocaine by reducing its absorption from the site of administration.

10. Suspension of Penicillin G slows the absorption from the site of injection and prolongs the action of Penicillin G (Benzathine Penicillin G).

BIOAVAILABILITY:

Bioavailability is concentration of drug available at the site of action.

If more absorption of a drug, then there will be more bioavailability of that drug at the site of action.

Absorption is proportional to bioavailability.

All the factors influencing the absorption of drugs will also influence the bioavailability of drugs.

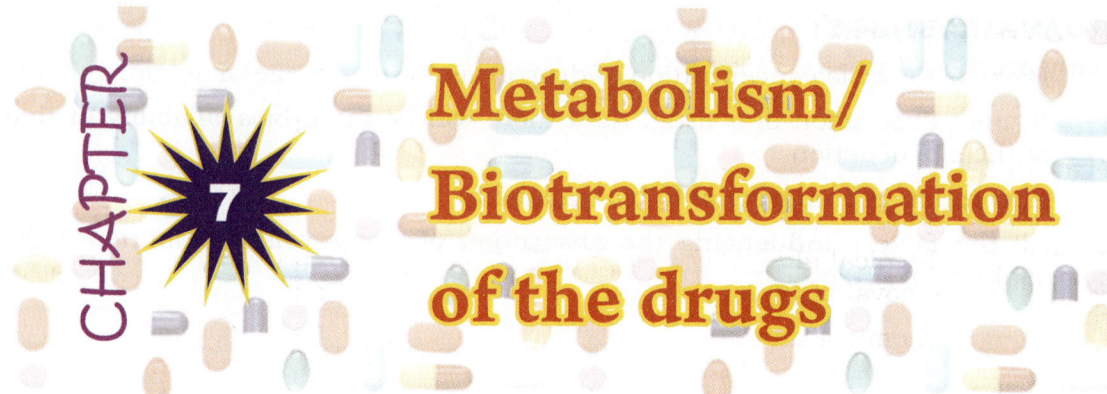

Metabolism/ Biotransformation of the drugs

CHAPTER 7

Both the terms are more or less similar, with slight difference.

Metabolism is a chemical alteration of drugs in which the active drugs are always converted into inactive metabolites.

Biotransformation is a chemical alteration of drugs in which the active drugs are converted into inactive form and active form also (inactive prodrug is converted into active drug inside the body).

L-Dopa (inactive prodrug) is converted to Dopamine (active form) in the liver and brain.

$$Active\ drug$$
$$\downarrow$$
$$Metabolism$$
$$\downarrow$$

Inactive drug →active drug → inactivation ← active metabolite ← active drug
$$\downarrow \qquad\qquad \downarrow$$
Excreted   Prolonged duration

Sites of metabolism: LIVER, intestinal wall, kidney, plasma etc.,

LIVER: The most important organ for the metabolism of more than 90% of drugs.

Enzyme: Microsomal enzymes (CYP-450/Mixed Function Oxidases/Drug metabolising enzymes) are responsible for metabolism/degradation of drugs.

CYP-450 has got many isoenzymes (more than 15-20), which are present in smooth endoplasmic reticulum of liver. Microsomal enzyme are also present in the intestinal wall and kidney. The isoenzymes are represented as CYP-3A4 (metabolise around 60% of the drugs) and other isoenzymes will metabolise the rest of the drugs.

Non-microsomal enzymes present in mitochondria of liver cells, plasma, cytoplasm etc., are Mono Amine Oxidase, Cyclooxygenase, Acetylcholine esterase, Xanthine Oxidase etc.,

Liver microsomal enzymes (most) are subjected to induction or inhibition by many drugs and produce Drug-Drug interactions, which are clinically significant.

The metabolism of drugs take place by the following chemical reactions:

PHASE I : Oxidation, Reduction and Hydrolysis.

Oxidation: Chemical alteration of a drug by addition of Oxygen atom to the drug molecule or removal of Hydrogen atom from the drug molecule.

Reduction: Chemical alteration of a drug by addition of Hydrogen atom to the drug molecule or removal of Oxygen from the drug molecule.

Hydrolysis: Chemical alteration of a drug by the addition of water molecule.

PHASE II: (Synthetic reaction):

Conjugation (chemical alteration of a drug by combining with one of the body ligands)

Glucuronide conjugation (common form) is the addition of glucuronic acid to the drug molecule.

Example :   Paracetamol, diazepam

N-acetyl conjugation- INH, Dapsone, OCP (Oral Contraceptive Pill)

Sulfate conjugation- corticosteroids

Aminoacid conjugation- Dopamine, Adrenaline

Enzyme induction: Some drugs increase the synthesis (not stimulation) of microsomal enzymes and increase their activity are called ENZYME INDUCERS.

Common enzyme inducers are: Rifampicin, Carbamazepine, Barbiturates, chronic smokers and chronic alcoholics, Griseofulvin etc., The common isoenzyme, induced by drugs is CYP3A4, which also metabolise more than 60% of the drugs.

Some of the common drugs metabolised by the same enzymes are Ritonavir, Macrolide antibiotics, oral contraceptives, Warfarin, Paracetamol etc.,

Clinical significances of enzyme induction:

1. The enzyme induces reduce the efficacy of many drugs because the metabolism of those drugs are increased. They also reduce the plasma concentration and lead to therapeutic failure of those drugs given along with enzyme inducers (including contraceptive failure for oral contraceptive pills).

2. They reduce the plasma concentration of antidiabetic and antihypertensive drugs. The dose adjustment will become difficult.

3. Plasma concentration of body Folic Acid and Vit D are reduced (due to increased metabolism) and lead to megaloblastic anaemia and osteomalacia.

4. Paracetamol poisoning in children: Paracetamol is metabolised into hepato toxic metabolite, N acetyl benzoquinoneimine. Enzyme inducers will increase the formation of the toxic metabolite. (Antidote is N-Acetyl cysteine) (Ref. Paracetamol)

5.   Enzyme induction increases the synthesis of porphyrin, leads to precipitation of acute intermittent porphyria (hereditary) (abdominal pain, gastrointestinal and neurological disorders in susceptible individuals).

6.   Enzyme inducers are not without Clinical uses : They are used in Cushing's syndrome (increase metabolism of Glucocorticoids). Also useful in kernicterus, the neonatal jaundice: (the enzyme inducers increase the foetal hepatic glucuronyl transferase enzyme activity, which conjugates the bilirubin to glucuronic acid and excreted, reduces the bilirubin concentration in plasma. Hence they are useful in kernicterus (Phenobarbitone).

Enzyme inhibition and the clinical significances:

1.   The drug interaction due to enzyme inhibition is more dangerous than the enzyme induction.

Enzyme inhibitors are: Erythromycin, Clarithromycin, Valproic acid, Ketoconazole, Metronidazole, Omiprazole, Calcium Channel Blockers like Verapamil and Diltiazem, Ciprofloxacin (except Ofloxacin)

Toxicity of concomitantly administered drug is increased (increased bleeding for dicumarol) cardiotoxicity with Cisapride (banned). In these situations, the clinicians should assess the clinical status. If it is possible, an alternate drug to be prescribed. If it is not possible, the dose of the drug to be reduced according to the clinical conditions.

Factors affecting drug metabolism:

1. Drug-Drug interactions: Enzyme inducers increase the metabolism of some drugs, when given along with them and lead to therapeutic failure of those drugs. Whereas the enzyme inhibitors reduce the metabolism of many drugs given along with the enzyme inhibitors and increase their toxicity for the same therapeutic dose.

The clinicians should remember the enzyme inhibitors. As far as possible, it is better to avoid prescribing the enzyme inhibitors when given along with 2 or more other drugs.

2. Genetic variations: Some individuals have got fast acetylating enzyme, which metabolise Isoniazid faster and reduce its efficacy. Some individuals have got slow acetylating enzyme, which metabolise Isoniazid slower and increase its toxicity.

3. Age: The glucuronyl transferase enzyme is deficient or absent in the neonates. Chloramphenical, which is metabolised by glucuronyl transferase produces toxicity in the neonates (gray baby syndrome).

4. Diseases: Liver disease, hypothyroidism reduce the metabolism of many drugs and lead to drug toxicity in normal therapeutic dose.

5. Nutritional deficiency reduces metabolism of many drugs.

First pass metabolism:

     After the oral administration, the drug reaches the liver first through portel vein before going to systemic circulation. Drugs are metabolised at that time.

Some drugs are metabolised faster and some drugs slower. This is referred as 'first pass metabolism'. The drugs which have got high first pass metabolism will not reach the site of action with desired therapeutic concentration after oral administration. There is no use of giving that type of drug orally. It has to be given parenterally. When the drugs are given parenterally, they bypass the liver **for the first time** and the drug directly goes to the systemic circulation and site of action before going to the liver.

Example: GTN (Glyceryl Tri Nitrate)

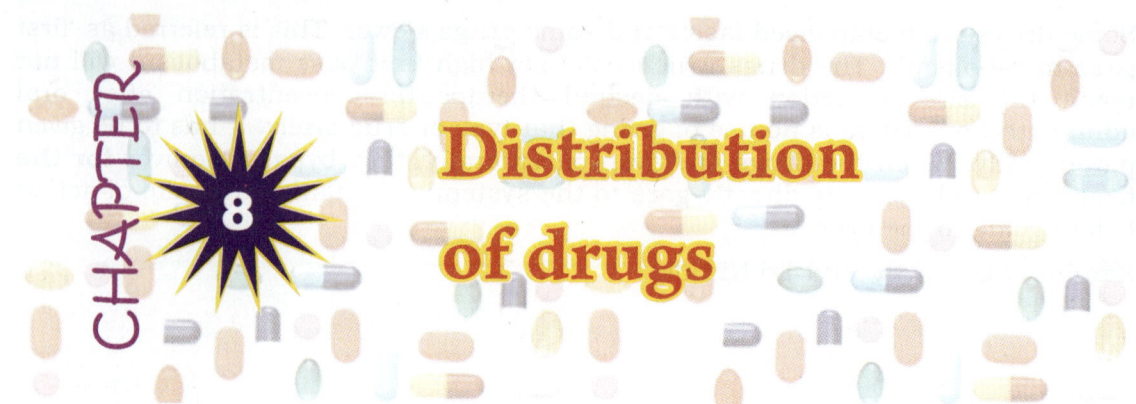

CHAPTER **8**

Distribution of drugs

DISTRIBUTION OF DRUGS:

The drugs always move (transported) in the fluid medium only (Fig.12). From the heart, the drug (with blood) is pumped out (during C.O.P) to the arteries and then to arterioles, which carry the drug and deliver to all the tissues in the body (Fig.13).

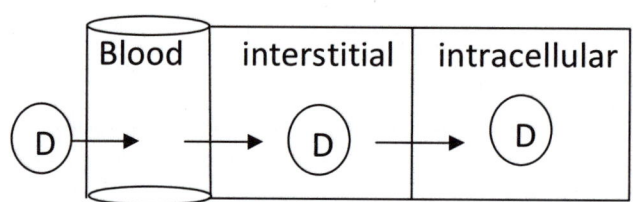

Fig.12 : Distribution of drugs in body fluids.

The drug crosses from arterioles →reaches interstitial fluid → reaches the receptors present on the cell membrane →and then the drug reaches intracellular to occupy receptors in the cytoplasm and in the nucleus.

The drug then stimulates the respective receptors present on the cell membrane, cytoplasm and nucleus and produces appropriate pharmacological actions.

The drug crosses the membranes in the distribution of drugs, depending on the medium of the fluid and characteristic features of the drugs (whether it is lipid soluble/water soluble, pH medium etc.,)

As a rule, all the lipid soluble drugs cross all biological membranes and reach intracellular structures (receptors).

Fig.13 Circulation of Drug in the body

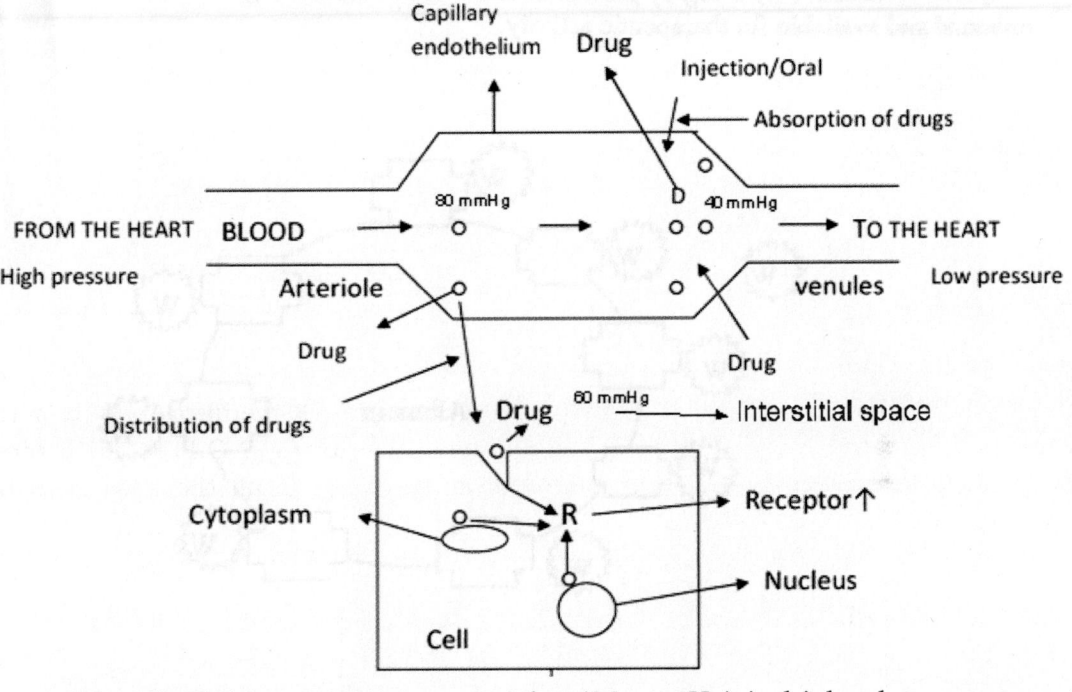

(Fig.13) Fluid pressure in arterioles (80 mmHg) is high when compare to interstitial fluid pressure (60 mmHg) – Hence the fluid from the arteriole (along with drug) is pushed out (filtered) into interstitial fluid. The drug acts on the receptors, and then reaches venule side. Fluid pressure in the interstitial fluid (60 mmHg) is high when compare to that of venules (40 mmHg). So the fluid is pushed back (along with drug) to the venules from the interstitial fluid and taken to heart for further round of distribution. So, the drug is going on circulating in the body till it is completely excreted.

Clinical significances of protein bound drugs:

Some drugs have affinity towards protein (albumin) in the blood and bind to it. They are called as protein bound drugs. The percentage of protein binding varies from drug to drug

1. The protein bound drugs will be circulating only in the blood (due to their big molecular structure after binding with protein, they cannot leave the blood).
2. The protein bound drugs will be having equilibrium with free drug (bound drug ⇌ free drug). Once the free drug concentration falls, then the protein bound drug will be dissociated to 'free drug', so the duration of the protein bound drug will be increased.
3. Protein bound drugs are pharmacologically inert.
4. Protein bound drugs do not cross BBB, placental barrier and are not metabolised or not excreted.

Fig.14A **Warfarin (W) is highly protein bound to albumin, leaving a small fraction unbound and available for therapeutic activity.**

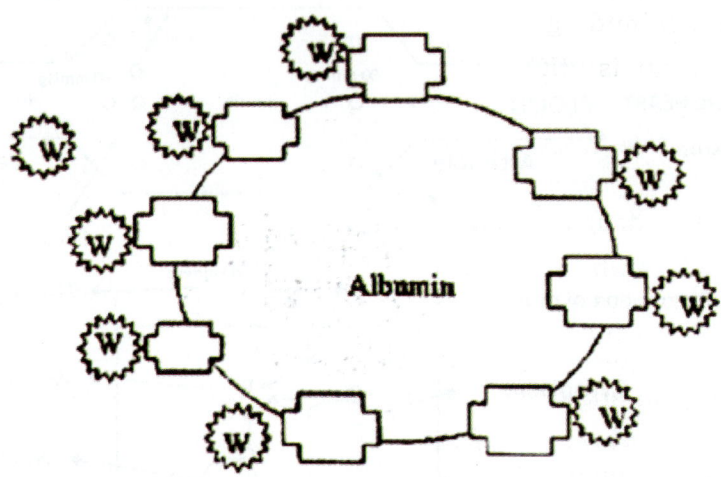

Fig.14-B The addition of the displacer drug salicylic acid (S) with a higher affinity for albumin and a higher serum concentration, displaces warfarin from the binding sites. A larger free fraction of warfarin with more biological activity occurs.

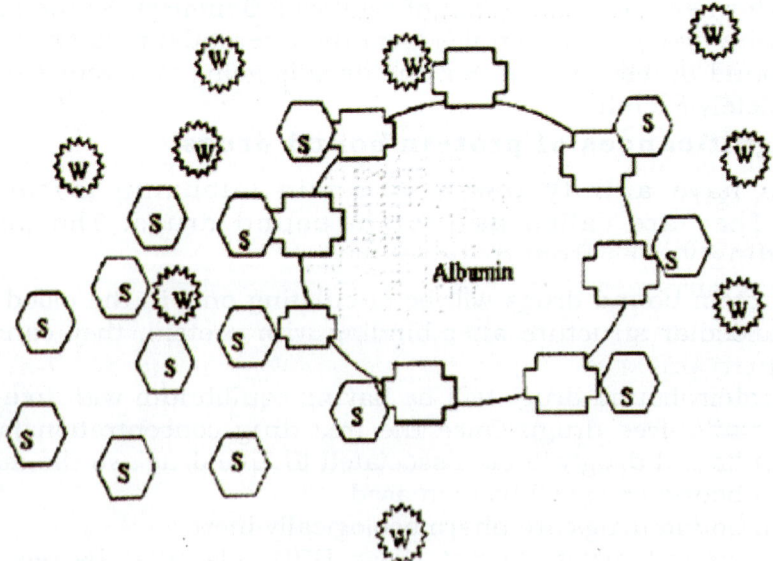

5. Drug interaction is common among the protein bound drugs. (Fig.14-A/14-B)

   Example: Basic drug displaces the basic drug from the basic sites. Like that the acidic drug also displaces acidic drug from acidic site. When both protein bound drugs are given together, the high affinity (towards protein) drug will displace the low affinity drug irrespective of the percentage of protein binding.

   Warfarin is HIGHLY protein bound (99%) but has WEAK affinity to the protein.

   Aspirin is WEAKLY protein bound (40%) but has HIGH affinity towards protein. So, Aspirin displaces warfarin from protein bound site.

   1% free drug of Warfarin is sufficient plasma concentration for action.

   When combined with Aspirin, which displace Warfarin from protein bound site and increases the free Warfarin level in the blood and the toxicity of Warfarin (bleeding). So this combination should be avoided (even the 1% free Warfarin release increases the blood concentration to double of Warfarin and hence the toxicity).

6. **Redistribution of drugs:** It takes place only for high lipid soluble drugs (Thiopentone). Thiopentone rapidly goes to brain and produces general anaesthesia action and immediately leaves the brain (short action). It gets deposited in the fatty tissues immediately, hence short duration of action of Thiopentone sodium. The short duration of action of Thiopentone is due to its rapid redistribution but not due to its increased metabolism or excretion. (the duration of action is 15-20 min.) If the surgery procedure requires more than 20 min, this drug cannot be repeated. Because repeated injection will lead to saturation of fat and once the fat gets saturated, the drug will leak out and plasma concentration of Thiopentone is increased and toxicity occurs (prolonged apnoea) If the surgical procedure requires more than 40 min, other IV general anaesthetic (Ketamine) can be preferred as repeated injection is possible to prolong the duration of action. Thiopentone sodium can be given as infusion in neurosurgery.

Factors influencing the distribution of drugs

1. Blood Brain Barrier (BBB) (Fig.15)

   Lipid soluble drugs are better distributed including CNS (lipid soluble drugs cross BBB better) Unlike the capillary endothelium of peripheral blood vessels, the endothelium of brain capillary has got tight junction (No intercellular aqueous pores). Water soluble drugs do not cross BBB. And also one more glial cells are present over the capillary endothelium. This structure of the capillary endothelium makes it a tight barrier to many drugs. This structure is called BBB. Only lipid soluble and actively transported drugs will cross BBB.

   The drug to produce actions on CNS must cross BBB.

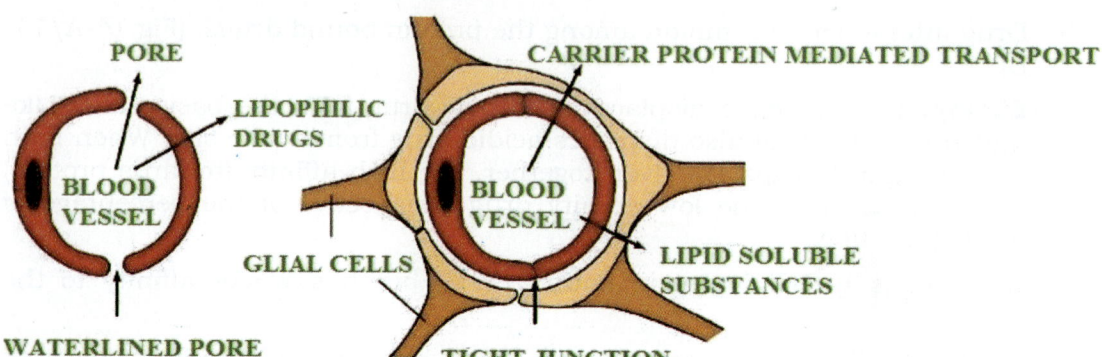

Fig.15 Blood Brain Barrier

2. CTZ (Chemoreceptor Trigger Zone). Even though it is situated in the CNS, it is not covered by BBB.

This anatomical structure is very much useful for the treatment of vomiting due to L-Dopa. Domperidone is given to prevent the vomiting due to L-Dopa without affecting the basal ganglia (antiparkinsonism action), since Domperidone does not cross BBB, but reaches CTZ, where it acts as antiemetic and does not reach Basal Ganglia. But metoclopramide, which cross BBB will produce antiemetic action as well as antagonising the anti-parkinsonism action of L-Dopa. (Ref. : Prokinetic agents under G.I.T.)

VOLUME OF DISTRIBUTION: (Fig.12) This is the volume of fluid, in which the active drug is distributed. The volume of distribution depends on apparent volume of distribution, which will be calculated as follows:

$$Vd = \frac{Total\ amount\ of\ drug\ administered\ IV\ (mg)}{Plasma\ concentration\ of\ drug\ mg/ml}$$

Vd= Apparent volume of distribution

The total body fluid is 40 L (approximate)

Plasma volume is 5 L

Interstitial fluid volume is 15 L

Intracellular fluid volume is 20 L

If the volume of distribution of a drug is 5 L and below, then the drug is distributed only in plasma (Heparin). The volume of distribution of Heparin is 5 L, that means, Heparin will be distributed only in the blood and act on blood.)

If the volume of distribution of a drug is 20 L, then the drug is distributed in plasma and in extra cellular fluid.

If the volume of distribution of a drug is 40 L, then the drug is distributed throughout the body fluid. If the volume of distribution is more than 40 L, then the drug is deposited in some organs.

CHAPTER 9

Excretion of drugs and kinetics of elimination

EXCRETION OF DRUGS: The process by which the drugs or their metabolites are eliminated from the body.

Organs of excretion: KIDNEY (through urine), skin (through sweat),mammary gland (through milk), GIT (through faeces), Liver (bile).

Kidney is the most important organ of excretion, through which more than 90% of drugs or metabolites are excreted.

Three processes are involved in the excretion of drugs through kidney.

Fig 16-A. Glomerular filtration

Fig 16-B. Tubular secretion

Fig 16-C. Tubular reabsorption

I. CLINICAL SIGNIFICANCES OF GLOMERULAR FILTRATION: (Fig.16-A) GFR is approximately 150 L. Many drugs are excreted in the active form. In normal kidney function, there won't be any problem for those drugs. But in renal failure, the GFR (Glomerular Filteration Rate) is low and so the elimination of the active drug is reduced and plasma concentration is increased and hence the toxicity of the drug.

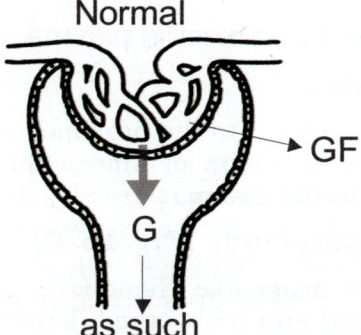

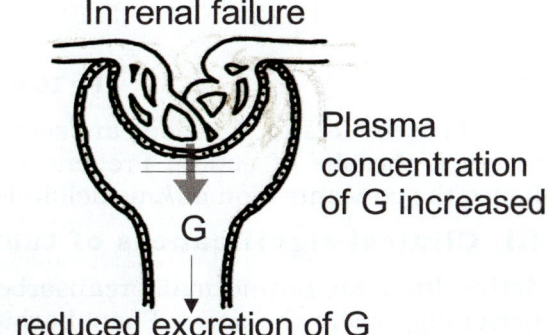

G - Gentamicin
GF - Glomerular Filtration

Fig. 16A Glomerular filtration

Precautions: Those drugs which are excreted in active form (Gentamicin) should be avoided in renal failure. If not possible, then the dose is proportionately reduced on the basis of creatinine (renal) clearance. Take it for granted, the creatinine clearance in normal is 100 ml/min. If the creatinine clearance is 50% (for the drug in question), then the dose of the drug should be 50% of the normal dose. Like this the dose of the drug is to be calculated.

$$Dose\ of\ the\ drug\ (in\ question) = \frac{Normal\ dose\ x\ creatinine\ clearance\ of\ drug\ ml/min}{Normal\ creatinine\ clearance\ 100\ ml/min}$$

II. Clinical significances of tubular secretion: (Fig.16-B)

1. Frusemide and Thiazides are secreted into the proximal tubule in active form and reach the site of action in the renal tubule to produce diuretic action.

2. There will be competition between drugs excreted through tubular secretion. Example : Ampicillin and Probenecid are secreted through the same sites. When those drugs are given together, Probenecid will inhibit the secretion of Ampicillin and increases the concentration of Ampicillin in the plasma, which is very much needed in the treatment of Gonorrhoea (To achieve high concentration in plasma, oral high dose of Ampicillin is needed, which will produce intolerable side effect like diarrhoea). So in the treatment of gonorrhoea both Probenecid and Ampicillin (normal dose) are given.

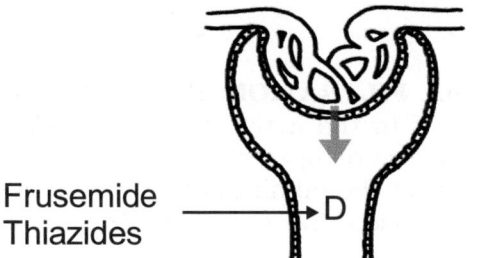

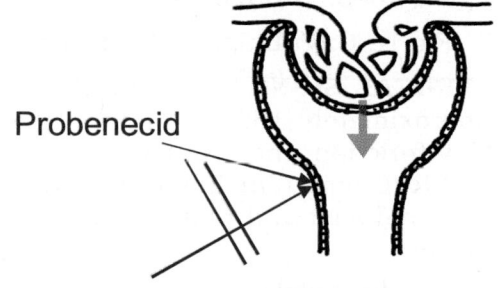

Probenecid + Amoxicillin

Probenecid

Frusemide Thiazides → D

Increased Amoxicillin plasma conc.

Fig 16-B. Tubular secretion.

Frusemide and Thiazides are secreted in active form into the proximal tubule to reach the site of action. Probenecid inhibits the secretion of Amoxicillin and hence the concentration of Amoxicillin is increased in the plasma.

III. Clinical significances of tubular reabsorption: (Fig.16-C)

Active drugs are not normally reabsorbed except few drugs like Phenobarbitone in poisoning, where the active Phenobarbitone is filtered and reabsorbed, being lipid soluble. Only lipid soluble drugs are reabsorbed and the plasma concentration is increased.

Phenobarbitone poisoning: Active drug appears in the urine. Phenobarbitone is a acidic drug. In the acidic urine, it gets unionized (lipid soluble) and reabsorbed and poisoning will be aggravated. To quicken the excretion of Phenobarbitone, the urine should be alkalanized by giving IV sodium bicarbonate. In the alkali medium of urine, Phenobarbitone gets ionized and will not be reabsorbed and then excreted. In the same way the basic drugs poisoning, the urine should be acidified by giving IV Ammonium chloride/Ascorbic acid.

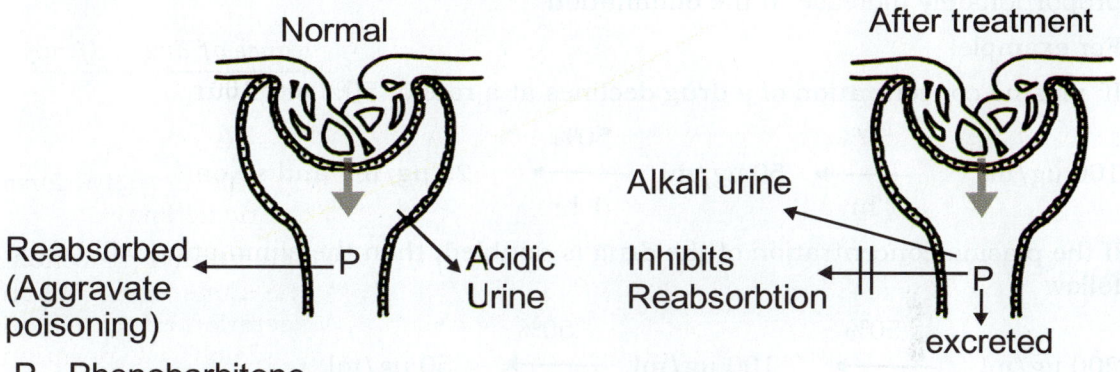

Fig 16-C. Tubular Reabsorption

Phenobarbitone in Alkali urine gets ionized, not reabsorbed and excreted.

Excretion of drugs through milk secretion: Many drugs are secreted in the milk in active form. In that adult dose it may produce toxic effects in the infants (breast feeding). Breast feeding should be avoided when the mother takes drugs that are excreted through milk. The breast feeding mother should consult the doctor before taking any drug.

Clinical significances of biliary excretion and enterohepatic circulation:

1. The drugs which undergo enterohepatic circulation prolong the duration of action of drugs.
2. From the liver→ OCP (Oral Contraceptive Pill) is secreted into the intestine through bile → In the intestine it is deconjugated by the intestinal bacterial flora into active form → reabsorbed back to liver. If the bacterial flora is inhibited by Ampicillin → prevent the deconjugation of OCP and back to liver → excreted in the faeces →↓ (reduce) plasma concentration of OCP → therapeutic failure (failure of contraception).
   Ampicillin or any other antibiotics that suppress the bacterial flora should not be given with OCP.

KINETICS OF DRUG ELIMINATION

The rate and the pattern of drug elimination follows any one of the following kinetics:

1. First order kinetic.
2. Zero order kinetic
3. Mixed order kinetic

1) First order kinetic :

Majority of the drugs obey First order kinetic

Here a CONSTANT FRACTION (PERCENTAGE) of the drug is eliminated at unit time. If the concentration of the drug is increased in the plasma, there is proportionately increase in the elimination

For example:

If plasma concentration of a drug declines at a rate of 50% per hour.

$$100 \; \mu g/ml \quad \xrightarrow[\text{1 hr}]{\text{50\%}} \quad 50 \; \mu g/ml \quad \xrightarrow[\text{1 hr}]{\text{50\%}} \quad 25 \; \mu g/ml \; \text{ and so on}$$

If the plasma concentration of the drug is doubled, then the elimination will be as follow

$$200 \; \mu g/ml \quad \xrightarrow[\text{1 hr}]{\text{50\%}} \quad 100 \; \mu g/ml \quad \xrightarrow[\text{1 hr}]{\text{50\%}} \quad 50 \; \mu g/ml$$

Here the plasma half life is not increased and remains CONSTANT, irrespective of the increase in the plasma concentration of the drug. In this kinetic, it needs approximately 5-6 half lives for complete elimination of the drug.

2) Zero order kinetic:

In this kinetic, a constant or fixed QUANTITY (AMOUNT) of the drug is eliminated per unit time. Say for example 50 $\mu g/ml$ in unit time (not 50%/ml in unit time) is eliminated.

If the initial plasma concentration is 100 $\mu g/ml$ and 50 $\mu g/ml$ is eliminated per hour, then the elimination will be as follow:

$$100 \; \mu g/ml \quad \xrightarrow[\text{1 hr}]{\text{50 } \mu g} \quad 50 \; \mu g /ml \quad \xrightarrow[\text{1 hr}]{\text{50 } \mu g} \quad \text{Nil}$$

If the plasma concentration is increased to double, then the elimination will be as follow:

$$200 \; \mu g/ml \quad \xrightarrow[\text{1 hr}]{\text{50 } \mu g} \quad 150 \; \mu g/ml \quad \xrightarrow[\text{1 hr}]{\text{50 } \mu g} \quad 100 \; \mu g /ml$$

Here the plasma half life is increased to 2 hrs, not constant.

3) Mixed order kinetic:

Low dose obey first order kinetic

High dose obey zero order kinetic.

Some drugs obey this kinetic of elimination. For example: Warfarin, Digoxin, Aspirin etc.,

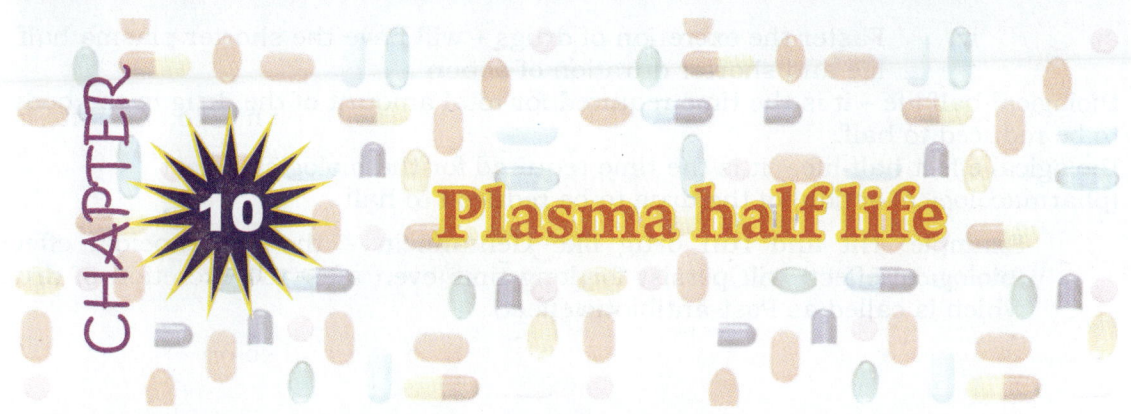

PLASMA HALF LIFE AND ITS CLINICAL SIGNIFICANCES:

The time taken for a drug to be reduced to half of its original concentration in plasm is referred as 'plasma half life $-t_{1/2}$'

1. If higher the plasma half life, longer the duration of action of drugs.
2. Dose interval depends on the plasma half life
3. Normally, after a single therapeutic dose, approximately 4-5 plasma half lives are needed for drugs following first order kinetic to eliminate the drug completely from the body. If the drug concentration is 100 mg at the beginning, then

1st half life 100 mg to 50 mg

2nd half life 50 mg to 25 mg

3rd half life 25 mg to 12.5 mg

4th half life 12.5 mg to 6.25 mg

5th half life 6.25 mg to 3.8 mg

6th half life 3.8 mg to 1.8 mg

Plasma half life of some important drugs
1. GTN – 1 hr (shorter duration of action)
2. Digoxin – 10 days (longer duration of action)

It is needed to calculate the loading and maintenance dose for digoxin
Factors affecting plasma half life
i) Protein binding of drug: Drugs binding to plasma proteins increases the plasma half life and hence the duration of action. (warfarin sodium)
ii) Entero-hepatic circulation: Drugs undergo enterohepatic circulation increases the plasma half life and hence increases duration of action.
iii) Faster the metabolism of drugs – will have the shorter plasma half life and shorter duration of action.

iv)   Faster the excretion of drugs – will have the shorter plasma half life and shorter duration of action..

Biological half life – it is the time required for total amount of the drug in the body to be reduced to half.

Biological effect half-life – it is the time required for the biological effect (pharmacological action) of the drug to be reduced to half.

Example: Hit and run drug like Gentamicin – the bacteriocidal effect (biological effect) will persist for long time even after the excretion of drug which is called as Post-antibiotic effect.

Methods of prolonging the duration of action of drugs, therapeutic index

CHAPTER 11

METHODS OF PROLONGATION OF DURATION OF ACTION OF DRUGS:

I. By slowing the absorption of drugs:
  1. Oral
  i. Sustained release (SR) formulation – examples: Diclofenac sodium, Nifedipine – each unit of drug particles have individual coating with different types of inert RESINS. So that each type of coating dissolves at different time intervals. Such tablets provide a steady and sustained release of the drug over the period of 12-24 hrs (long duration of action) and have a lesser side effects.
  2. Parenteral : To prolong the duration of action of drugs, there are given as follows
  i. Oily suspension - By reducing the solubility (Procaine + Penicillin).
  ii. By increasing the particle size of the drug – Insulin Zinc Suspension.
  iii. By reducing the systemic absorption due to vasoconstriction – Adrenaline + Lignocaine
  iv. By increasing the protein binding capacity of the drug – the drug is slowly released from the protein binding site (by reducing the absorption) and hence prolong the duration of action of drugs ex: Protamine + Zinc + Insulin.
  v. Transdermal patch – GTN - the drug is incorporated into the adhesive patch, which is fixed on the skin. The drug is slowly released and absorbed which prolongs the duration of action of drugs.
  vi. Transmucosal (ocusert) – Pilocarpine ocusert, which is kept in eye. The drug is slowly released and absorbed which prolongs the duration of action of drugs.

II. Distribution – refer protein bound drugs - warfarin

III. By inhibiting metabolism
  a. Anticholinesterase – (Ref: Neostigmine)
  b. Cilastatin + imipenem (Ref : Imipenem)

IV. By reducing excretion – Probencid + Ampicillin, Probencid + Amoxicillin (Fig.16B)

Probenecid competitively ↓ (inhibits) the secretion of Ampicillin and amoxicillin → ↑ (increases) the concentration of those drugs in the plasma, which is very much useful in the treatment of gonorrhoea. The high concentration of Ampicillin in the plasma cannot be achieved for the treatment of gonorrhoea by giving high oral dose, since it produces intolerable diarrhoea). So, Ampicillin (in normal therapeutic dose) is combined with Probenecid only for the treatment of gonorrhoea.

Therapeutic index

Therapeutic Index is the ratio between ED_{50} (the dose effective in 50% of the animal) and LD_{50} (the dose effective to kill 50% of the animal)

$$\text{Therapeutic Index} = \frac{LD_{50}}{ED_{50}}$$

LD = Lethal dose
ED = Effective dose
Clinical significance
The higher the therapeutic index, the safer is the drug.
The drug is considered to be safe if the T/I is above 1.

Digoxin, lithium are having low margin of safety and hence they are highly toxic, if there is a slight increase in plasma concentration.

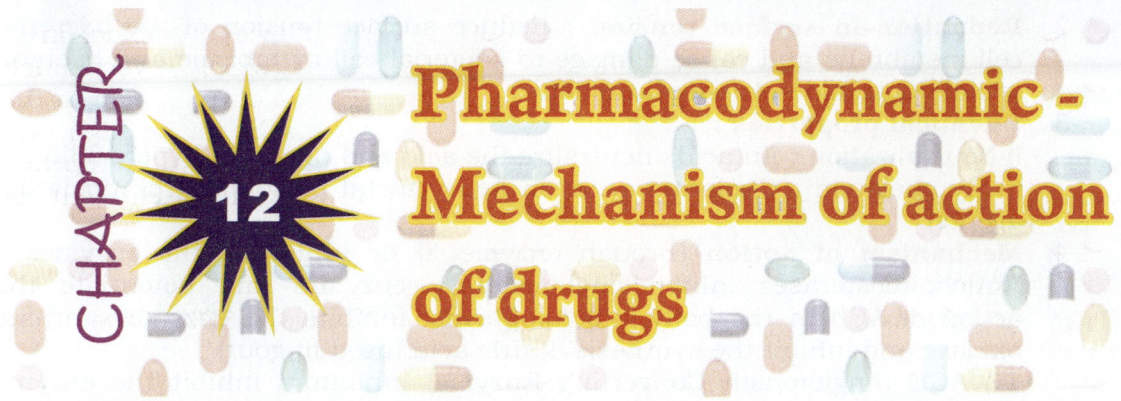

Pharmacodynamic – Mechanism of action of drugs

PHARMACODDYNAMIC (dynamic=power) is the power of the drugs, which include the pharmacological actions and the mechanism of actions of drugs (how drugs act?).

Types of pharmacological actions:

1. Stimulant action: Stimulation of particular tissues/organs; CNS stimulants, cardiac stimulants to produce excess action.

2. Depressant action: Inhibition of particular tissues/organs: CNS depressants, cardiac depressants etc., to produce less action.

3. Irritant action: Irritation of particular tissues/organs → Bisacodyl and Senna produce purgative action by their irritant action on intestinal smooth muscles.

4. Counterirritant action: Turpentine oil, menthol (Iodex).They are used in headache and muscular pain. They irritate the skin. The irritant impulses and pain impulses are carried by the same nerve fibre. Here the irritant impulse will compete with the pain impulse and prevent the pain impulse passing through the nerve and the individuals feel skin irritation and forget the pain impulse.

5. Action on microbes: There is static action or cidal action on microbes. Static means drugs that inhibit the growth and multiplication of microbes. Cidal action means that drugs kill the microbes.

6. By replacement action: In adrenal insufficiency (Hydrocortisone), Insulin in Type-1 Diabetes Mellitus.

7. By modifying the immune status: Immunosuppressive drugs in autoimmune diseases.

Mechanism of actions of DRUGS (HOW DRUGS ACT?)

1. **Physical properties :** Drugs may act due to their physical properties: Osmotic diuretic- Mannitol, Osmotic purgative- Magnesium sulphate (ref: diuretics and purgatives)

2. **Reduction in surface tension :** Reduce surface tension of the bacterial cell membrane and cause damage to bacterial cell membrane and bacteria will die(Cetrimide- Antiseptic action)

3. **Chemical properties :**
   i) Neutralization : Antacids neutralize the acid and useful in hyperacidity.
   ii) By chelation : Chelating agent in heavy metal poisoning (ref: chelating agents)

4. **Mechanism of action** through enzyme: i) by inhibiting the enzymes – Anticholinesterases inhibit cholinesterase enzymre and potentiate the action of ACh in the body. ii) Allopurinol inhibits the enzyme xanthine oxidase and inhibit the synthesis of uric acid (used in gout)
   iii) ACE (Angiotensin Converting Enzyme) inhibitors inhibit the enzyme ACE and produce fall in BP and they are used in hypertension (ref: Antihypertensive drugs)

5. **Radio isotopes:** ^{131}I destroys thyroid gland and is useful in throtoxicosis. (Ref: Radioactive Iodine)

6. **Radio opacity:** It is also called as contrast media, used for diagnostic purpose by visualizing the blood vessels (by organic Iodide), GIT (by Barium meal) etc.,

7. **Adsorption** is, the surface absorption. i) Kaolin adsorbs bacteria and toxin, used in non- specific diarrhoea.

8. **Demulcent:** Pharyngeal demulcent act by soothening the pharynx and used in cough.

9. **Electrical charge:** Heparin by its strong electro negative charge combines with clotting factors with strong electro positive charge and neutralize (inhibit) them to produce anticoagulant action.

10. **Through receptors:** Receptor mechanism is very important, because most of the drugs act through their respective receptors. The drugs stimulate /inhibit the receptors and produce pharmacological actions.

Receptor is a macromolecular, active site present on the cell membrane or intracellularly. The receptors are specific in binding the drug. The drug and receptor are considered as 'lock' and 'key'. One particular key only opens the particular lock. Likewise, one particular drug can combine only with particular receptors (ACh-muscaranic and nicotinic receptors, Insulin with Insulin receptor, Glucocorticoids with glucocorticoid receptors).

• Receptor proteins are synthesized by the cells
• Receptors have definite life span, after which the receptors are degraded and new receptors are synthesized by the cells.
• Receptors are present on the cell membrane, in the cytoplasm or in the nucleus.

Functions of receptors:

1. Recognition and binding of ligand

2. Propagation of message

For the above functions, the receptor has two functional domains (sites)
1. A ligand binding domain – the site to bind the drug molecule (affinity of the drug)

2. An effector domain – which undergoes a change to propagate the message (intrinsic activity of the drug)

Drug + receptor → drug receptor complex →pharmacological action

There are thousands of receptors present in the body.

Example of receptors: Muscaranic receptors, Nicotinic receptors, α receptors, β receptors etc.,

Affinity: The ability of the drug to bind with the receptor to form drug-receptor complex. Like key (drug) enters into key hole (receptor) of the lock.

Intrinsic activity: The ability of the drug to stimulate the receptor. Like the key (drug) opens the lock (stimulate the receptor) after entering into the key hole (receptor) of the lock.

Drug + Receptor ⟶ DR complex ⟶ Pharmacological actions

Agonist: is a drug which has got both affinity towards the receptor and intrinsic activity (stimulate the receptor). Example: ACh, Adrenaline, Histamine etc.,

A	IA
Affinity	Intrinsic activity

Antagonist: is a drug which has got only affinity to the receptor but no intrinsic activity.

Example: Atropine, α - adrenergic blockers, β - adrenergic blockers etc.,

Only Affinity No intrinsic activity

Partial agonist/antagonist: is a drug which has got affinity but has got submaximal intrinsic activity. Example: Pentazocine.

Affinity   Submaximal intrinsic activity

Up regulation of receptor: The number of receptors are increased. Sudden withdrawal of β adrenergic blockers, increases the number of receptors causes an exaggerated response to agonist (rebound hypertension, exaggerated angina pectoris).

Down regulation of receptors: Due to repeated administration of an agonist, there is reduced response for the same dose. This may be due to less number of receptors are available for action. This is termed as 'tolerance' Example : GTN (Glyceryl Tri Nitrate), Hypnotics, etc., produced tolerance.

Drug+ Receptor complex → Drug Receptor complex → stimulate receptor → stimulate second messenger → affect various enzymes → transport of ions across cell membrane. If Na+ enters into the cell,then there will be stimulant action. If Cl⁻ enters into the cell, then there will be inhibitory action.

Receptor mediated mechanism are of four types: (Fig.17A, 17B)

1. Ion channel receptors.
2. G-protein coupled receptors.
3. Enzyme kinase linked receptor
4. Enzyme as receptor.

1. Ion channel receptor: These receptors are present on the cell membrane and are coupled directly to an ion channel (also known as ligand gated ion channel) open only when the receptor is occupied by an agonist (Ca++, Na+, K+, Cl-) Channel blockers act by closing the channels, blocking the ion movement and produced antagonist action to the agonist.

2. G-protein coupled receptors (Fig.17A): These are membrane bound receptors which are coupled to the effector system (enzyme/channel) through GTP binding proteins called G-protein
Examples: Muscarinic receptor, adrenergic receptor, dopaminergic receptor etc.,
Gs = stimulatory, stimulate adenylyl cyclase.
Gi= inhibitory, inhibits adenylyl cyclase.
Go= inhibits Ca++ channel
Through adenylyl cyclase, c-AMP path way:

Agonist occupies and stimulates receptors
↓
Activation of G-protein
↓
activation of adenylyl cyclise
↓
accumulation of intracellular second messenger, c-AMP
↓
stimulate protein kinase
↓
alter the functions of many enzymes, ion channels, transporters
↓
increased contractility of heart, impulse generation, relaxation of smooth muscles etc.,

Fig.17A G-Protein mediated mechanism of drugs

AGONIST

R

Gs

AC

GTP   GDP

ATP

CAMP

PKA

PHOSPHORYLATION

PHARMACOLOGICAL ACTIONS

ENZYMES CARRIERS PROTEINS

TROPONIN

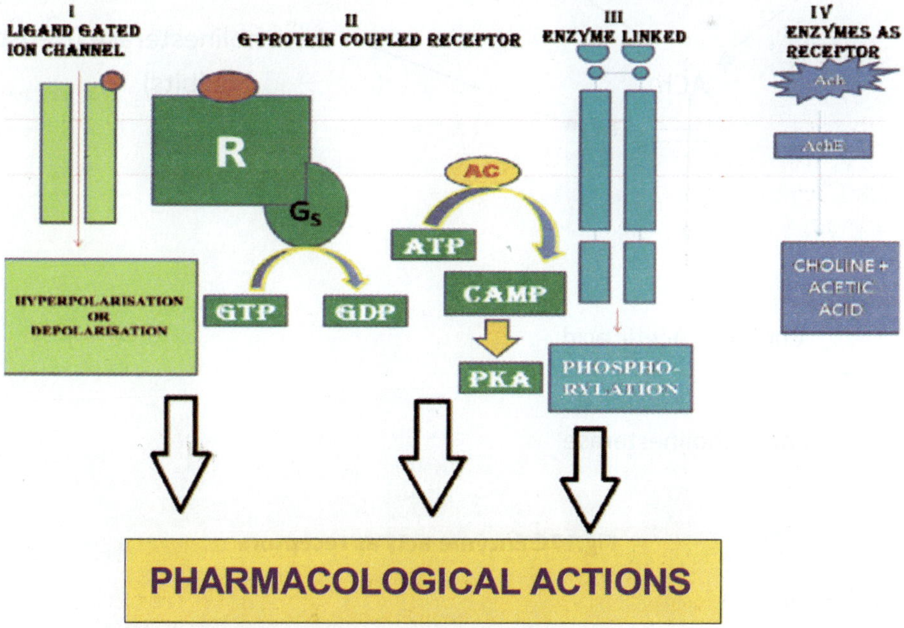

| I
LIGAND GATED ION CHANNEL | II
G-PROTEIN COUPLED RECEPTOR | III
ENZYME LINKED | IV
ENZYMES AS RECEPTOR |

HYPERPOLARISATION OR DEPOLARISATION

R

Gs

AC

GTP   GDP

ATP

CAMP

PKA

PHOSPHO-RYLATION

Ach

AchE

CHOLINE + ACETIC ACID

PHARMACOLOGICAL ACTIONS

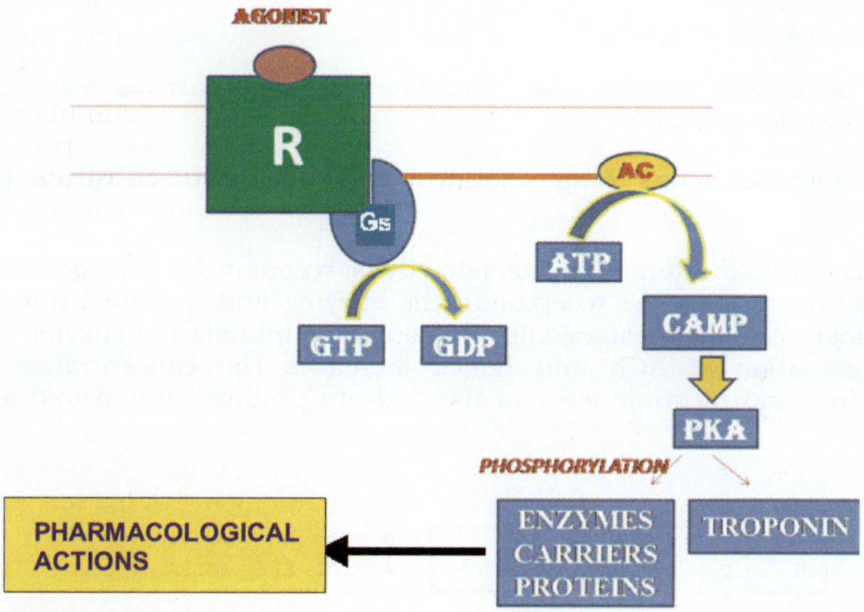

Fig.17B Receptors mediated mechanism of drugs

3. Enzyme kinase linked receptor (Fig.17B): These receptors are directly linked to tyrosine kinase. These are the receptors that are ligand(agonist) activated transmembrane enzymes having catalytic activity.

Example: Insulin receptor.

Insulin binds with receptor ⟶ stimulate tyrosine kinase ⟶ responsible for various cellular effects

4. Some enzymes act as receptor for drug and endogenous substrate. (Fig.17-B/17-C)

Example: Cholinesterase is considered as receptor for endogenous substrate, ACh. ACh occupies the receptor in the enzyme and degraded into choline and acetic acid. Anticholinesterase like Neostigmine inhibits the enzyme and prevents the degradation of ACh and hence increases the concentration of ACh at muscarinic and nicotinic sites in the body to produce muscarinic and nicotinic actions.

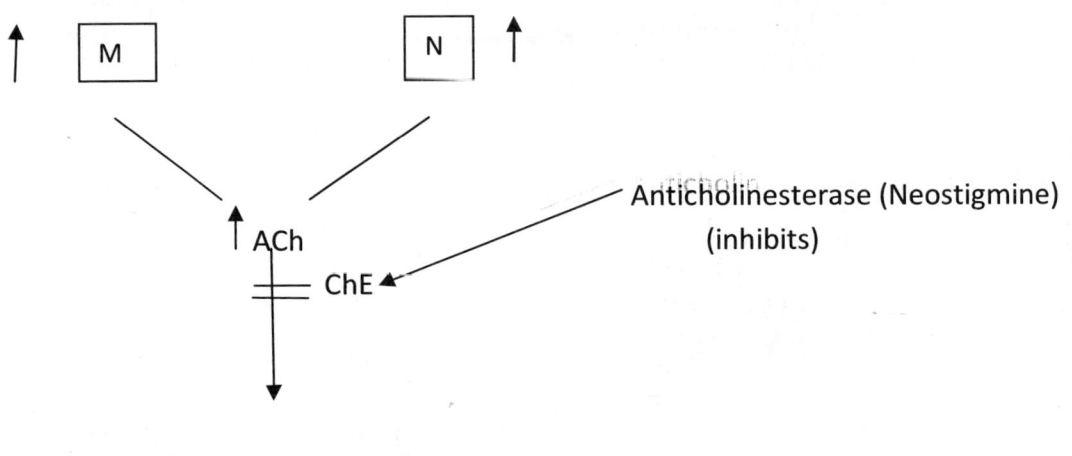

Choline + Acetic acid

ChE – Cholinesterase

Fig.17C Enzyme acts as receptors

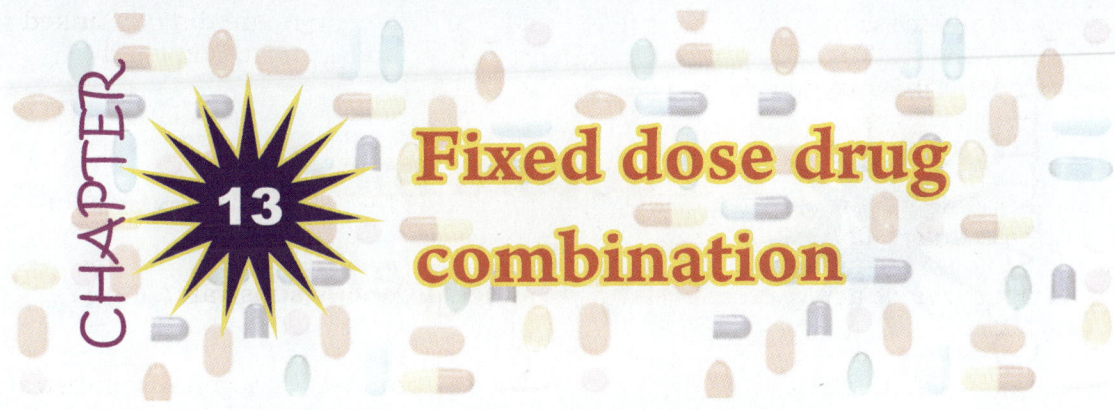

Fixed dose drug combination

CHAPTER 13

The fixed dose drug combination is, the combination of two different drugs in a single pharmaceutical formulation.

As a rule, if two drugs to be combined in a single pharmaceutical formulation, they should have approximately same plasma half life.

1. Cotrimoxazole : It is the combination of Sulfamethoxazole (plasma half life is 10 hrs) and Trimethoprime (plasma half life is 11 hrs)
2. L-dopa(plasma half life is 1.7 hrs) and Carbidopa (Plasma half life is 2 hrs)
3. Augmentin : Amoxicillin and clavulanic acid

The examples of Fixed-Dose drugs combination

(1) Sulfamethoxazole + Trimethoprim (cotrimoxazole)
        400 mg + 80 mg
         800 mg + 160 mg (DS) Double strength

(2) Levo dopa   + Carbidopa (Syndopa)
        250 mg + 25 mg
        100 mg + 10 mg

(3) Amoxacilin   + Clavulamic acid (Augmentin)
        250 mg + 125 mg

(4) Neostigmine   + Atropine in the treatment of myasthenia gravis
        15 mg   + 1 mg

The ratio of the doses depends on the volume of distribution of the drug.

Advantages of the combination

1. Patience's compliance is good
2. Enhanced effect of the combination (Ref: Cotrimoxazole)
3. Reduced side effect (Neostigmine and atropine)
4. Increased bioavailability (Ref: L-dopa)

Disadvantages of the combination:

1. It becomes difficult to confirm the toxicity is due to which drug.
2. If desired/needed, it is very difficult to alter the dose of individual drug

Thus, the therapeutic aim should be clear that the patient is in need of that combination

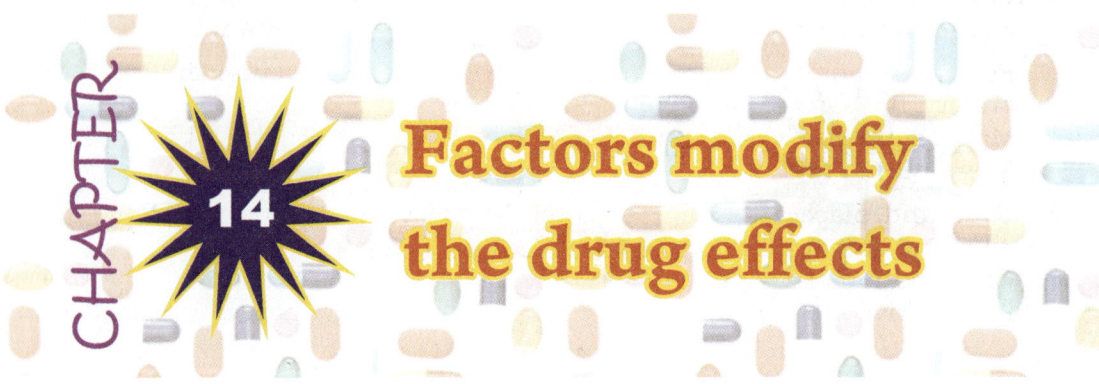

Factors modify the drug effects

CHAPTER **14**

FACTORS MODIFYING THE DRUG EFFECTS:

There are many factors modify the effects of drugs either qualitatively or quantitatively.

First you write the factors and then explain.

1. Age
2. Sex
3. Body weight/body surface area
4. Route of administration of drugs
5. Time and place of administration of drug
6. Combination with other drugs
7. Tolerance and tachyphylaxis
8. Pathological states (diseases)
9. Pharmacogenetics
10. Teratogenicity
11. Substance abuse.
12. Drug interaction
13. Drug resistance
1. Age: The adult dose in children will produce toxic effect. The dose for a child is to be reduced and calculated as follows:

    i)   Young's formula: Child's dose = $\frac{\text{Age in years}}{\text{Age+12}}$ X Adult dose

    ii)   Dilling's formula: Child's dose = $\frac{\text{Age in years}}{20}$ X Adult dose

2. Body weight and BSA (Body Surface Area): At the same age, there may be lean or fatty children. So this calculation is somewhat dependable.
$$\text{Child's dose} = \frac{\text{Weight of child (lb)}}{150} \text{ X Adult dose}$$

3. Sex: There is variation in drug actions in men and women- Alpha methyl dopa, clonidine will cause loss of libido in men. Female oral contraceptives are effective only in females. α-adrenergic blockers produce impotence only in male.

4. Route of administration of drug: Change of ROA (Route of Administration), will change the effects of drugs either qualitatively or quantitatively.

   Parenteral administration will produce more potent action than that of the oral for the same dose (quantitative change).
   Magnesium sulphate – oral – purgative | qualitative change
   Magnesium sulphate -- parenteral-CNS depressant | "

5. Time and place of administration: Hypnotics in noisy surroundings or in day time do not produce full effect.

6. Combination of drugs:
   i) Additive action: The combined effect of the drugs is equal to the addition of the individual drug effect. (1+1=2)

   ADDITIVE EFFECT : Both act at the same site .

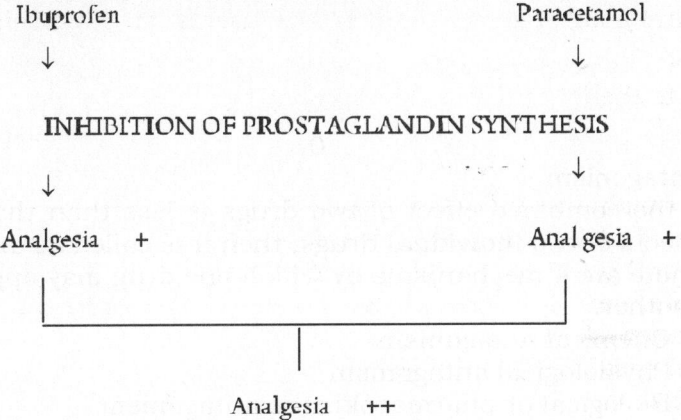

   ii) Synergism: The combined effect of the drugs is more than the addition of the individual effect of drugs (1+1= >2)
   SYNERGISTIC EFFECT : Both act at different sites.

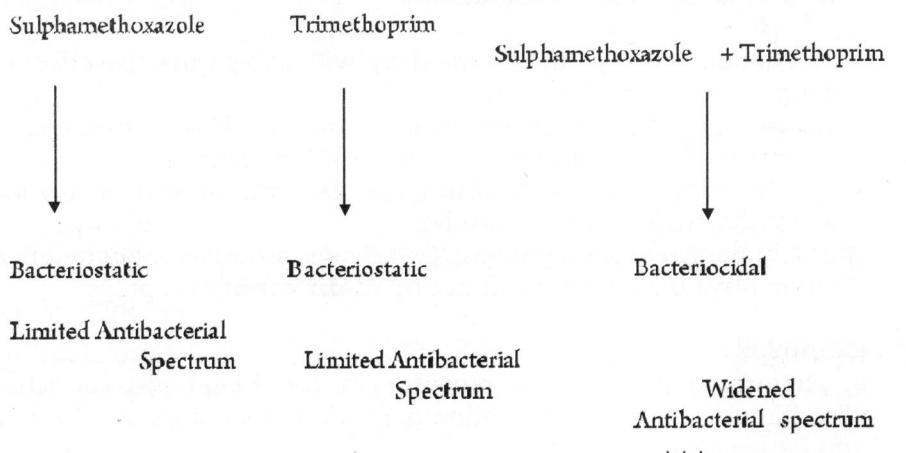

iii) Potentiation: The combined effect of the drugs is more than the addition of the individual effect of drugs. But here one drug is pharmacologically inert. (1+0=>2)

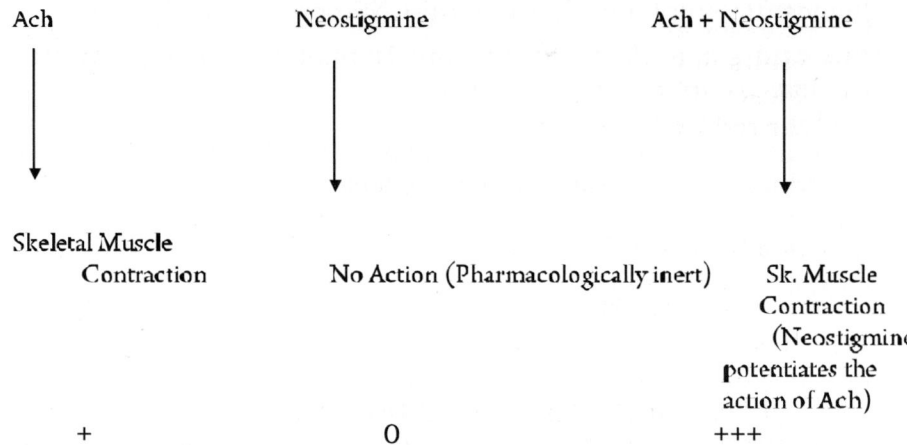

POTENTIATION : (Ref: Fig: Mechanism of action of Anti-cholinesterases)

Ach	Neostigmine	Ach + Neostigmine
↓	↓	↓
Skeletal Muscle Contraction	No Action (Pharmacologically inert)	Sk. Muscle Contraction (Neostigmine potentiates the action of Ach)
+	0	+++

iv) Antagonism

If the combined effect of two drugs is less than that of the sum of the effects of two individual drugs, then it is called as drug antagonism. There are 4 mechanisms by which one drug may oppose the action of another.

1. Chemical antagonism
2. Physiological antagonism
3. Biological or pharmacokinetic antagonism
4. Pharmacological (Pharmacodynamic) antagonism
I. Competitive antagonism
i) Reversible (equilibrium)
ii) Irreversible (non-equilibrium)
II. Non-competitive antagonism

1. Chemical antagonism: One drug will antagonize the effect of another drug by chemical reaction.
i). Antacid – alkalies (Aluminium hydroxide, Magnesium trisilicate) – neutralize the acid in the treatment of hyperacidity.
ii). Chelating agents – chelating agents combine with heavy metals to form non-toxic soluble complex.
2. Physiological antagonism: Two drugs produce opposite effect on the same physiological system acting at **different** receptors

Example:
i). Histamine acts on H_1 receptor in the blood vessels which lead to vasodilatation, while Adrenaline acts on a_1 receptors on the blood vessels and cause vasoconstriction.

ii). CNS stimulants and CNS depressants

3. Biological or pharmacokinetic antagonism: One drug antagonizes the effect of another drug due to pharmacokinetic properties

Example:
i). Decreases absorption of one drug by another drug → Tetracyclines + Ca++ salts ii) Increased metabolism of one drug by another drug → reduce the efficacy (Rifampicin (Enzyme inducer) + Warfarin). The enzyme inducer reduce the anticoagulant effect of warfarin.

4. Pharmacological antagonism (Pharmacodynamic antagonism) – antagonism between two drugs by acting on the **same** receptor.
i) Reversible competitive → ACh + Atropine - antagonize each other by acting on muscarinic receptor, depending upon the concentrations.
→ Morphine + Naloxone - antagonize each
other by acting on μ receptors
ii). Irreversible competitive → antagonist binds to the receptor strongly by covalent bond and cannot be easily replaced by agonist, even in higher concentration of agonist.
Adrenaline + Phenoxybenzamine on α_1 receptor.

7. Tolerance and Tachyphylaxis: Reduced response to the normal dose of the drug due to repeated administration of that drug.

Types of tolerance:

1. Natural tolerance – Black races tolerant to mydriatics
2. Acquired tolerance(common)-tolerance due to repeated administration of drugs
    i)   Pharmacokinetic tolerance: due to pharmacokinetic properties (reduced absorption, increased metabolism, increased excretion etc.,)
    ii)   Pharmacodynamic properties: The tissue at the site of action is less responsive to the normal dose of a drug (Alcohol, Barbiturates, opioids etc.,)
    iii) Cross tolerance: Tolerance among the drugs with related chemical structure (Example : Benzodiazepines). If the individual is tolerant to one drug in the BDZ group, he will be tolerant to all other drugs in that group.
    iv)   Tachyphylaxis: Acute tolerance (tolerance develops within hours)- due to the down regulation of receptors or due to the exhaustion of storage, which is released by the drug for action. Example : Ephedrine, Amphetamine

8. Pathological states (diseases): In liver diseases and in hypothyroidism, the metabolism of drugs is reduced and the toxicity of many drugs increased.

9. Genetic factor

Pharmacogenetic : The effects of the drugs vary from individual to individual due to variation in genetic materials in the body. Pharmacogenetic deals with the study of the variation in the effects of drugs due to genetic factors variation (genetically determined abnormal responses to drugs)

Example

(1) Deficiency of G6PDH (Glucose 6-Phosphate Dehydrogenase) - G6PDH is essential for the integration of cell wall of RBC. If there is deficiency of Glucose 6-Phosphate Dehydrogenase due to genetic factor, the cell wall of RBC becomes weak and the RBC will burst which will lead to haemolysis. Primaquin, Dapsone inhibit G6PDH. These drugs will easily produce haemolysis (anaemia) in the individual having deficient G6PDH. These drugs are also contraindicated in pregnancy, because in the foetus there is deficiency of G6PDH. So there will be haemolysis in foetus.

(2) Atypical pseudocholinesterase: Pseudocholinesterase degrades succinylcholine in the body. Atypical pseudocholinesterase is formed due to genetic variation in some individual. The Atypical pseudocholinesterase is not capable of degrading succinylcholine. Hence the concentration of succinylcholine is increased in plasma and lead to toxicity like prolonged apnea.

(3) Rapid and slow acetylator status: The acetylation enzyme degrades INH. In slow acetylator the INH produces toxicity like peripheral neuritis. In fast acetylator the therapeutic effect of INH is reduced.

(4) Acute intermittent porphyria : precipitated by enzyme inducers is due to genetic defect, which increase porphyrin synthesis. There will be accumulation of porphyrin, which is called as porphyria, characterized by neurological, gastrointestinal and behavioural abnormalities.

(5) Pharmacogenomic : Ref. Gene therapy

10. Teratogenicity (Ref : Adverse effects of drugs)

11. Substance dependence

Substance dependence will affect the effects of drugs. Some substances produce euphoria (pleasurable effects or feeling of well being) and hence some individual would like to experienc that effect (not on medical ground), will start taking the drug repeatedly. The repeated use of that particular substance will lead to dependence of that substance in that individual. Example: coffee, cigarette, LSD, marihuana, alcohol etc.,

Psychological dependence: If any individual depends on a particular substance (not on medical ground) psychologically (not compulsorily) is called psychological dependence. Even if he stops taking that substance, there won't be any harm to that individual.

Physical dependence: On the contrary to psychological dependence, the individual depends on the substance compulsorily, without which he will experience some unwanted (harmful) effects like withdrawal syndromes. The body undergoes physiological changes to adapt itself to the continued presence of the drug in the body. Stopping of the drug will lead to rebound increase of the physiological changes, which the individual experience as withdrawal syndromes (irritation, palpitation, sweating, tremors, dysphoria, etc.,) like that of sudden withdrawal of β-adrenergic blockers or sudden withdrawal of anti-epileptic drugs will lead to rebound increase in epilepsy symptoms called as status epilepticus.

Example: Opioids, barbiturates, alcohol in heavy use – (severe)

And overuse of LSD, marihuana – (mild) withdrawal syndromes are seen.

Substance abuse is misuse of the substances for pleasurable purpose (not on medical ground)

12. Drug interaction (ref: drug interactions)

13. Drug resistance : Many organisms develop resistance to drugs due to repeated administration of drugs (ref: chemotherapy-drug resistance)

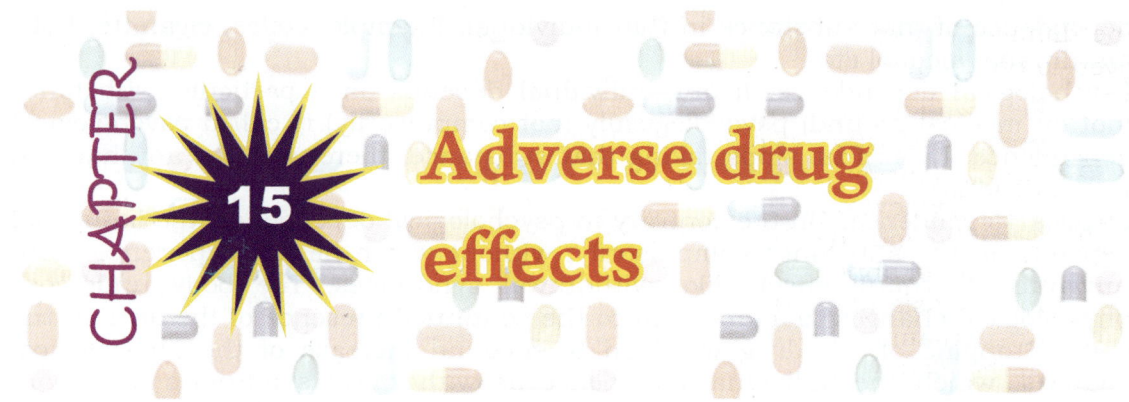

CHAPTER **15** Adverse drug effects

Adverse Drug effects:

Adverse effects of a drug is unwanted pharmacological actions in therapeutic or in over dose.

They are of two types

TYPE – A –PREDICTABLE   TYPE B -UNPREDICTABLE
Insulin-(hypoglycaemia)   (allergy, idiosyncrasy)
(drug related)   (patients related)

Type A Predictable:

1. Side effects are unwanted effects of a drug in THERAPEUTIC DOSE

2. Toxic effects are unwanted effects of a drug in OVER DOSE

3. Poisoning means that a drug endangers the life by affecting the vital functions like respiration and BP.

4. Drug intolerance: Some persons are hyperactive to a drug (Chloroquine in therapeutic dose will produce nausea and vomiting But in some it produces excess vomiting for the same therapeutic dose)

5. Teratogenicity: The drug is capable of producing foetal abnormalities, when given to pregnant women is called 'teratogenicity'

Possible mechanism of teratogenicity:

i) direct effect on differentiation of foetal tissues (Vit A analogue, Isotretinoin).

ii) they interfere with placental oxygenation or supply of nutrients in the foetal tissues.

iii) the drugs may act directly on some specific foetal organs to produce their damage (antithyroid drugs will produce hypothyroidism in foetus). Folic acid is to be given to minimise the teratogenic effect.

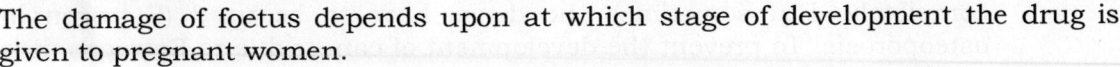

The damage of foetus depends upon at which stage of development the drug is given to pregnant women.

1. Fertilization and implantation (from conception to 17 days)- failure of pregnancy, which is often unnoticed.
2. Organogenesis (18th day to 55th day of gestation)- It is the most vulnerable period, where deformities are produced.
3. Growth and development (56th day onwards)-The developmental and functional abnormalities can occur in this period (ACE inhibitors can cause hyperplasia of organs, specially lungs and kidneys. NSAIDs (Non Steroidal Anti Inflammatory Drug) will cause premature closure of ductus arteriosus in the foetus.

Some drugs cause abnormalities in foetus when the drugs are given to pregnant women.

1. Thalidomide – phocomelia (absence of limbs)
2. Phenytoin – cleft palate
3. Antithyroid drugs – Foetal Hypothyroidism
4. Tetracyclines – abnormalities in bone and teeth
5. Morphine – respiratory depression in foetus
6. Chloramphenicol – Gray baby syndrome

Example of some safe drugs in pregnancy:

1. Insulin in diabetes mellitus
2. Heparin as anticoagulant
3. Pethidine as absteric analgesia
4. G^{+ve} infection – Ampicillin, Amoxicillin
5. In hypertension – α – Methyldopa, Hydralazine
6. In schizophrenia – Atypical antipsychotic drugs
7. In epilepsies – Newer antiepileptic drugs

6. Carcinogenicity and mutogenicity: carcinogenicity is the ability to produce cancer. Mutogenicity is the ability to mutate DNA and so GENE (alter the structure). This leads to alteration of particular protein structure → abnormalities, including development of cancer (Estrogen can cause breast cancer)

Drug → free radicals are released → reactive and damage different cellular structure including DNA molecule → mutation of gene → cancer. However, the carcinogenic effect of a drug is not proved completely. But sometimes the drugs have to be used (Estrogen in osteoporosis. To prevent the development of cancer due to Estrogen, it is combined with Progesterone.)

7.   Photosensitivity: i) Phototoxic and ii) Photoallergy

8.   Substance dependence (ref: substance abuse)

9.   Drug withdrawal symptoms: (Acute adrenal insufficiency is due to sudden withdrawal of Glucocorticoids and unstable angina is due to sudden withdrawal of β adrenergic blockers)

Type b (unpredictable reactions)

I.   Allergy: is a hypersensitive reaction to drugs.

   1. Type I (immediate type reaction)- Example : Anaphylactic shock (Fig.18). Mechanism: The drug (allergen) sensitizes in the body → antibodies are produced → when the drug is introduced for the second time into the body → antigen and antibody reaction takes place on mast cells → degranulation of mast cells → release of mediators like Histamine, PAF, SRS-A, kinins etc., All are powerful bronchoconstrictors and vasodilators (fall in BP) → Anaphylactic shock and death.

Fig. 18 Type I Hypersensitivity Reaction

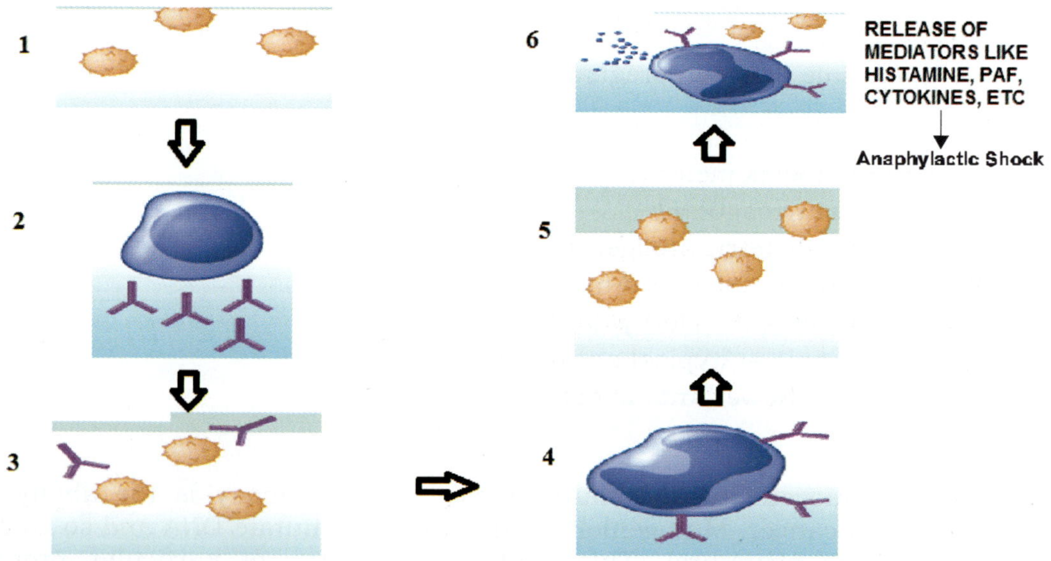

1 - ANTIGENS ENTER BODY
2 - DIFFERENTIATED B CELL SECRETES IgE ANTIBODIES
3 - ANTIGEN–ANTIBODY INTERACTION NEUTRALISES ANTIGEN
4 - EXCESS IgE ANTIBODIES BIND TO TISSUE MAST CELLS AND BLOOD-BORNE BASOPHILS
5 - ANTIGEN RE-ENTERS BODY (MAY BE AFTER A PERIOD OF TIME)
6 - ANTIGEN–ANTIBODY INTERACTION TRIGGERS MAST CELL/BASOPHIL DEGRANULATION

Treatment: Adrenaline, (IM inj. 0.5 ml of 1 in 1000) which is a powerful bronchodilator and vasoconstrictor (rise BP). This is the only drug simultaneously dilate the bronchi and rise BP and save the life.

2. Type II (Cytotoxic reaction)- haemolysis, thrombocytopenia, SLE (Systemic Lupus Erythematosus).

3. Type III (Arthus reaction): large antigen-antibody complexes → bind with a complement and precipitate on vascular endothelium and resulting in vasculitis (serum sickness, lymphadenopathy and joint pain are common clinical signs) Stevens-johnson syndrome is another manisfastation.

4. Type IV (delayed type hypersensitivity): Unlike the previous 3 types, it is 'T' cell mediated (CMI). Example: contact dermatitis

II. Idiosyncrasy: It is genetically determined abnormal reaction to a drug. Few drugs produce uncharacteristic reactions in some. (Example : Barbiturates in some individual cause excitement. Normally Barbiturates are CNS depressant). Quinidine in some causes cramps, purpura, asthma and vascsular collapse.

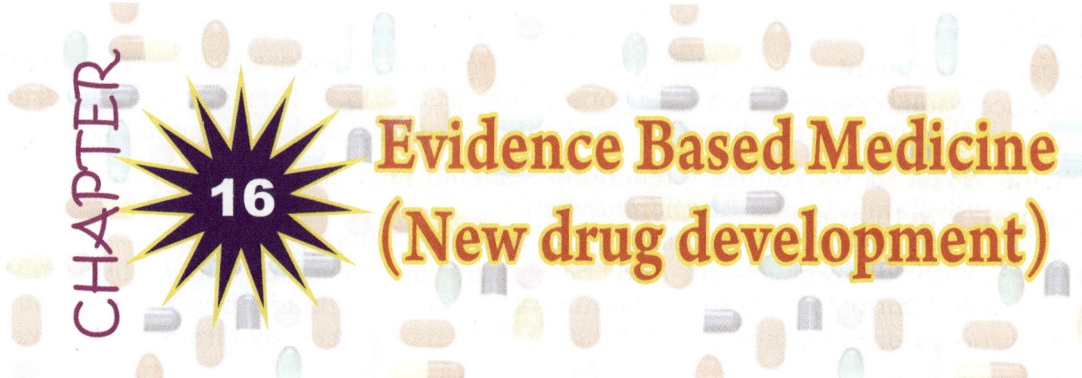

CHAPTER 16

Evidence Based Medicine (New drug development)

In the recent times new drugs are introduced in a rapid pace and the usage of older drugs becomes declining. The medical students must know how the newer drugs are developed? and also the various steps involved in the development of new drugs. Drug development has become a tedious, complex, prolonged and highly expensive procedure. Approximately new drug development from the initial stage takes 10 years and costs 500-1000 million US dollars.

Drug invention approaches :

1. Exploration of natural resources is still an important avenue for the new drug development. Opium, Cinchona, Digitalis, Belladonna, newer antimalarial Quinghaosu (artemisinin) are outstanding examples of plant sources. Animal sources such as Adrenaline, Thyroxine, Insulin, Antisera etc., and minerals like Iron, Calcium etc., are important medicines derived from natural resources.

2. Synthetic drugs 3. Molecular modelling 4. Biotechnology using DNA recombinant technology. 5. Gene therapy. These are the important new drug invention approaches adopted.

Preclinical Studies:

After identifying a suitable compound it is tested on animals to establish the pharmacological profile before introducing to human beings. Generally experiments are carried out in mouse, rat, guinea pig and then on larger animals. The following are the tests performed in animals screening tests, tests on isolated organs, animal models of human disease,toxicity tests etc., The aim of preclinical study is to determine the safety of the drug. Toxicity tests such as acute toxicity, subacute toxicity, chronic toxicity, reproductive and Teratogenicity, mutagenicity, carcinogenicity etc., are done.

EVIDENCE BASED MEDICINE:

Earlier, a new drug was introduced for treatment of diseases only based on experience by clinicians' observation Only herbals are used as medicine. But now a days, drugs are manufactured in large quantities. For that evidence based medicine replaced the experience based medicine. That means, a new drug is introduced into treatment only after confirmed by evidence based medicine.

Evidence based medicine is the process of systematically finding, evaluating and using contemporary research findings as the basis of clinical decisions. Therapeutic evaluation of a drug includes clinical studies which are basically clinical trials (testing the test drug on human) healthy human volunteer and diseased.

Clinical trials :

The suitable compound selected based on the animal study will be approved by the regulatory authorities as "investigational new drug" (IND) licence. This drug is formulated into suitable dosage form and undergoes the 4 phases of clinical trial. Standards for the design, ethics, conduct, monitoring, auditing, recording and analyzing data and reporting of clinical trials are laid down by Good Clinical Practice (GCP) guidelines by International Conference of Harmonization (ICH). National agencies such as ICMR in India also framed ethical guidelines for clinical trials. This provides accurate data and results which are credible. The rights of the subjects, integrity and confidentiality of trial subjects are protected as per the Helsinki Declaration of the World Medical Association.

First the inclusion and exclusions criteria to be decided depending upon the clinical trial drug

Exclusion criteria: 1. Generally the elderly persons, pregnant ladies, children, patients suffering from any other diseases

Others are included in the trial, depending upon the drug trial

There is every possibility of bias either by participants or by investigators in favour of or against the test drug. To minimise the bias, the following procedures are followed:

1. Randomization: The subjects are allocated to either group using a preselected random number table or computer programme, so that any subject has equal chance of being assigned to the test or the control group.
2. Blinding: This refers to concealment of the nature of treatment (test or control) from the subject (single blind), or both the subject and the investigator (double blind) For this purpose, the two medications should appear similar in appearance and taste. The randomized controlled double

blind trial is the most credible method of obtaining evidence of efficacy, safety or comparative value of treatment.

3. End point: The primary and secondary (if any) end points (cure, degree of improvement, symptom relief etc.) of the trial must be specified in advance.

CONSENT LETTER:

A letter of consent is written (in English or local language known to the volunteers) is a legal document, which binds both the parties (drug firm or clinicians who is handling clinical trial and volunteers, who is willing to participate in the drug trial)

The consent letter contains the following rules and regulations like,

1. The letter discusses the possible risks, side effects the volunteers encounter if he/she does agree to push through the clinical trial procedure.
2. Adequate compensation is to be given to volunteer in case of death (to the family) or any disability the trial causes.
3. The duration of validity of consent letter should be specific periods.

The consent letter should be signed by concerned parties before starting the clinical trials.

Following are the 4 phases of clinical trials with characteristics of each phase.

Phase I : Human Pharmacology and safety

The administration of drug in human is done by qualified clinical pharmacologist/ trained physician. There must be adequate facility to monitor vital functions and handle any drug related emergencies. Subjects are healthy volunteers. The number of patients are from 20-80. Starting from low dose increased to optimum effective dose. Safety, tolerability and adverse drug reactions and vital signs are monitored. Human pharmacokinetic parameters of the new drug is recorded.

Phase 0 : (microdosing) This new method is introduced to reduce time and cost of the drug development process.FDA also encouraging novel cost cutting approaches in new drug development. Microdosing human study is undertaken before phase -1 trial. Very low doses about 1/1000 of the estimated human dose administered to the healthy volunteers and pharmacokinetic studies done using sophisticated instruments such as Accelerated mass spectrometry (AMS) with radiolabelled drug or LC –Tandem mass spectrometry (LC-MS-MS).These studies yield very good pharmacokinetic information.

PHASE I	PHASE II	PHASE III	PHASE IV
First in Human (Healthy volunteers)	First in patient	Multi centre Trial	Post-marketing Surveillance
1-100 participants	50- 500 participants	Few hundred to few thousand participants	Many thousands of participants
Healthy volunteers Occasionally advanced or rare disease	Patient-subjects receiving experimental drug	Patient-subjects receiving experimental drug	Patients in treatment with approved drug
Open label	Randomized and controlled (Can be placebo-controlled) may be blinded	Randomized and controlled (Can be placebo-controlled)or uncontrolled, may be blinded	Open label
Safety and Tolerability	Efficacy and dose ranging	Confirm efficacy in larger population	Adverse events, compliance, drug-drug interactions
Months- 1 year	1-2 years	3-5 years	No fixed duration
U.S dollars 10 million	U.S. dollars 20 million	U.S.dollars 50-100 million	-No fixed rate
Success rate : 50%	50%	25-50%	--

Phase II: Therapeutic exploration and dose ranging

Conducted by physicians who are trained as clinical investigators. Involves 100-500 patients. Primary aim is to study the therapeutic efficacy, dose range and ceiling effect of the drug. Generally carried out in 2-4 centres. Mostly it is a controlled randomized study.

Phase III : Therapeutic confirmation and Comparision

These are randomized double blind comparative trials conducted in a large group of patients 500-3000 by several physicians in many cetres. The goal is to establish the efficacy of the drug in comparision with the existing therapy. Safety and tolerability also are also assessed in a bigger population. Indications and guidelines for therapeutic usage are formulated. "New drug application" (NDA) is submitted to licensing authority once it is accepted, approval will be given for marketing.

Phase IV : Post marketing surveillance

After the drug has been marketed and used in general population, through practicing physicians, data are collected regarding efficacy, acceptability, and adverse effects of the drug. Uncommon, idiosyncratic advesre reactions ,drug interactions are detected. Patterns of drug utilization and other indications of the drug may be found out in this phase. Special groups clinical trials such as children, elderly, pregnant/lactating women may be undertaken at this stage to establish the safety of the new drug.

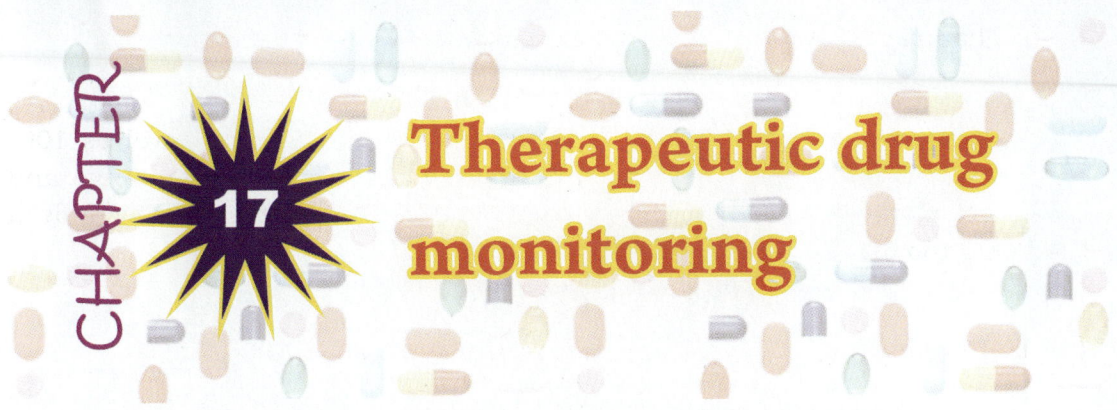

Therapeutic drug monitoring

CHAPTER 17

THERAPEATIC DRUG MONITORING
(Monitoring of plasma concentration of drugs)

Measurement of plasma drug concentration for some drugs is needed to know about their efficacy and the patient's compliance. So that appropriate adjustments in the dosage regimen can be made.

For example : In grand mal epilepsy, the plasma concentration of anti-epileptic drugs should be measured periodically and the plasma concentration of that drug should be kept within the necessary range throughout the treatment.

The plasma concentration of valproic acid in grand mal epilepsy should be kept between 80-100 mg/ml to prevent the attack of epilepsy.

Therapeutic drug monitoring (TDM) is particularly useful in the following situations:

1. Drugs with low margin of safety
   Example: Digoxin, antiepileptic drugs, lithium
2. To check patient's compliance
   Example: Anti psychotic drugs, antidepressent drugs
3. In case of poisoning to know how much severe.
4. Potentially toxic drugs used in the presence of renal failure.
   Example: Aminoglycoside antibiotics.

Monitoring of plasma concentration is of no value for

1. Drugs with irreversible action – Anticholinesterase
2. 'Hit' and 'run' drugs like Gentamicin, Mono amino oxidase inhibitors.
3. Drugs activated in the body – Levo dopa
4. Drugs whose response is easily measurable – anti hypertensive, antidiabetic, oral anticoagulants etc.,

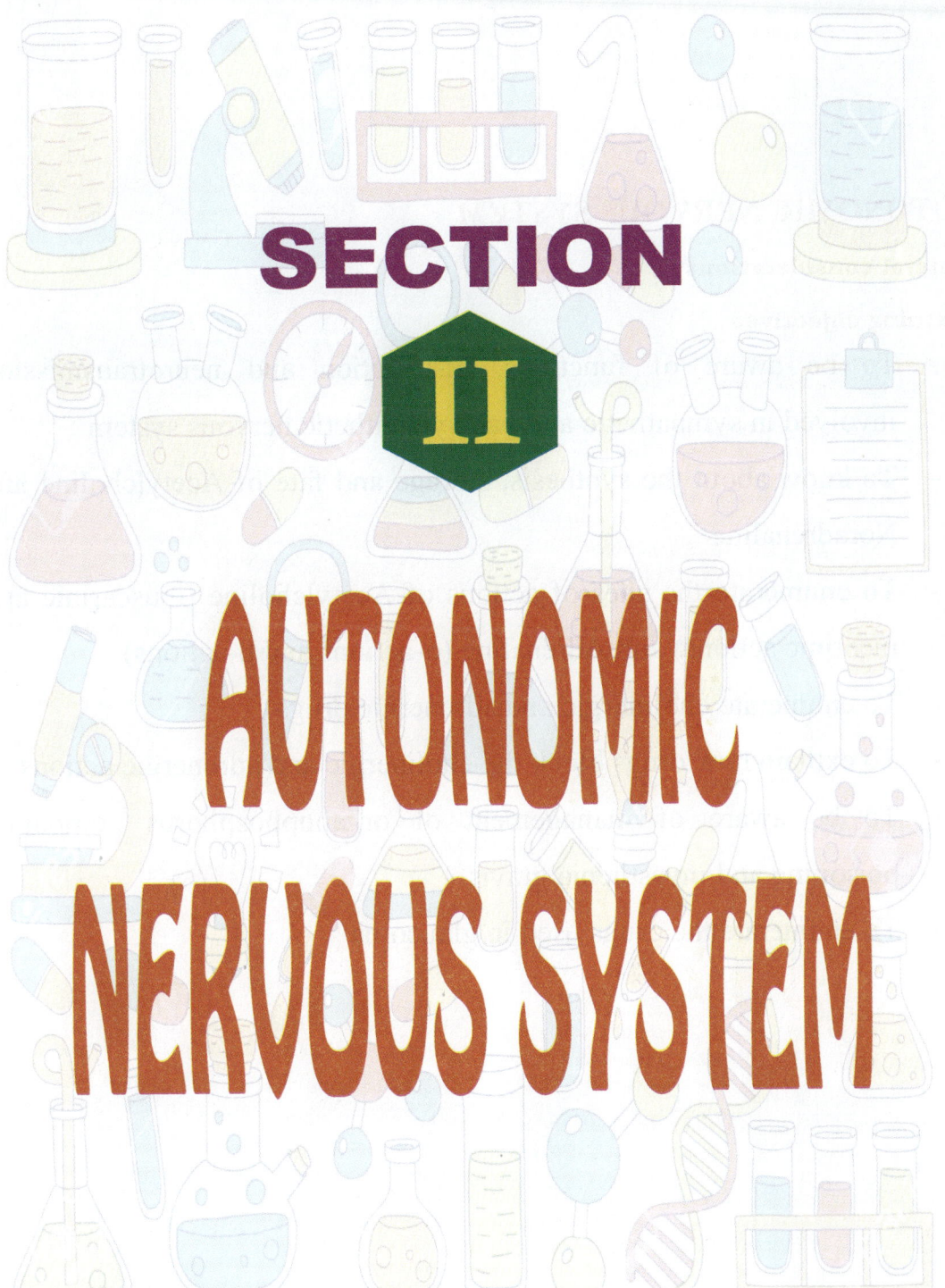

SECTION

II

AUTONOMIC NERVOUS SYSTEM

AUTONOMIC NERVOUS SYSTEM

General considerations

Learning objectives

- To be aware of functions, distribution and neurotransmission involved in sympathetic and parasympathetic nervous system
- To know about the synthesis, storage and fate of Acetylcholine and Noradrenaline
- To enumerate the sites of actions of Acetylcholine (muscarinic and nicotinic actions) and Adrenaline (α-actions and β-actions)
- To enumerate cholinergic and adrenergic drugs
- To explain how drugs block the cholinergic and adrenergic actions
- To be aware of management of organophosphorus compound poisoning and myasthenia gravis
- To enumerate the drugs used in glaucoma

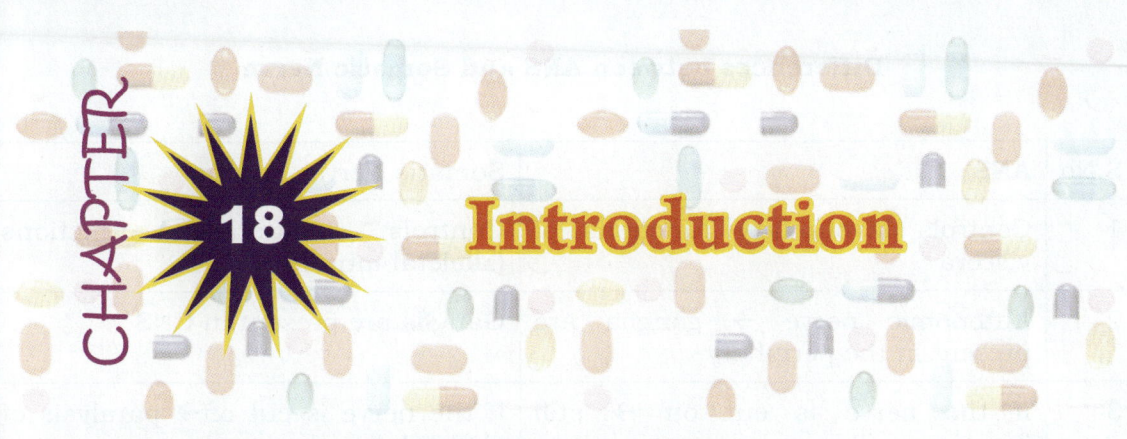

CHAPTER 18

Introduction

"Auto" means "Automatic functions / involuntary functions". ANS maintains/ controls the involuntary functions of the viscera – Viscera include smooth muscles (GIT, urinary bladder, bronchi), exocrine glands (sweat, salivary, tracheobronchial, parietal cells, which secrete acid), blood vessels, heart, eye (iris muscle and ciliary muscles)

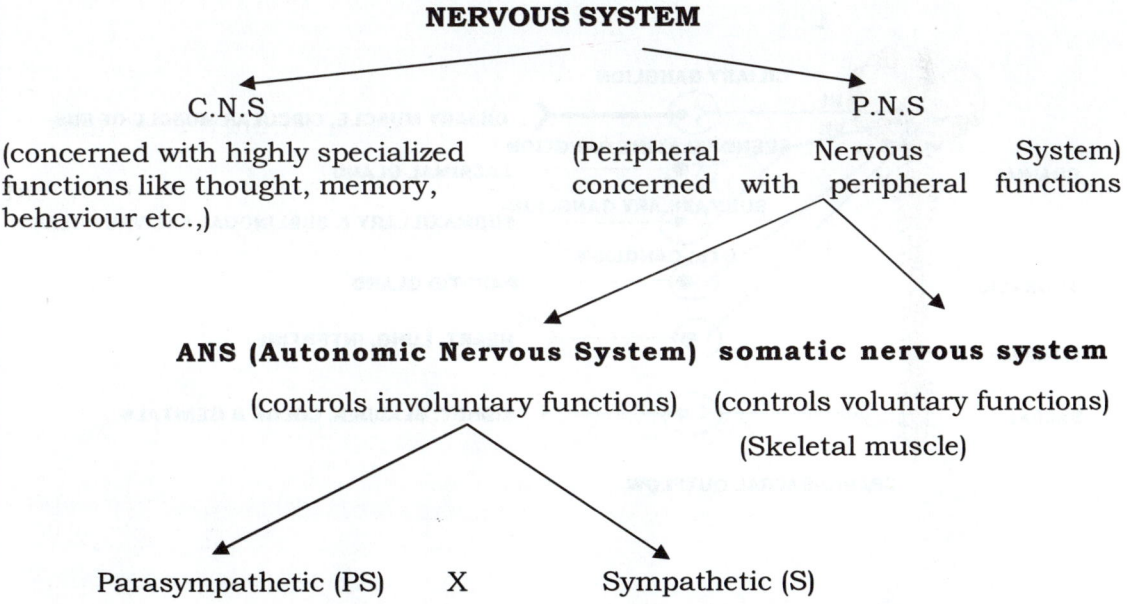

NERVOUS SYSTEM

C.N.S

(concerned with highly specialized functions like thought, memory, behaviour etc.,)

P.N.S

(Peripheral Nervous System) concerned with peripheral functions

ANS (Autonomic Nervous System)
(controls involuntary functions)

somatic nervous system
(controls voluntary functions)
(Skeletal muscle)

Parasympathetic (PS)   X   Sympathetic (S)

Differences between ANS and Somatic Nerve

S.No	ANS	Somatic Nerve
1	Controls involuntary functions of viscera	Controls voluntary functions (skeletal muscles)
2	Autonomic nerve → ganglia are present in the periphery	Ganglia are present in CNS
3	If the nerve is cut off → still functions will be going on	If the nerve is cut off→ paralysis of skeletal muscles occur

Fig. 19-A PARASYMPATHETIC NERVOUS SYSTEM AND ITS INNERVATION IN VARIOUS ORGANS

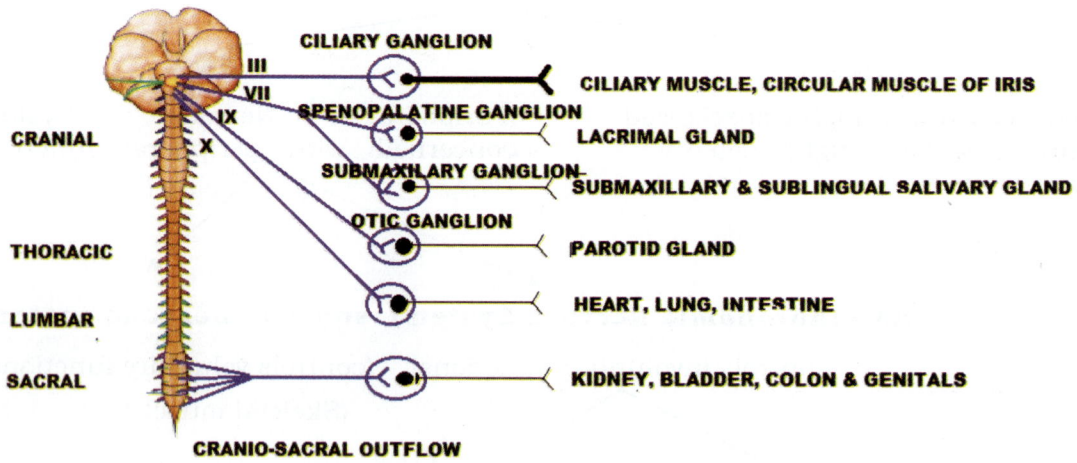

Fig.19-B SYMPATHETIC NERVOUS SYSTEM AND ITS INNVERVATION IN VARIOUS ORGANS

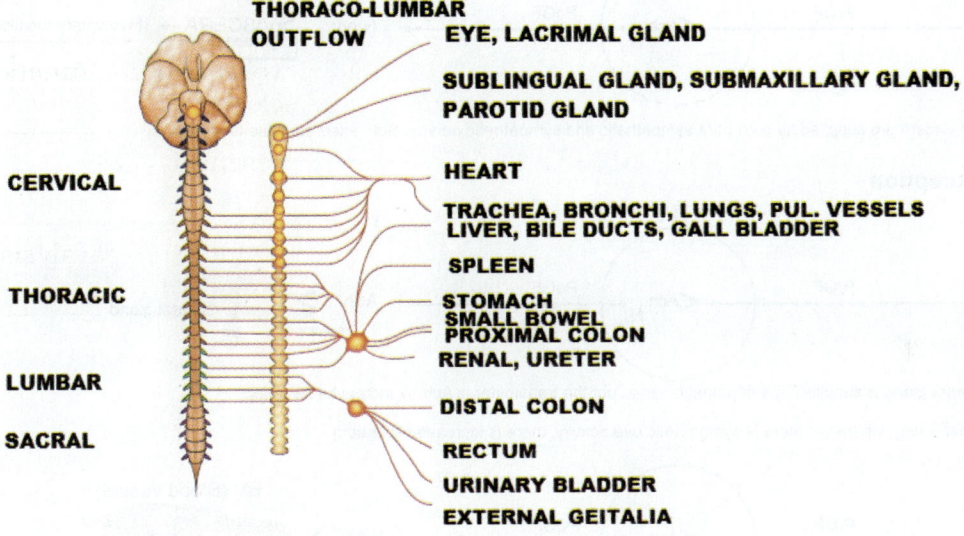

THORACO-LUMBAR
OUTFLOW

EYE, LACRIMAL GLAND

SUBLINGUAL GLAND, SUBMAXILLARY GLAND,
PAROTID GLAND

CERVICAL

HEART

TRACHEA, BRONCHI, LUNGS, PUL. VESSELS
LIVER, BILE DUCTS, GALL BLADDER

SPLEEN

THORACIC

STOMACH
SMALL BOWEL
PROXIMAL COLON
RENAL, URETER

LUMBAR

DISTAL COLON

SACRAL

RECTUM

URINARY BLADDER

EXTERNAL GEITALIA

Fig.20 STRUCTURE OF AUTONOMIC NERVES AND SOMATIC NERVE

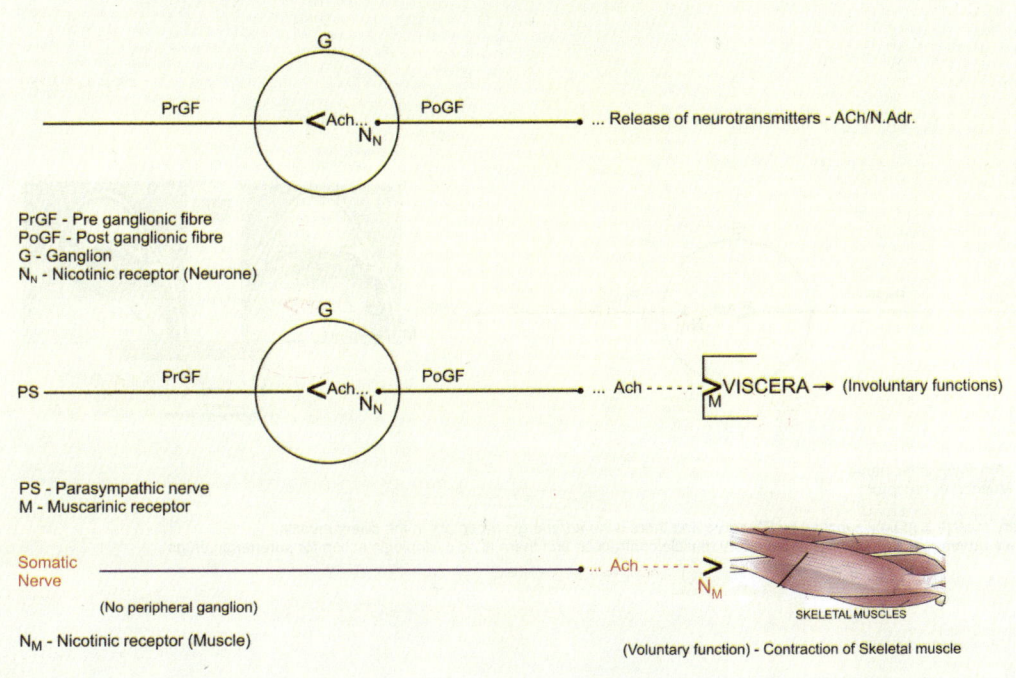

PrGF — Pre ganglionic fibre
PoGF — Post ganglionic fibre
G — Ganglion
N_N — Nicotinic receptor (Neurone)

PS — Parasympathic nerve
M — Muscarinic receptor

Somatic Nerve   (No peripheral ganglion)

N_M — Nicotinic receptor (Muscle)

... Release of neurotransmitters - ACh/N.Adr.

... Ach - - - - - VISCERA → (Involuntary functions)

... Ach - - - - - SKELETAL MUSCLES

(Voluntary function) - Contraction of Skeletal muscle

Fig.21 EXCEPTIONS IN ANS

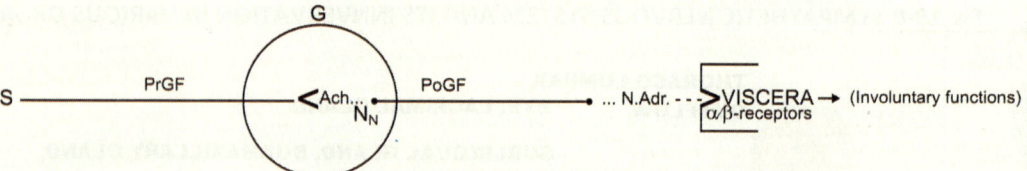

All viscera are supplied by both para sympathetic and sympathetic nerves. Both exert opposite functions.

Exception

1)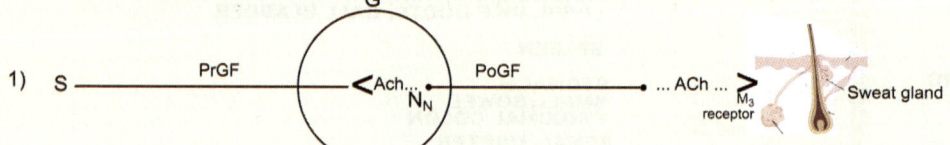

Sweat gland is supplied by sympathetic nerve, but the transmitter is Ach → increases sweating

That is why, whenever there is sympathetic overactivity, there is increased sweating

2)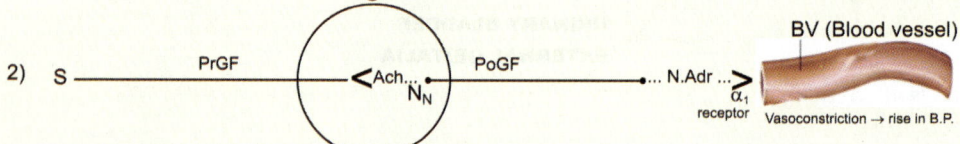

Blood vessels are only under the sympathetic constrictor tone. (There is no parasympathetic nerve supply to the blood vessel.)

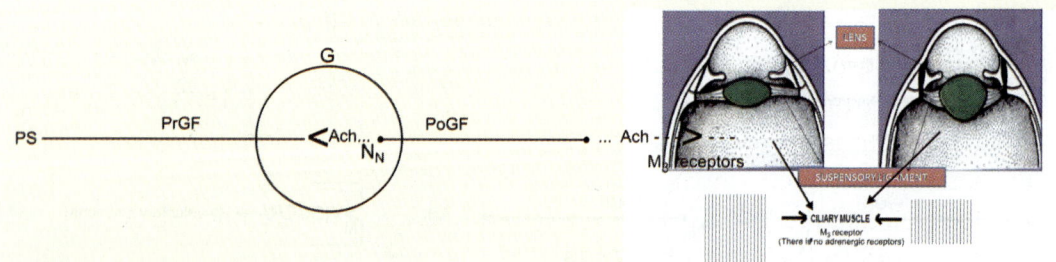

PS - Parasympathic nerve
M - Muscarinic receptor

Ciliary muscle is mainly supplied by PS nerve and there is no adrenergic receptors in the ciliary muscle.
Hence adrenergic drugs do not affect ciliary muscle contraction and there is no cycloplegic action for adrenergic drugs.

Differences between Parasympathetic nervous system and Sympathetic nervous system (Fig.19A/19B)

S.No		Parasympathetic	Sympathetic
1	**ORIGIN**	Cranio (3,7,9,10) and Sacral outflow (S2,3,4) Only these cranial nerves are PS, because they have ganglia in the periphery and they release neurotransmitter, ACh (Acetylecholine).	Thoroco lumbar outflow (T1-T12, L1,2,3)
2	**TRANSMITTER**	ACh	Noradrenaline
3	**RECEPTORS**	Cholinergic (muscarinic & nicotinic)	Adrenergic (α & β)
4	**ACTIVITY**	Active during rest and digestion	Active during FFF (Fight, Freight, Flight)

- All the autonomic drugs act through neurotransmitters and respective receptors
- All the viscera are supplied by both Parasympathetic and Sympathetic nerves (exception – (Fig.21) Blood vessels are supplied by only Sympathetic nerve, sweat gland is supplied by Sympathetic nerve but the transmitter is ACh)
- Ciliary muscles is mainly supplied by Parasympathetic nerve

Synthesis, storage, release and fate of ACh: (Fig.22)

- Choline is taken up by the cholinergic nerve ending
- Acetyl-Co-A (Acetyl coenzyme A) is present in the cholinergic nerve ending
- Choline combines with Acetyl coenzyme A and is converted into ACh
- Then ACh is stored in the granules at the nerve ending
- ACh is released in responds to stimulus from CNS
- The released ACh travels in the synaptic cleft and occupies the cholinergic receptors in the effector organs
- Then ACh stimulates the receptors and produces respective pharmacological actions
- After that, the ACh is destroyed in the body by the enzyme cholinesterase in a fraction of seconds into choline and acetic acid.

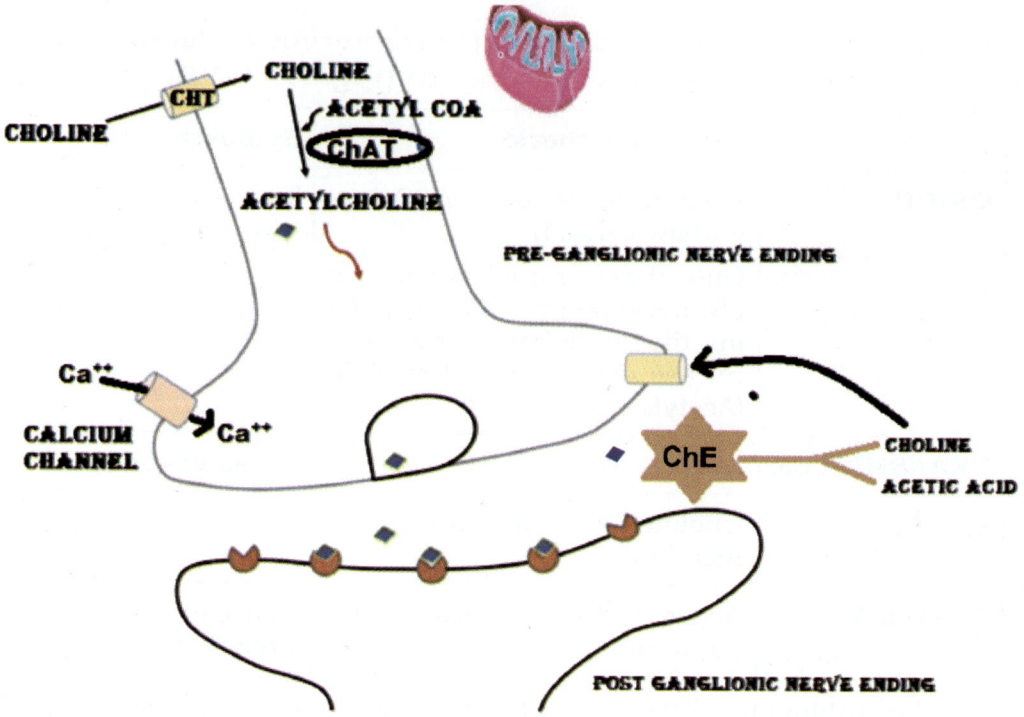

ChE - Cholinesterase

Fig.22 ACETYLCHOLINE (ACh) SYNTHESIS, STORAGE, RELEASE AND METABOLISM

- Choline is taken up by the nerve ending to resynthesis ACh
- That is why ACh is not suitable for therapeutic use, since it is destroyed by the enzyme in a fraction of time
- If cholinergic action is required, other cholinergic drugs, which are slowly destroyed or anticholiesterase are preferred.

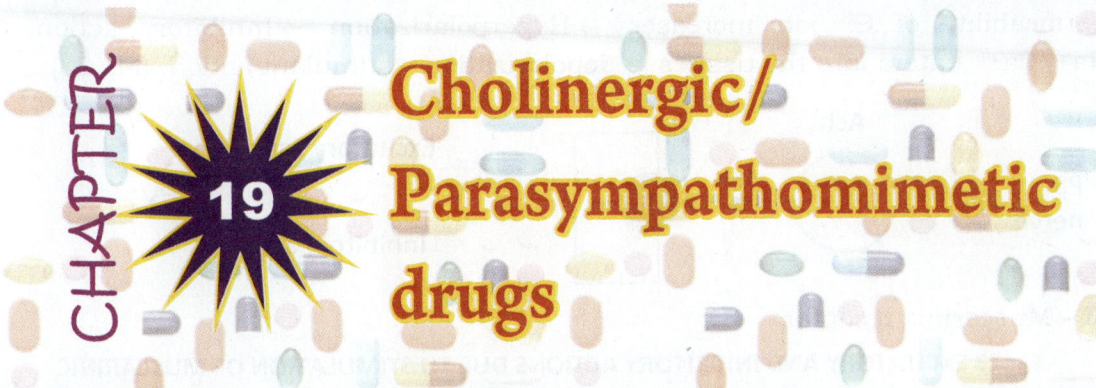

Cholinergic/ Parasympathomimetic drugs

Cholinergic drugs produce the actions similar to that of Acetylcholine exerted through muscarinic receptors mainly.

Parasympathomimetic drugs produce the actions similar to that of actions due to stimulation of all parasympathetic nerves.

More or less both terms are similar.

I. DIRECTLY ACTING
- Pilocarpine (Alkaloid)
- ACh (it is an important neurotransmitter in the body but clinically not useful, since the drug is quickly destroyed in the blood (fraction of seconds))

II. INDIRECTLY ACTING (anticholinestarases)
- They do not occupy the receptors directly, but they act through ACh in the body. They are called anticholinestarases. They are of 2 types:
  - ➢ Reversible anticholinestarases
  - ➢ Irreversible anticholinestarases

1. **REVERSIBLE ANTICHOLINESTARASES**
   i. Neostigmine
   ii. Physostigmine
   iii. Pyridostigmine
   iv. Edrophonium
   v. Tacrine
   vi. Rivastigmine

2. **IRREVERSIBLE ANTICHOLINESTARASES** (Organophosphorous compounds)
   i. Malathion ⎤ insecticides
   ii. Parathion ⎥
   iii. Tabun   ⎥ nerve gas
   iv. Sarin   ⎦

Pharmacological actions of CHOLINERGIC DRUGS / ACETYLCHOLINE (ACh)

Acetylcholine is an important neurotransmitter in the body. But it cannot be used clinically, because of rapid destruction of acetylcholine in the body. Anticholinesterases are preferred if acetylcholine like actions required.

Stimulation of receptor → IPSP (Inhibitory Post Synaptic Potential) develops → permeability of Cl⁻ ion increases → Hyperpolarization → Inhibitory action. If Na+/Ca++ enters into the tissues → depolarization – stimulant action. (Fig.23)

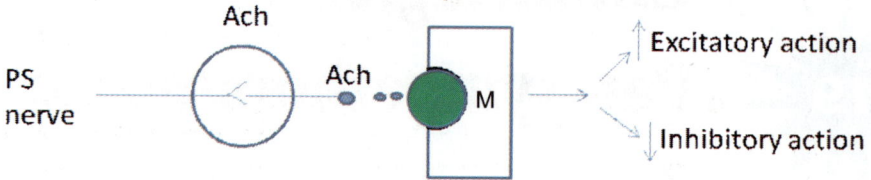

M – Muscarinic receptor

Fig.23 EXCITATORY AND INHIBITORY ACTIONS DUE TO STIMULATION OF MUSCARINIC RECEPTORS

Muscarnic actions	Nicotinic actions
1. ↑ stimulation of smooth muscles	↑ stimulation of skeletal muscles
2. ↑ stimulation of exocrine secretions	Blocked by neuromuscular blocking agents
3. ↓ inhibition of heart	
4. On eye : miosis, ↓ (reduce) I.O.P.	
5. ↓ (fall) in B.P. – due to vasodilatation	

Blocked by anticholinergic / antimuscarinic drugs like Atropine

I. MUSCARINIC ACTIONS (Fig.24)

1) Stimulation of smooth muscles (M_3)
- Stimulation of gastrointestinal smooth muscles → stimulate gastrointestinal motility → increase tone of gastrointestinal smooth muscle and relaxation of sphincters → diarrhoea.
- Stimulation of smooth muscles of urinary bladder → stimulation causes contraction of detrusor muscle and relaxation of sphincters, leading to voiding of urinary bladder (urination)
- Stimulation of bronchial smooth muscle causes bronchoconstriction.

2) Stimulation of exocrine glands (M_3)
   Stimulation of exocrine glands cause increased sweating, salivation, tracheobronchial secretion, lacrimation and acid secretion from parietal cells (M_1) of stomach

3) Inhibition of heart (M_2) will lead to decreased heart rate (Bradycardia), reduced cardiac output, reduced conduction velocity.

4) On Eye (M_3) (Fig.25A/25B)

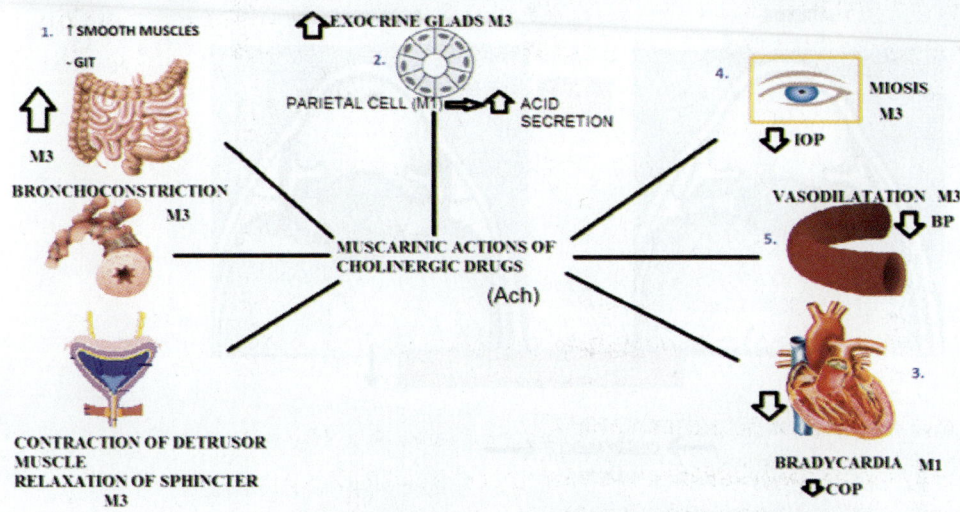

Fig.24 Muscarinic action of Cholinergic drugs

1. Stimulation of all smooth Muscles Diarrhoea, Micturition, Bronchoconstriction
2. Stimulation of Exocrine Glands Increase Salivation, Lacrimation, Sweating, Gastric Acid Secretion (M_1) and Tracheobronchial Secretion
3. Inhibition of Heart - Reduces the heart rate, force of contraction and conduction
4. On eye - moisis, reduces the IOP, spasm of accomodation
5. Vasodilatation → Fall in BP

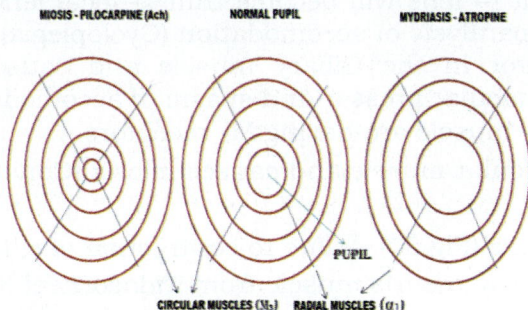

Fig.25A Illustration of Iris Muscle and action of Miotics and Mydriatics

Cholinergic drugs (Pilocarpine) stimulates M_3 receptors in the circular muscle and causes constriction of pupil (miosis). Atropine blocks M_3 receptors in the circular muscles and causes dilatation of pupil (Mydriasis).

Adrenergic Drugs stimulate α_1 receptors in the radial muscle and causes mydriasis

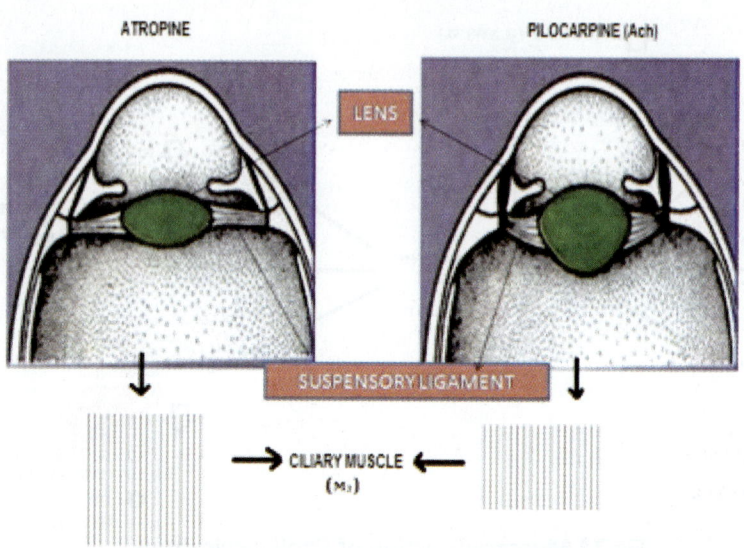

Fig.25B Action of Pilocarpine and Atropine on Ciliary Muscle

Atropine → Inhibits M₃ receptor in Ciliary muscle → Relaxation of Ciliary muscle → Narrowing of canal of schlemn ad decreasing of the patency of trabecular mesh → Decreases the flow of Aqueous humour → Accumulation of Aqueous humour in the aterior chamber of the eye → increase the Intraocular pressure.

Pilocarpine produces opposite action of Atropine and causes reduction of intraocular pressure.

Atropine - blocks M₃ receptor in Ciliary muscle → Relaxation of Ciliary muscle → Tightening of suspensory ligament → lens will become thin → focal length will be away → near vision is difficult → paralysis of accomodation (Cycloplegia).

Pilocarpine stimulates M₃ receptor in the Ciliary muscle and causes actions opposite to atropine (reduces intraocular pressor and spasm of accomodation).

- Circular muscle and ciliary muscle are having M₃ receptors.
- Acetylcholine constricts circular muscle and causes miosis (Constriction of pupil)
- Reduces intraocular pressure (Fig.30) → due to contraction of ciliary muscle and miosis (pulls away the iris muscle from iridocorneal junction → widen the canal of schlemn → increases the drainage of aqueous humour → reduces intraocular pressure
- On ciliary muscle: ACh contract ciliary muscle and relaxes suspensory ligament → lens will become more convex → lens is fixed for near vision → spasm of accomodation.
5) On Blood vessels (M₃)
   Blood vessels are not supplied by parasympathetic nerves. But M₃ receptors are present. Exogenously administered cholinergic drugs stimulate the M₃ receptors and cause vasodilatation → fall in B.P.

II. NICOTINIC ACTIONS (Fig.26)

Somatic
Nerve ⟶ •···· Ach ····> >
NM

(No peripheral ganglion)

SKELETAL MUSCLES

NM - Nicotinic receptor (Muscle)

(Voluntary function) - Contraction of Skeletal muscle

Fig.26 – Stimulation of N$_M$ receptor (Muscle) and contraction of Skeletal muscle

- On skeletal muscle (N$_M$)
- Stimulation of skeletal muscle → fasciculation and twitching. Very high dose causes relaxation of skeletal muscles.

III. ACTIONS ON CNS

1. Basal ganglia → overactivity of cholinergic system will cause parkinsonism.
2. Deficiency of acetylcholine will cause alzheimer's disease.
3. Stimulation of M$_1$ receptor in inner ear will lead to vomiting. (motion sickness)

PILOCARPINE

- Pilocarpine is a cholinergic drug.
- It is directly acting cholinergic drug
- The actions on eye:
- Miosis, Reduce intraocular pressure and hence useful in glaucoma
- **Mechanism of action** as miotic: (Fig.25A/25B/30)
- It stimulates muscarinic receptor present in the circular muscle(sphincter papillae), constriction of pupul.
- **Mechanism of action** in reducing intraocular pressure:

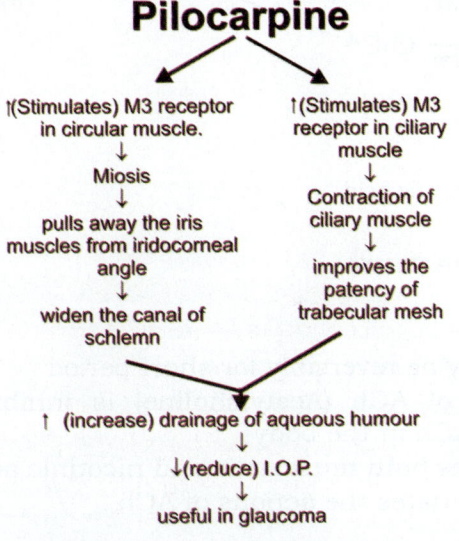

Pilocarpine

↑(Stimulates) M3 receptor in circular muscle.
↓
Miosis
↓
pulls away the iris muscles from iridocorneal angle
↓
widen the canal of schlemn

↑(Stimulates) M3 receptor in ciliary muscle
↓
Contraction of ciliary muscle
↓
improves the patency of trabecular mesh

↑ (increase) drainage of aqueous humour
↓
↓(reduce) I.O.P.
↓
useful in glaucoma

- **Clinical uses** as Miotic: 1. In glaucoma 2. To reverse the unwanted mydriatic action after the use of Tropicamide in testing of refractory error. 3. It is used alternate with mydriatic in inflammatory conditions of the eye(iritis, iridocyclitis) to prevent the adhesion between iris and cornea.

For prolonged action, it is used in the form of ocusert (Refer : Ocusert under dosage forms of drugs)

Adverse effects when used in glaucoma:

Due to the spasm of ciliacy muscle and iris muscle, it causes brow pain.

NEOSTIGMINE

- It is a commonly used anticholinesterase.

Mechanism of action

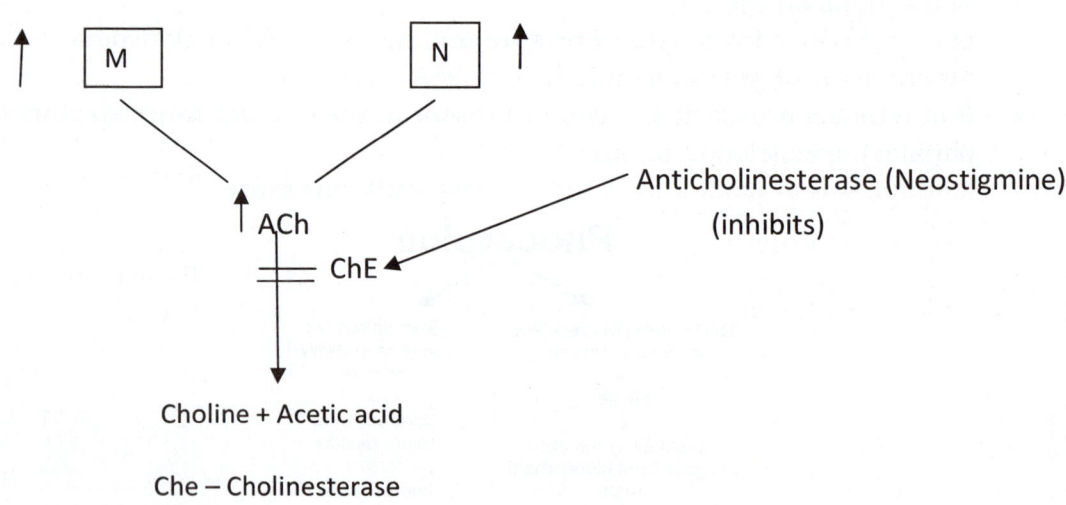

Che – Cholinesterase

- It inhibits the enzyme reversibly for short period
- The degradation of ACh (Acetylcholine) is inhibited and increases the concentration of ACh in the body
- That ACh increases both muscarnic and nicotinic actions
- Neostigmine potentiates the actions of ACh.

Pharmacological actions

Neostigmine has got both muscarinic and nicotinic actions like that of ACh (Ref: before for detail)

Clinical uses of NEOSTIGMINE

1. In myasthenia gravis (Ref: Treatment of myasthenia gravis) along with Atropine (Atropine antagonizes all the unwanted muscarinic actions without affecting the wanted nicotinic action of Neostigmine).
2. In curare like drugs (skeletal muscle relaxants)overdose/poisoing
3. To reverse unwanted action of the skeletal muscle relaxant after surgery.
4. In Cobra poisoning (it is believed that Neostigmine neutralises poison)
5. In post operative paralytic ileus and urinary retention (in some there will be excess smooth muscles relaxation after surgery)

Adverse effects (all muscaranic actions)

Diarrhoea, increased frequency of urination, bronchoconstriction, increased sweating, salivation, tracheobronchial secretion, gastric acid secretion (gastric irritation), bradycardia, fall in BP, miosis.

Dose 10-15 mg/3 times /daily

OTHER DRUGS

- Pyridostigmine- It is long acting and given once daily
- Physostigmine is suitable for Atropine poisoning, since it effectively crosses Blood Brain Barrier and antagonises the central toxicity of Atropine
- Edrophonium is suitable for diagnostic purpose: (To differentiate between cholinergic crisis and myasthenia gravis). If there is an improvement in skeletal muscles performance (ptosis is relieved) after giving Edrophonium, then the patient is suffering from myasthenia gravis and if it worsens then the patient is suffering from cholinergic crisis (ptosis).
- Tacrine: useful in Alzheimer's disease. (Alzheimer's disease is due to deficiency of ACh in CNS).

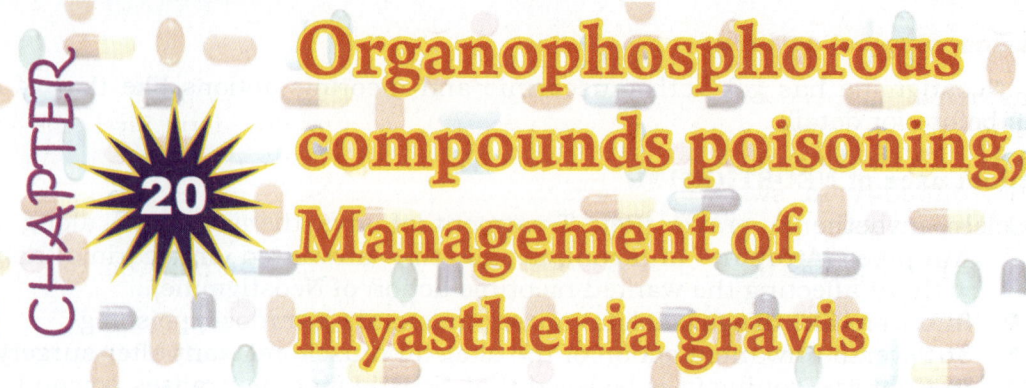

CHAPTER 20

Organophosphorous compounds poisoning, Management of myasthenia gravis

ORGANOPHOSPHOROUS COMPOUND POISONING

CAUSES:

1. Due to accidental poisoning, while spraying insecticides in the field.
2. In suicidal attempt (since the compound is available freely in the fertilizer's shop and in farmer's house)

Symptoms: (will be useful for diagnostic purpose)

- Excess muscaranic and nicotinic actions
- Excess muscaranic actions: excess salivation, sweating, lacrimation, tracheobronchial secretion, acid secretion, inhibition of heart (bradycardia), vasodilatation (fall in BP), miosis, involuntary urination.
- excess nicotinic actions:initial fasciculation followed by respiratory muscles paralysis.

Management :

1. Remove all the clothes of the patient and wash the entire body, since the poison is absorbed freely through skin.
2. Support BP and respiration.
3. Gastric lavage is given to remove unabsorbed poison in the GIT, if the patient consumed poison orally.
4. Specific antidotes: Atropine 1 mg/IV is repeated in every two hours till pupils dilate (to antagonise all the muscaranic effects).
5. Pralidoxime: choline esterase reactivators (to antagonise the nicotinic effects-It hydrolyses the enzyme-cholinesterase and free the enzyme. The enzyme becomes active. So, the excess ACh at the nicotinic site is degraded).

Mushroom poisoning (Excess muscarinic actions)

Treatment : Atropine 1 mg/IV repeated till pupil dilates.

TREATMENT OF MYASTHENIA GRAVIS

Myasthenia gravis is an autoimmune disorder characterised by progressive loss of skeletal muscles tone, skeletal muscle weakness and fatiguability. First, the small and rapidly moving muscles are affected leading to ptosis, slow movement of limbs, difficulty in swallowing and difficulty in speech and lastly respiratory muscles paralysis.

In myasthenia gravis the nicotinic receptors are considered as 'non-self'

- Anti nicotinic receptors antibodies are produced
- Antigen (nicotinic receptors)-antibody reaction takes place on nicotinic receptors
- The nicotinic receptors are destroyed and the number of nicotinic receptors reduced for the action of ACh. There is a progressive loss of skeletal muscles tone

Treatment

1. Increase the concentration of ACh in the nicotinic sites by giving Neostigmine along with Atropine-Ref: Neostigmine.
2. Prevent the destruction of nicotinic receptors by giving immuno - suppressive drugs like Glucocorticoids, Cyclosporin, Methotrexate (Ref : Immuno-suppressant drugs)
3. If not controlled by the above drugs, plasmaphresis (infusion of fresh blood) is performed.
4. Lastly thymectomy (removal of thymus gland, which release immune cells) is performed.

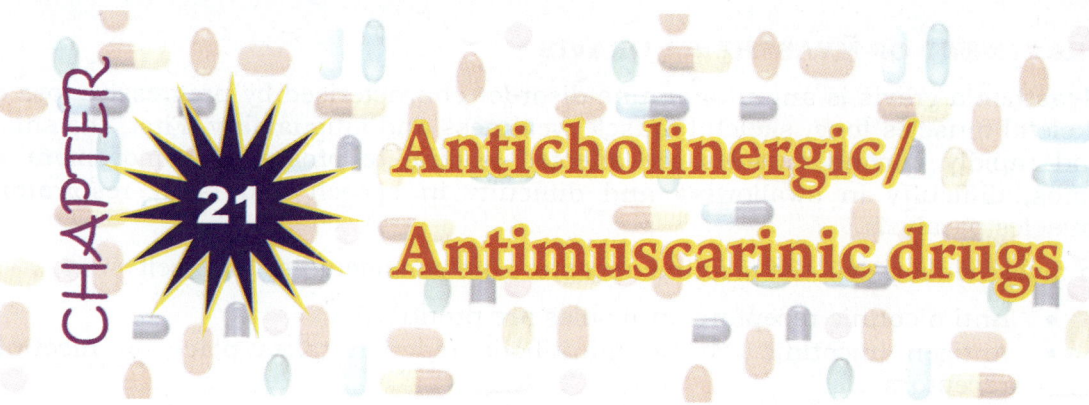

Anticholinergic/ Antimuscarinic drugs

CHAPTER 21

ANTICHOLINERGIC DRUGS (MUSCARANIC BLOCKERS)

The drugs which inhibit/reverse the actions of cholinergic drugs by blocking the muscaranic receptors are called anticholinergic or muscaranic blockers.

CLASSIFICATION OF DRUGS:

I.   Natural alkaloids: (Belladona alkaloids): Atropine, Hyoscine (Scopalamine)

II. Atropine substitutes (Atropine like drugs but have more specific useful actions and less toxic effects) – Synthetic drugs. Atropine produces non-specific actions and hence many side effects.

1. Drugs used on eye: Tropicamide, Cyclopentolate

2. Drugs used as antispasmodic: DICYCLOMINE, Oxyphenonium, Propanthelene, Clidinium, Isopropamide

3. Drugs used as antisecretory: Glycopyrrolate, Pirenzepine

4. Drugs used in parkinsonism: Benzhexol (Trihexyphenidyl), Benztropine

5. Vasico active drugs – oxybutynin, tolterodine, drotaverine

ATROPINE

It is an alkaloid from the plant Atropa belladona.

It is an anticholinergic drug

Mechanism of action: (Fig.27) Atropine has got high affinity towards muscarinic receptors. But it has got no intrinsic activity. It blocks all the muscarinic receptors and prevents acetylcholine to occupy and act.

Atropine reverses all the actions of acetylcholine.

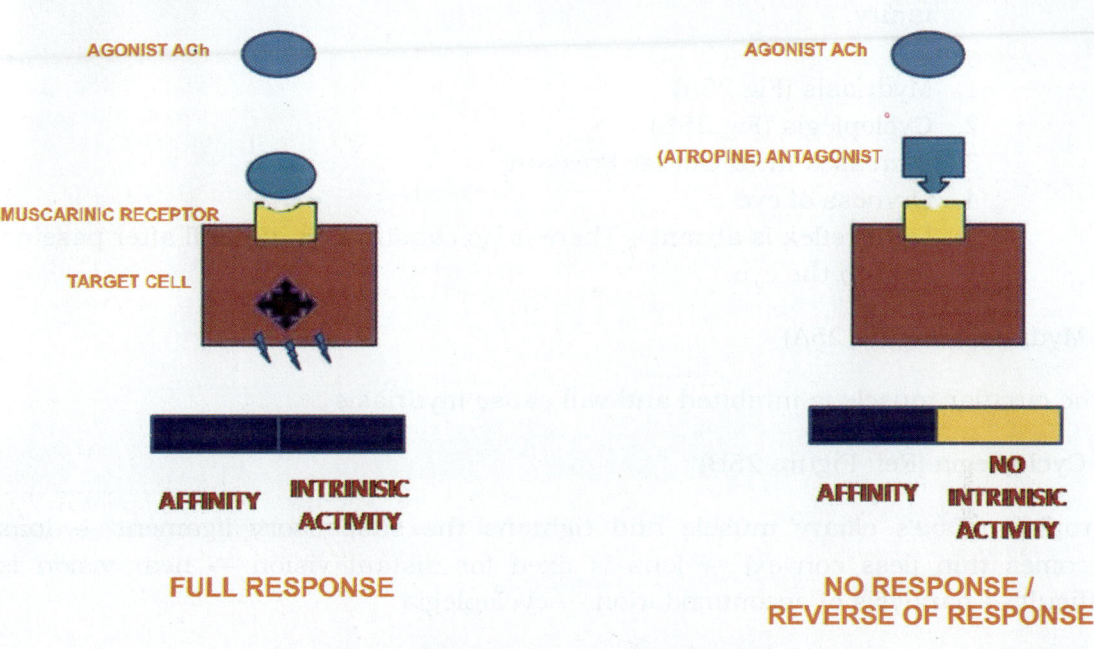

Fig.27 Mechanism of action of Atropine

Pharmacological actions of ATROPINE (opposite to thet of acetylcholine)

I. On smooth muscles
1. Gastrointestinal smooth muscles:
    Atropine decreases the tone and motility. It produces constriction of
    sphincters. Gastric emptying is delayed. Intestinal transit time is
    increased. All the actions cause constipation.
2. Genitourinary system. The muscles of ureter and urinary bladder
    wall are relaxed. Voiding is slowed down (urinary retention)
3. Bronchial muscle: Smooth muscles of pulmonary airway are relaxed
    and hence bronchodilatation.

II. On Exocrine secretion - Atropine
1. inhibits all the exocrine secretions
2. inhibits sweating will cause dryness of skin and increases body
    temperature.
3. inhibits salivation leads to dry mouth and difficult in swallowing.
4. inhibits acid secretion, useful in peptic ulcer
5. inhibits tracheobronchial secretion. The respiratory tract becomes
    dry. The Mucus becomes thick and plugs, which lead to infection.

6. inhibits lacrimation causes dryness of eye and is prone to dust injury.

III. On eye
1. Mydriasis (Fig.25A)
2. Cycloplegia (Fig.25B)
3. Increases Intra Ocular Pressure
4. Dryness of eye
5. Light reflex is absent – There is no constriction of pupil after passing light to the eye.

1) Mydriasis (Figure 25A)

- the circular muscle is inhibited and will cause mydriasis

2) Cycloplegia (Ref: Figure 25B)

Atropine relaxes ciliary muscle and tightens the suspensory ligament → lens becomes thin (less convex) → lens is fixed for distant vision → near vision is difficult → paralysis of accommodation → cycloplegia.

3) Intraocular pressure

Atropine produces mydriasis → Iris muscle pushes towards iridocorneal junction → obstructs canal of schlemn → reduces the drainage of aqueous humour → increases the concentration of aqueous humour in the anterior chamber of eye → increases intra ocular pressure. It is contraindicated in glaucoma.

IV. **On Heart:**
Atropine reverses cholinergic drugs/vagus induced cardiac inhibition. It is not effective in reversing cardiac inhibition due to other causes.
Stimulation of heart causes increase in heart rate (tachycardia), increases cardiac output, increases the conduction velocity of myocardium.

V. **Blood vessels:**
Atropine produces vasoconstriction only in cholinergic drugs induced vasodilatation. Blood vessels are not supplied by parasympathetic nerve. But blood vessels have got M_3 receptors.

VI. **On CNS:**
1. Antiparkinsonism action: Parkinsonism is partly due to overactivity of cholinergic system in basal ganglia.
2. Anti motion sickness action: M_1 receptors are present in semicircular canal of inner ear. M_1 receptors are stimulated →

vomiting impulse is carried to vomiting centre and produce vomiting (motion sickness). Hyoscine inhibits M_1 receptor and is effective in motion sickness by preventing the vomiting impulse reaching the vomiting centre.

Clinical uses of ATROPINE AND ATROPINE SUBSTITUTES

USES of Atropine:

1. In Organophosphorous compound poisoning
2. To reverse the unwanted muscaranic effects of Neostigmine in Myasthenia gravis
3. In motion sickness (Hyoscine is used-given half an hour before performing journey)

USES of Atropine substitutes:

I. On eye: (Cyclopentolate, Tropicamide). The duration of action of these drugs is short. The adverse effects are also short lasting. But Atropine is long acting and the adverse effects are also long lasting.

1. For testing refractory error (cycloplegic action is needed. That is why mydriatic like Phenylephrine is not useful for this purpose, since it does not have cycloplegic action)

2. To give rest to eye in some inflammatory conditions

3. To prevent adhesion between iris and cornea in inflammatory conditions, it is given alternate with miotic

II. As antispasmodic: (Dicyclomine)

1. To relieve pain in intestinal,ureteric and biliary colic

2. In urinary incontinence and nocturnal enuresis in children

3. In non-specific diarrhoea

4. In bronchial asthma and in COPD (Chronic Obstructive Pulmonary Disease) - (Ipratropium bromide)

5. In irritable bowel syndrome

III. As antiseretory and vagolytic action: (Glycopyrrolate) As preanaesthetic medication, and in hyper-hydrosis (excess sweating) and in peptic ulcer.

IV. In parkinsonism. (Ref: antiparkinsonism drug) – Anticholinergic antiparkinsonism drugs

V. As vasicoactive drugs are used for detrusor instability resulting in urinary frequency and urge incontinence. Useful in nocturnal enuresis. It does not affect heart. (Oxybutynin)

Adverse effects of ATROPINE:

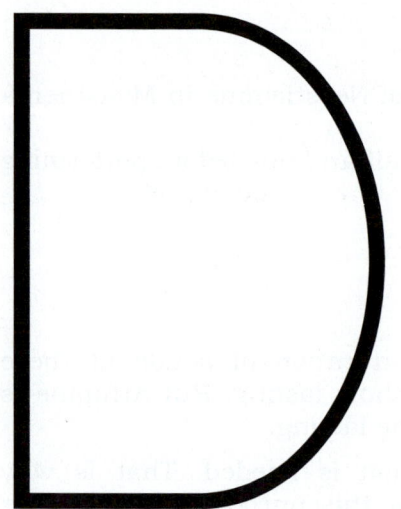

- Dilatation of pupil (mydriasis) and cycloplegia
- Dryness of mouth, skin, eye
- Difficulty in micturition(urinary retention)
- Difficulty in defaecation (constipation)
- Difficulty in swallowing
- Difficulty in speech
- Delirium

Atropine poisoning (Belladona poisoning) – symptoms are adverse effects of Atropine

Physostigmine is given (IV), which effectively crosses BBB and antagonises the central toxicity of Atropine as well as peripheral toxicity.

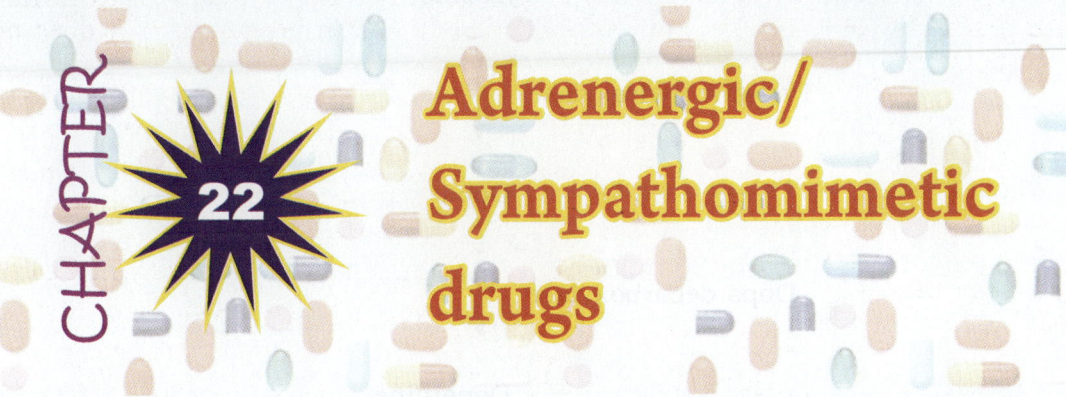

Adrenergic/ Sympathomimetic drugs

CHAPTER 22

Adrenergic drugs resemble Adrenaline and produce α and β actions exerted through α and β receptors.

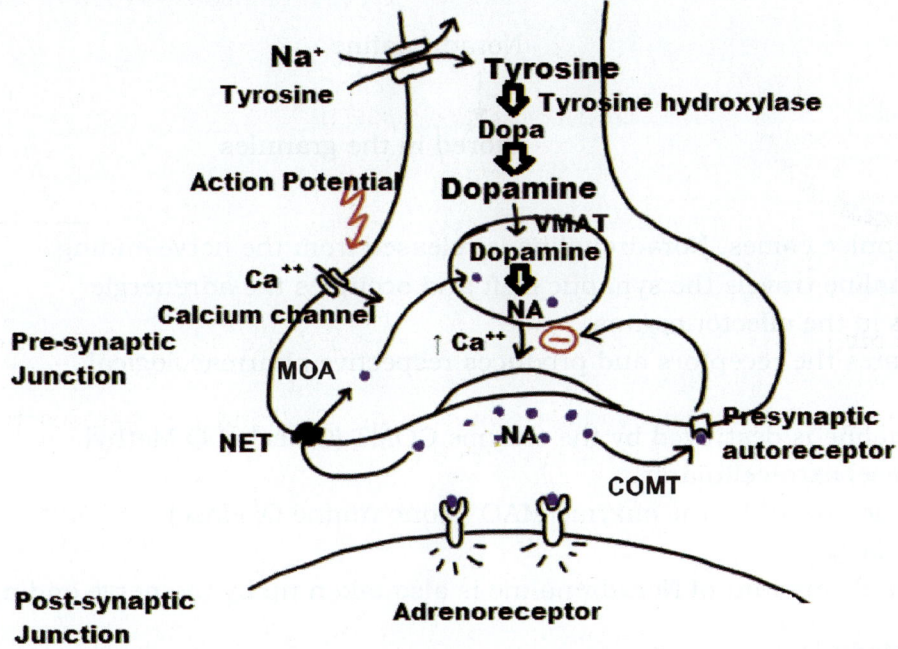

Fig.28 Synthesis, Storage and Release of Norepinephrine

- Phenylalanine which is present in the blood is converted into Tyrosine
- Then Tyrosine is taken up by the sympathetic nerve.
- Inside the sympathetic nerve ending, Tyrosine → Dopa → Dopamine → Noradrenaline

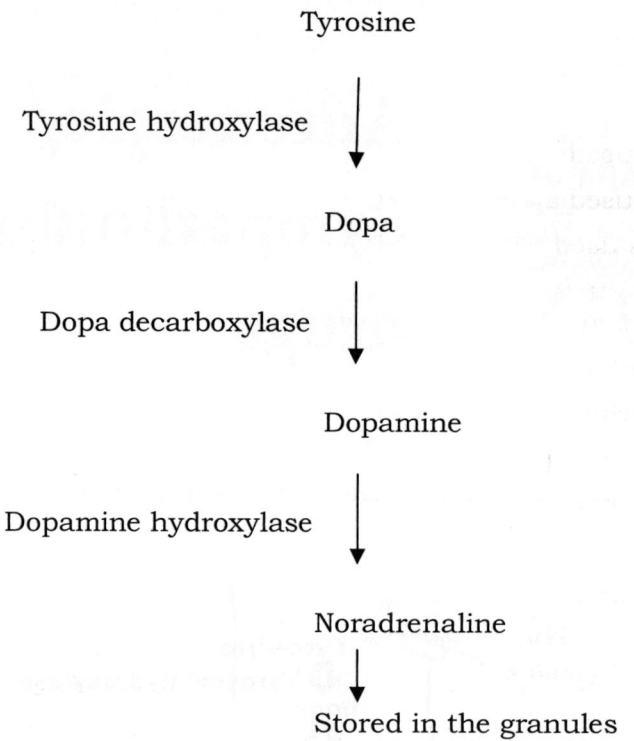

Tyrosine

Tyrosine hydroxylase

Dopa

Dopa decarboxylase

Dopamine

Dopamine hydroxylase

Noradrenaline

Stored in the granules

- If any impulse comes, Noradrenaline is released from the nerve ending
- Noradrenaline travels the synaptic cleft and occupies the adrenergic receptors in the effector organs
- It stimulates the receptors and produces respective pharmacological actions
- Noradrenaline is destroyed by the enzyme COMT (Catechol O Methyl Transferase) extracellularly
- It is also destroyed by the enzyme MAO (Mono Amine Oxidase) intracellularly
- Considerable amount of Noradrenaline is also taken up by the nerve ending

In the Adrenal Medulla

- Noradrenaline further is converted to Adrenaline by the enzyme N-Methyl transferase, which is present in large quantity in Adrenal Medulla (not present in the sympathetic nerve ending)
- In Pheochromocytoma (tumour of the adrenal medulla) large amount of Adrenaline is synthesized and released which will lead to excess α actions and β actions.

CLASSIFICATION OF ADRENERGIC DRUGS ACCORDING TO THEIR Clinical Uses

I.   Drug used in anaphylactic shock: Adrenaline (I.M.)

II.   Drug used along with local anaesthetic: Adrenaline (1:10,000 dilution)

III.   Drugs used in hypotension: Methoxamine, Mephentermine, Ephedrine

IV.   Drugs used in bronchial asthma and COPD (Chronic Obstructive Pulmonary Disease) : β_2 agonists:

1. Salbutamol

2. Terbutaline

3. Salmeterol

V.   Drugs used as uterine relaxants : β_2 agonists:

1. Salbutamol

2. Nylidrine

3. Isoxuprine

VI.   Drugs used as nasal decongestants: | These drugs produce
1. Xylometazoline | vasoconstriction, reduce
2. Naphazoline | nasal secretion, shrinkage
3. Pseudoephedrine | of mucous membrane and
4. Phenylephrine | relieve nasal congestion.

VII.   Drug used for funduscopic examination: Phenylephrine

VIII. Drug used in glaucoma: α_2 agonist: Dipivefrine

IX.   Drugs used as CNS stimulants: Amphetamine, Ephedrine

X.   Drugs used as anorexic agents: Fenfluramine, Sibutramine

XI.   Drug used in prophylaxis of migraine: α_2 agonist: Clonidine

XII.   Drugs used in cardiogenic shock: Dopamine, Dobutamine

ADRENALINE (PROTOTYPE)

- It is a sympathomimetic drug
- It is secreted from adrenal medulla and circulating in the blood

Actions of Adr → both α actions and β actions

α Actions	β Actions
1. Vasoconstriction (α_1) → veins and arterioles (rise in B.P) 2. Mydriasis (contraction of radial muscle of Iris) α_1 3. Contraction of neck muscles of bladder and prostate (α_1) → decreases urine flow 4. Inhibits Synthesis of aqueous humour (α_2) 5. Ejaculation **X** **α adrenergic blockers**	1. **Stimulate Heart (β_1). It is a powerful cardiac stimulant, increases heart rate (tachycardia), force of contrac-tion and conduction – increases oxygen demand, increases work load on the heart, toxic dose increases automaticity and reduces refractory period of ventricles lead to ventricular fibrillation** 2. Stimulates Secretion of renin (β_1) from Juxta glomerular apparatus in kidney 3. Increases aqueous humour secretion/synthesis (β_2) 4. **Bronchodialatation (β_2) – powerful action** 5. Relaxation of uterus (β_2) 6. Relaxation of skeletal muscle blood vessels (β_2) 7. Hyperglycemia (β_2) 8. Stimulates skeletal muscle (β_2) → tremor **X** **β adrenergic blockers**

Sympathetic overactivity causes thick salivation and increased sweating acting through Acetylcholine at sweat glands

Adrenaline on B.P

Both Vasoconstriction and vasodilatation → rise in B.P followed by fall in B.P → biphasic response for adrenaline is seen

Dale's vasomotor reversal phenomenon

There will be a fall in B.P for Adrenaline after α adrenergic blocker. This is called Dale's vasomotor reversal phenomenon for Adrenaline. Rise in B.P. is due to α-action and fall in B.P. is due to β_2 action

Clinical uses of ADRENALINE

1. In anaphylactic shock (1ml of 1:1000 dilution/I.M) Adrenaline is the drug of choice. In anaphylactic shock → there is bronchoconstriction and hypotension → if it is not treated immediately → lead to death. Adrenaline is life saving drug because it simultaneously increases the B.P and produces bronchodilatation.
2. Along with local anaesthetic (1 : 10000 dilution) → vasoconstriction at the local site → reduces systemic absorption of local anaesthetic → prolongs the duration of action of local anaesthetic and reduces the systemic toxicity of local anaesthetic. It also reduces the bleeding at the field of surgery.

3. In cardiac resuscitation (intracardiac injection)
4. To control epistaxis as local haemostatic
5. Adrenaline is used in ENT surgery as spray to have clear vision.

DOG'S B.P

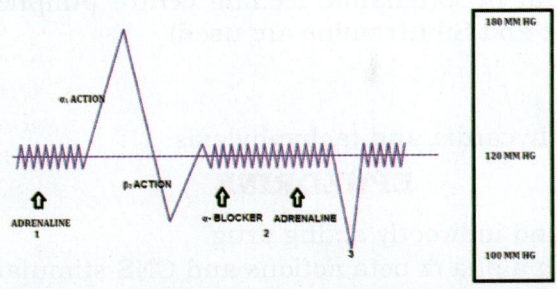

DALES VASOMOTOR REVERSAL PHENOMENON

1. Adrenaline stimulates a1 receptors in blood vessel - vasoconstriction - raise in BP and followed by slight fall in BP (b2 action)
2. Adrenaline +a Adrenergic blocker - Alpha blocker inhibits alpha action of adrenaline without affecting beta action.
3. Beta action - fall in BP.
This reversal of raise in BP to fall in BP for adrenaline after alpha blocker is called Dale's Vasomotor reversal phenamenon.

Adverse effects of ADRENALINE

Increases cardiac work precipitates angina, arrhythmia (increased automaticity) tachycardia, palpitation, anxiety, tremor, sweating, which occur due to sympathetic overactivity.

C/I – Angina, hypertension, hyperthyroidism, arrhythmia, with Halothane general anaesthtic (Halothane sensitizas the myocardium to adrenergic drugs, produces ventricular arrhythmias)

NORADRENALINE

It differs from adrenaline as it has got only alpha actions. It is the neuro-transmitter from sympathetic nerve endings. It causes reflex bradycardia. It will not produce dale's vasomotor reversal phenomenon after α–adrenergic blocker

Clinical use : Not much. It is not useful in anaphylactic shock. Sometimes it is used with local anaesthetic (to prolong the action of local anaesthetic).

Adverse effects : Increases B.P. It causes extravasation and necrosis at the site of infusion.

AMPHETAMINE

- It is a sympathomimetic drug
- It is a CNS stimulant
- It is indirectly acting sympathomimetic drug by releasing Noradrenaline from the sympathetic nerve ending
- It has got mainly alpha actions and CNS stimulant action

Clinical uses

1. In narcolepsy, it postpones sleep.
2. In Attention Deficit Hyperactivity Disorder (ADHD) in children
3. Weight reduction due to anorexic action.
   Inhibits the lateral hypothalamic feeding centre (Amphetamine analogues like Fenfluramine and Sibutramine are used)

Adverse effects

- Insomnia, tachycardia and tachyphylaxis

EPHEDRINE

- It is directly and indirectly acting drug
- It has got both alpha & beta actions and CNS stimulant actions

Clinical uses

1. In hypotension due to spinal anaesthesia
2. In bronchial asthma (combined with other drugs)
3. As nasal decongestant (pseudoephedrine)
4. In narcolepsy

Adverse effects

- Insomnia, tachycardia & tachyphylaxis

DOPAMINE/DOBUTAMINE

DOPAMINE:

- Dopamine is a naturally occurring catecholamine of adrenergic drug.
- It is the precursor for Adrenaline, Noradrenalline.

Mechanism of action:

- In low dose (2-5 µg/kg/IV infusion), it stimulates specifically DA_2 receptor in the kidney and produces vasodilatation of the renal blood vessels. It increases glomerular filtration and excretion of sodium. It increases the blood flow to the kidney. It prevents renal failure in cardiogenic shock.
- In higher dose, it will also stimulate α and β receptors (which will antagonize the vasodilatory action in the kidney.

Clinical uses of Dopamine:

- 1. In cardiogenic shock resulting from MI (myocardial infarction) : It is effective only in low dose (it increases the blood flow to the vital organs like kidney)
- 2. In heart failure (increase cardiac output) and in renal failure (in low dose)

Adverse effects of Dopamine: tachycardia, hypertension, cardiac arrhythmias etc.,

DOBUTAMINE:

- It is a catecholamine.
- Its main action is on β_1 receptor stimulation in the heart.
- It increases the cardiac output without affecting heart rate (useful action in heart failure)

Clinical uses:

1. In heart failure, associated with MI, cardiac surgery.

Adverse effects:

rise in B.P. (aggravate hyper tension) and increases heart rate, increases oxygen demand (aggravate angina pectoris).

NASAL DECONGESTANTS: Xylometazoline, pseudoephedrine, phenylephrine, Naphazoline and Oxymetazoline.

- They are sympathomimetic drugs

Mechanism of action:
- They cause vasoconstriction and reduce nasal secretion.
- They cause shrinkage of the mucous membrane.
- They relieve nasal congestion.

Clinical uses:

1. In nasal congestion due allergic rhinitis or any other causes. They are not antihistamines.

Caution in hypertensive individuals.

PHENYLEPHRINE

- It is an adrenergic drug.
- It produces mydriatic.
- **Mechanism of action** as mydriatic: It stimulates the α_1 receptor in the radial muscle (dilator papillae), contracts radial muscle of iris to produce mydriasis.(Fig 25A)
- **Clinical uses of Phenylephrine as mydriatic:** 1. Only for the funduscopy examination. (No cycoplegia side effect). It is not contraindicated in glaucoma. But it is not suitable for testing refractory error of lens, for which the cycloplegic action is necessary. There is no prolonged mydriatic side effect because of its shorter duration of action.
- 2. As nasal decongestant (oral).

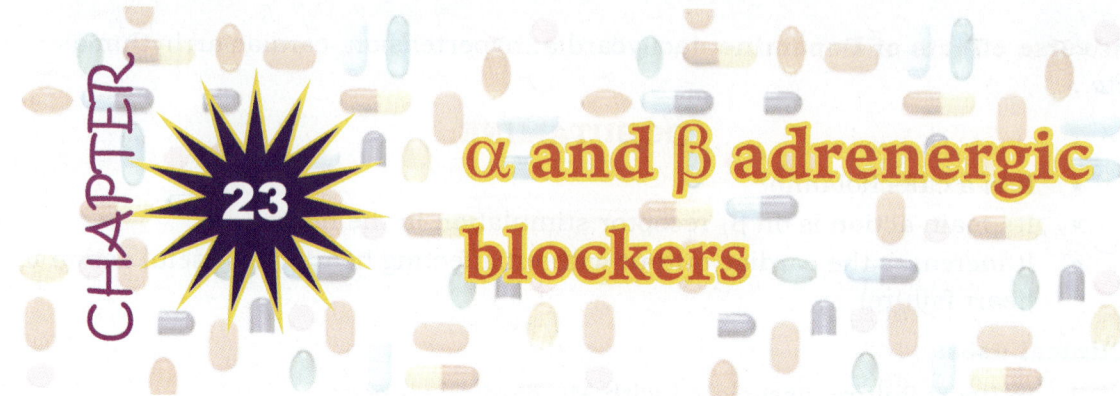

CHAPTER 23

α and β adrenergic blockers

α ADRENERGIC BLOCKERS

DRUGS: Prazosin and Terazosin-They are specific α $_1$ blockers

These drugs occupy and block the α-receptors to reverse all the α-actions of adrenergic drugs. They do not affect the β-receptors.

Actions of α- adrenergic blockers:

1. On blood vessels: Reverse the vasoconstrictor action of adrenergic drugs and produce vasodilatation, fall in B.P.
2. On sex organs: They cause failure of ejaculation and Impotency
3. On urinary bladder and prostate: relaxation of bladder and prostate neck muscles and increase the urine flow in BHP (Benign Hypertrophy of Prostate)

Clinical uses: 1. The first and important use is in BHP. They increase the urine flow. There will be better result if it is combined with Finasteride, a 5 α reductase inhibitor, which reduces size of the enlarged prostate, (androgen dependent) by inhibiting the conversion of inactive androgen to active Dihydroandrogen.

2. In pheochromocytoma along with β-adrenergic blocker.

3. In peripheral vascular diseases (little benefit)

Adverse effects: POSTURAL HYPOTENSTION, IMPOTENCY (both side effects affect the quality of life of hypertensive patients and hence not suitable), miosis, nasal stuffiness. First dose effect → faint → within half an hour of taking the drug. The drug should be given at bed time.

Dose : Prazosin (Minipress – 2 to 5 mg/daily)

β ADRENERGIC BLOCKERS.

- These drugs inhibit/reverse the β actions of adrenergic drugs by blocking β adrenergic receptors.

CLASSIFICATION OF β ADRENERGIC BLOCKERS:

I.   Non selective (inhibit both β_1 and β_2 receptors)
   1. Propranolol
   2. Timolol
   3. Sotalol
II.   Cardioselective (Block only β_1 receptors)
   1. Atenolol
   2. Esmolol
   3. Metoprolol
   4. Betaxalol
   5. Nabivolol
III. Both α and β receptors blockers:
   1. Labetalol
   2. Carvedilol

Useful in pheochromocytoma, (adrenal medullary tumour), where excess Adrenaline is released, which produces excess α actions and β actions.

β- ADRENERGIC BLOCKERS (PROPRANOLOL)

Mechanism of action: (Fig.29) β- adrenergic blockers have got high affinity towards adrenergic receptors. But they have got no intrinsic activity. They block the adrenergic receptors and will not allow the adrenergic drugs to occupy and act. They reverse all the β actions of Adrenaline and other adrenergic drugs.

Pharmacological actions of Propranolol

i.   On Heart (β_1)
      β-adrenergic blockers will decrease heart rate, myocardial contractility, conduction velocity and force of contraction. They decrease work load on the heart, O_2 demand and consumption are reduced. They produce fall in B.P.

ii.   Renin (β_1)
      β_1 receptors are present in the juxta glomerular apparatus of kidney. β-adrenergic blockers block β_1 receptor in the juxta glomular apparatus and inhibit the release of renin and inhibit the conversion of Angiotensinogen to ATI → reduce the production of

AT II, (powerful vasoconstrictor) → vasodilatation → fall in B.P. Renin is the important enzyme responsible for the genesis of hypertension.

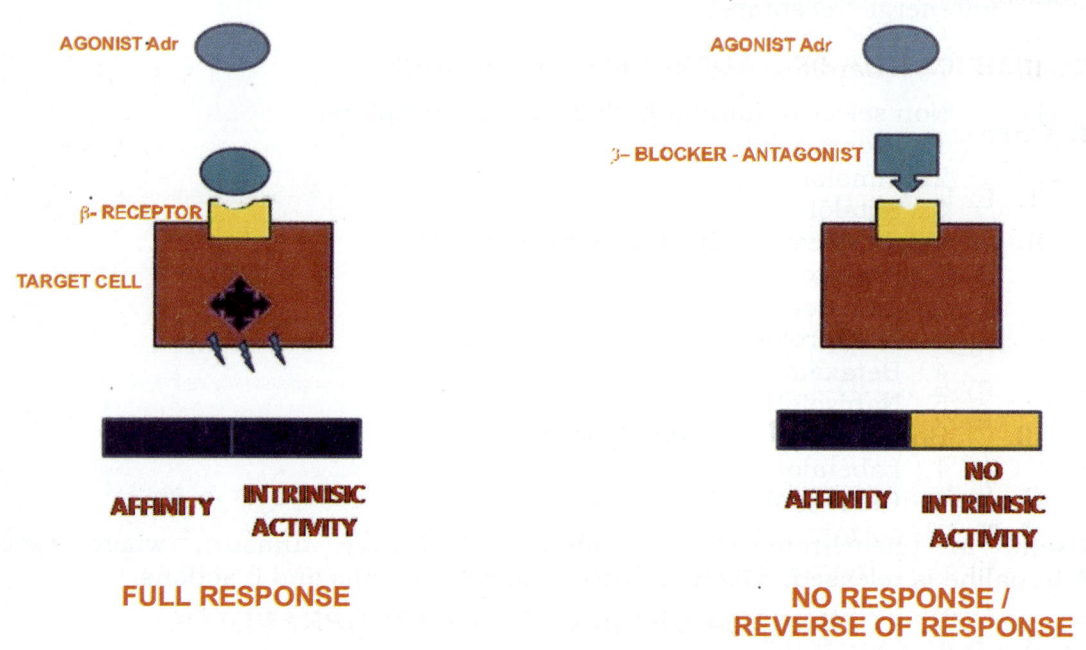

Fig.29 Mechanism of action of β-adrenergic blockers

iii. On Respiratory Tract (β_2):
They cause bronchoconstriction. However, cardio selective β-adrenergic blockers will not produce / less bronchoconstriction.

iv. On Metabolism:
Insulin like effect will cause hypoglycaemia.

v. On Eye:
β-adrenergic blockers inhibit the synthesis of aqueous humour and reduce the intraocular pressure. β-adrenergic blockers are first line drug in the treatment of glaucoma.

vi. On Skeletal muscle : Skeletal muscles contain β_2 receptor, stimulation of which causes tremor. β – adrenergic blockers will inhibit tremor.

Clinical uses of β ADRENERGIC BLOCKERS (13 USES) / Propranolol

I.   CARDIAC USES (Cardioselective β adrenergic blockers are preferred)

Clinical uses of   β adrenergic blockers:
- I.   Cardiac uses (cardioselective blockers are preferred)
- II.   Non Cardiac uses: (mainly the non selective blockers are preferred)

I. Cardiac uses:

1. In hypertension: i) β-adrenergic blockers inhibit renin secretion from the juxtaglomerular apparatus in the kidney. They inhibit the conversion of Angiotensinogen to Angiotensin I, inhibit the production of Angiotensin II, which is a powerful vasoconstrictor and also decrease the release of Aldosterone. Renin is the most important substance in the genesis of hypertension. β-Adrenergic blockers inhibit the renin secretion and reduce the B.P. and useful in hypertension. ii) Inhibit the COP and reduce B.P. iii) They also reduce the central sympathetic outflow

2. In Heart Failure: i) they antagonize the reflex tachycardia (which is one of the important symptoms of Heart Failure), which aggravates Heart Failure ii) they inhibit renin, which is another important factor in aggravating Heart Failure

3. In Angina pectoris: Useful only in classical angina (reduce oxygen demand and reduce work load on heart), they produce coronary vasoconstriction (contraindicated in Prinzemetal angina)
   Ref: Angina pectoris

4. In cardiac arrhythmia: Mainly useful in adrenergic drugs induced arrhythmias. They decrease automaticity and prolong the refractory period of myocardium.

5. In myoardial infarction: they prevent reocclusion and prevent spread

6. In cardiomyopathy: Force of contraction is an aggravating factor in this condition. Beta adrenergic drugs inhibit the FOC and are useful in this conditdion.

II. Non cardiac uses:

7. In prophylaxis of migraine

8. In glaucoma (First line drug. Mainly useful in wide angle glaucoma). They reduce the synthesis of aqueous humour.

9. In anxiety: The main symptoms of anxiety are due to sympathetic over activity (tachycardia, tremor, sweating) Beta adrenergic blockers antagonise all the symptoms

10. In tremor: The skeletal muscles contain β_2 receptors, stimulation of which lead to tremor, Beta adrenergic blockers inhibit tremor.

11. In pheochromocytoma: it is the condition due to adrenal medullary tumour. There is excess synthesis and release of Adrenaline, which will produce excess actions of α and β. Beta adrenergic blockers are given along with alpha adrenergic blocers or Labetalol alone, which has got both α and β adrenergic blocking activity.

12. In thyrotoxicosis: The symptoms of thyrotoxicosis are due to sympathetic overactivity to the heart. All those symptoms are antagonized by Beta adrenergic blockers.

13. In oesophageal varices bleeding: They produce splanchnic vasoconstriction and reduce bleeding.

Dose :

Propranolol (Inderal) 40-160 mg/daily
Atenolol (Betacard) 12.5-50 mg/daily
Metoprolol (Betaloc) 25-50 mg/daily

Adverse effects

- Bronchoconstriction (cardio selective drug produce less brochoconstriction)
- Bradycardia
- Cold extremities
- Heart Failure
- Hypoglycemia (mask the warning symptoms of hypoglycemia with Insulin)
- Sudden withdrawal → rebound hypertension & angina

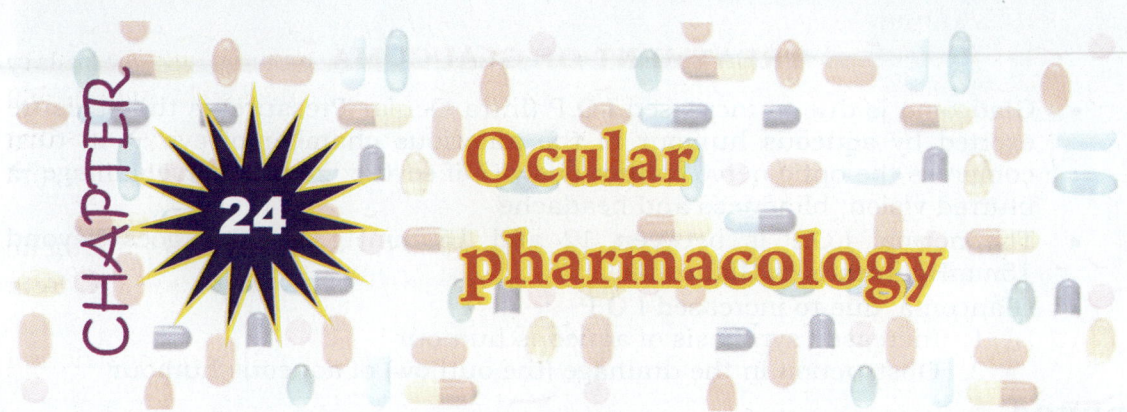

Ocular
pharmacology

It deals with the drugs which are acting on eye.

I.   Drugs used in Glaucoma
II.   Miotics and their clinical uses
III.   Mydriatics and their clinical uses
IV.   Antiinflammatory drugs used on eye
V.   Vit.A in night blindness (Nyclotopia)

I.   Drugs used in glaucoma: (Ref: drugs used in Glaucoma)
II.   Miotics: means constriction of pupil. There is only one miotic used
       clinically is Pilocarpine(Ref: Pilocarpine}
III.   Mydriatics: which dilate the pupil. There are two groups of mydriatics.
       1. Anticholinergic drugs: Tropicamide, cyclopentolate
           Mechanism of action and clinical uses (Ref: Atropine substitute used
           on eye)
       2. Adrenergic drugs: Phenylephrine (Ref: mechanism of action and
           clinical uses of Phenylephrine)

IV   Antiinflammatory drugs on eye: (Ref: Clinical uses of Glucocortdicoids
on eye)

V   Vit.A in Vit.A deficiency (night blindness, xerophthalmia) : (Ref: Vit.A)

TREATMENT OF GLAUCOMA

- Glaucoma is due to increased I.O.P (Intra Ocular Pressure) is the pressure exerted by aqueous humour in the anterious chamber of eye → in turn compress the optic nerve continuously → if severe → optic nerve damage → blurred vision, blindness and headache
- The normal I.O.P is between 12 and 15 mmHg. If I.O.P goes beyond 15mmHg it leads to Glaucoma.
- Glaucoma, due to increased I.O.P
  1. Increased synthesis of aqueous humour
  2. Obstruction in the drainage (the outflow) of aqueous humour

DRUGS

They act either by decreasing the synthesis of aqueous humour or by improving its drainage.

TYPES OF GLAUCOMA

1. Open angle (chronic simple Glaucoma) – genetic in nature – slowly the patency of trabecular meshwork is gradually lost → increase I.O.P is mainly due to increased synthesis of aqueous humour
2. Narrow angle (acute congestive) Glaucoma – It occurs in narrow iridio corneal angle→ due to obstruction of canal of schlemn by iris muscle → increase I.O.P & attack is usually precipitated by mydriatics.

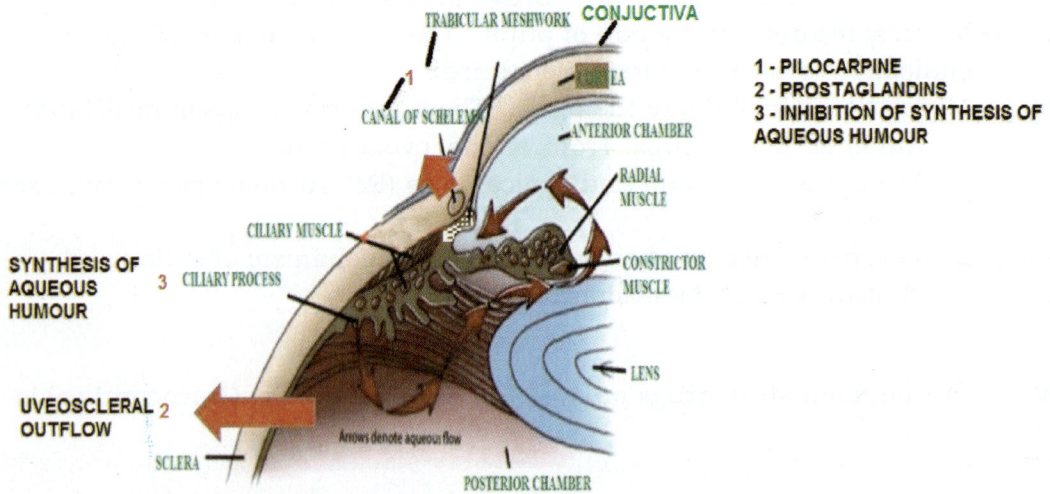

1 - PILOCARPINE
2 - PROSTAGLANDINS
3 - INHIBITION OF SYNTHESIS OF AQUEOUS HUMOUR

Fig.30 Synthesis, drainage of aqueous humour and sites of action of Antiglaucoma drugs

Aqueous humour is synthesized and secreted into posterior chamber of eye → passess through pupil → reaches anterior chamber → drained through trabecular mesh and canal of schlemn.

1. Pilocarpine - constriction of sphincter muscle, and contraction of ciliary muscle → increases the drainage of aqueous humour by widening canal of schlemn and trabecular mesh work → reduces IOP.

2. PGs increase uveoscleral outflow and reduce IOP.

3. β blockers, carbonic anhydrase inhibitors, α_1 agonists reduce the synthesis of aqueous humour form the ciliary body epithelium and reduce IOP.

DRUGS USED IN WIDE ANGLE GLAUCOMA (Fig.30)

- The drugs which inhibits secretion/synthesis of aqueous humour are useful.

Beta adrenergic blockers (Timolol, Betaxolol)

- They are first line drugs
- They do not affect the pupil's size
- They do not affect the tone of ciliary muscle or aqueous humour outflow
- They block β_2 receptors, which increase the synthesis of aqueous humour and also reduce blood flow to the ciliary body epithelium (inhibit the synthesis of aqueous humour)→ reduce the I.O.P → useful in wide angle Glaucoma

Advantages

- No headache (no persistent spasm of iris and ciliary muscle)
- Betaxolol (inhibit the β_1 receptor only) is less potent than Timolol (inhibits β_2 receptors)

PROSTAGLANDINS (Latanoprost)

- Prostaglandin receptors are present in ciliary body epithelium, stimulation of which lead to inhibition of synthesis of aqueous humour
- Now they become first line drug. They also increase uveoscleral outflow → reduce I.O.P

ALPHA ADRENERGIC AGONIST (Dipivefrin)

- Block α_1 receptors in the blood vessels of ciliary body epithelium,where the aqueous humour is synthesised. Dipivefrin stimulate the α_1 receptors in the blood vessels →vasoconstrition → reduced blood flow to the ciliary body epithelium → reduce synthesis of aqueous humour → reduce the I.O.P

CARBONICANHYDRASE INHIBITORS (Acetazolamide – oral & Dorzolamide – topical)

- Carbonic anhydrase enzyme is present in the ciliary body epithelium → produces bicarbonate ion which is essential for the formation of aqueous humour →carbonic anhydrase inhibitors → reduced formation of bicarbonate ion → less formation of aqueous humour synthesis → reduce I.O.P

DRUGS USED IN NARROW ANGLE GLAUCOMA (Fig.30)

- Miotics are useful (Pilocarpine)
- Miosis → retracts iris muscle away from iridocorneal angle → widen the Canal of Schlemn → increase the drainage of aqueous humour → reduce I.O.P
- Contraction of ciliary muscle→ patency of trabecular meshwork is improved → improve the drainage of aqueous humour → reduce I.O.P
- Normally beta blockers are also given as adjuvant.
- In emergency → iridectomy is the choice of treatment
- Mannitol : reduces I.O.P. by its osmotic action (Ref : Diuretics)

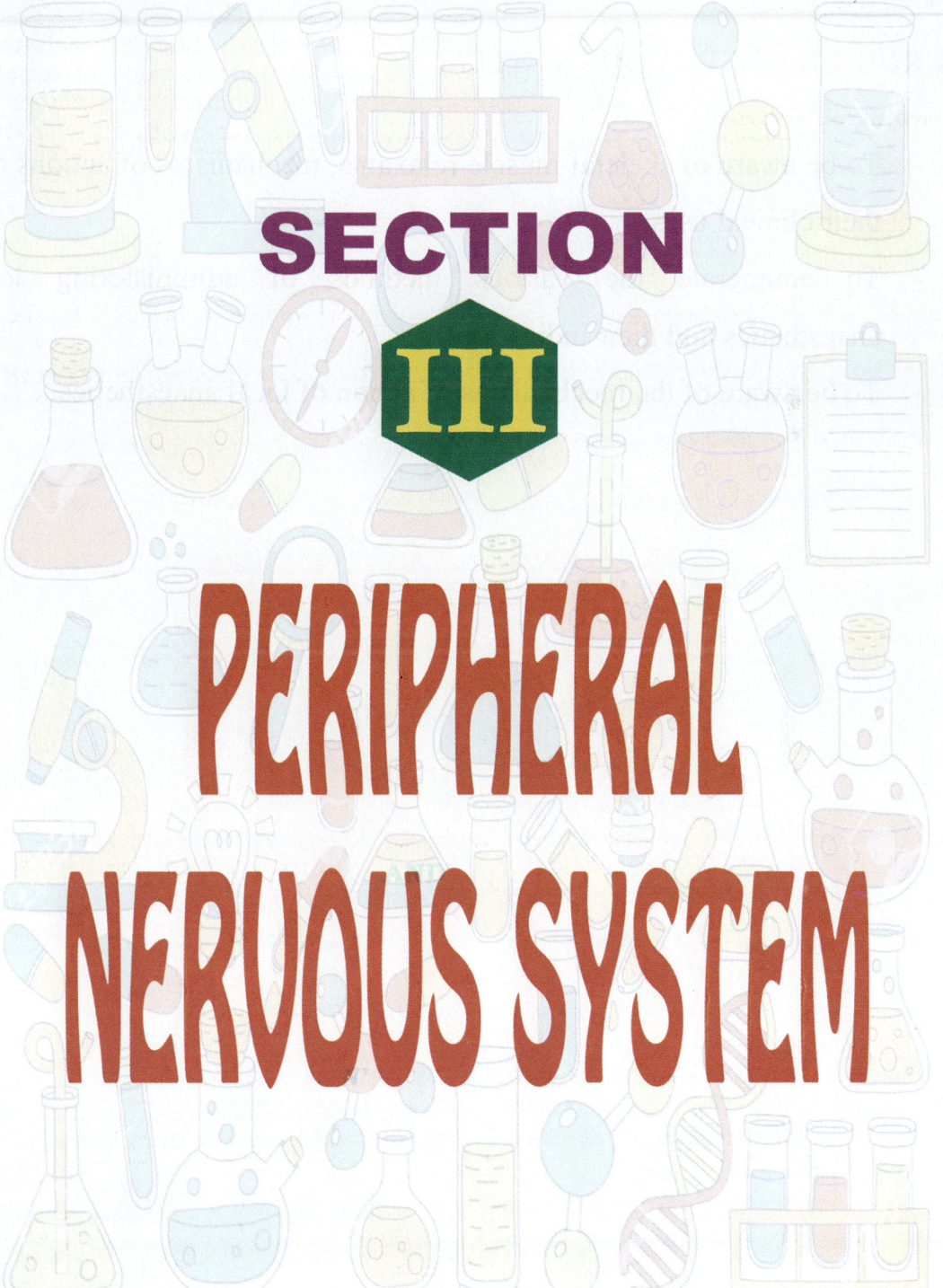

SECTION

III

PERIPHERAL NERVOUS SYSTEM

PERIPHERAL NERVOUS SYSTEM

Learning objectives

- To be aware of skeletal muscle relaxants, mechanisms of actions and their clinical uses.

- To enumerate the various methods of administering local anaesthetics and their indications.

- To be aware of the mechanisms of action of local anaesthetics.

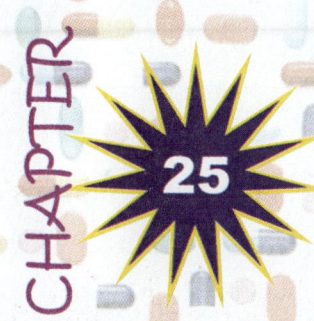

Peripherally and centrally acting skeletal muscle relaxants

CHAPTER 25

Peripherally acting skeletal muscle relaxants

The drugs that relax the skeletal muscles by acting on neuromuscular junction (motor end plates) or by acting directly on skeletal muscle.

- I.   NEUROMUSCULAR BLOCKING AGENTS
- II.   DIRECTLY ACTING
- I.   NEUROMUSCULAR BLOCKING AGENTS
  - 1. Non depolarizing Blockers:
    - i)   Long acting: Pancuronium, Pipecuronium, Doxacurium
    - ii)   Intermediate acting: Vecuronium, Atracurium, Rocuronium
    - iii)   Short acting: Mivacurium
  - 2.   Depolarizing Blockers:
    - i)   Succinylcholine
- II.   Directly acting
  - i)   Dantrolene sodium

Mechanism of action of Non depolarizing Blockers: (Fig.31A/31B)

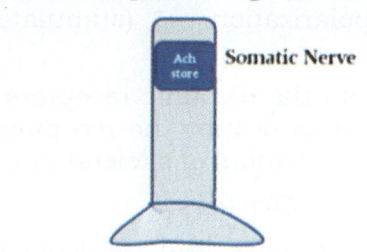

Somatic Nerve

Ach store

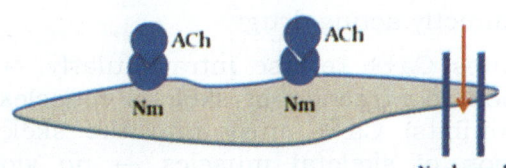

ACh   ACh

Nm   Nm

Na channel

Fig.31A Contraction of Skeletal Muscle

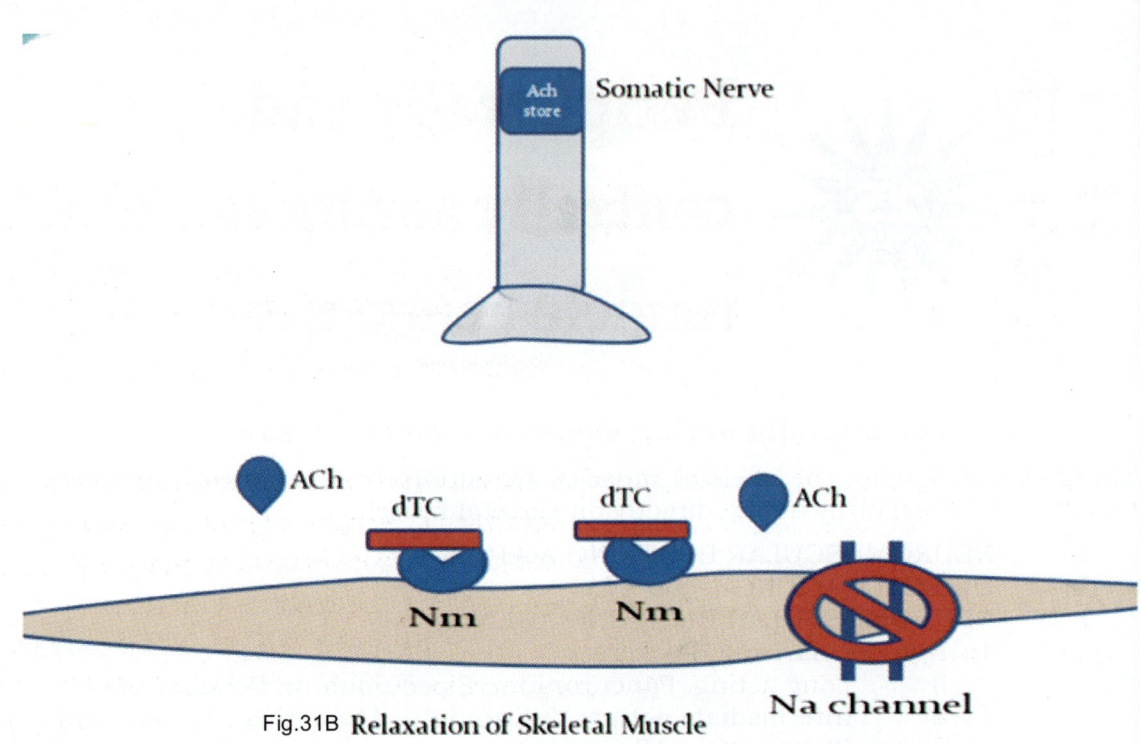

Fig.31B **Relaxation of Skeletal Muscle**

(Contraction)

ACh stimulates the nicotinic receptors in the skeletal muscle (N_M receptors) → opening of Na+ channel → Depolarization →↑ (stimulates) skeletal muscle → contracts skeletal muscle

Non depolarizing blockers ↓ (inhibit) the nicotinic receptors in the skeletal muscle competitively with ACh → ACh cannot occupy the receptors → No depolarization → No conduction of impulse →↓ (relaxation) of skeletal muscles

Mechanism of action of Depolarizing Blockers:

Drug → occupies the Nicotinic receptors (N_M) → depolarization like ACh, but persistent depolarization (no repolorization) → impulse cannot be transmitted → initial stimulation followed by relaxation of skeletal muscle.

Mechanism of action of directly acting drug:

Certain condition stimulates Ca++ release intracellularly → Ca++ →entry into skeletal muscles → violent contraction of skeletal muscles → hyperthermia. After Dantroline → ↓(inhibits) Ca++ entry into the skeletal muscles → no depolarization → relaxation of skeletal muscles → no violent contraction of skeletal muscle → temperature will come down.

NON DEPOLARIZING AGENTS

All the drugs are having similar Mechanism of action

All drugs are having similar Clinical uses

They differ only in pharmacokinetic properties (according to the conditions, the drugs have to be selected)

- They are skeletal muscle relaxants.
- They are peripherally acting neuromuscular blockers.

Mechanism of action : (Ref above before)

Pharmacological actions

I. Action on skeletal muscle: Intravenous injection of non-depolarizing drugs rapidly produce muscle weakness followed by flaccid paralysis. Fast moving smaller muscles (fingers, extraocular) are affected first, paralysis spread hands, feet → arm, leg, neck, face → trunk→ intercostal muscles → finally diaphragm. Recovery occurs in the reverse sequence. Diaphragmatic contractions resume first.

II. On Histamine release → slight histamine release will cause slight fall in B.P.

III. On CVS → reduced venous return

IV. Autonomic ganglia (N_N). Some degree of ganglion blockade → Fall in BP

Dose:

Pancuronium - 0.05 – 0.1 mg/kg

Vecuronium - 0.05 – 0.1 mg/kg

Pipercurium - 0.05 – 0.1 mg/kg

Clinical uses :

1. The most important use of neuromuscular blockers is as adjuvant to general anaesthetic. Adequate skeletal muscle relaxation can be achieved in higher planes (less anaesthetic dose is required) to produce adequate skeletal muscle relaxation. In major surgery adequate skeletal muscle relaxation is needed, which cannot be achieved by general anaesthetics alone in therapeutic dose. Adequate skeletal muscle relaxation is useful for the surgeon and the patients (small incision is sufficient, so small wound → less infection → healing will be quick, less painful). Also reduce the reflex muscle contraction in the region undergoing surgery.

2. To assist maintenance of controlled ventilation during anaesthesia
3. They are useful in major surgery, intubation, endoscopies and orthopaedic manipulations
4. For assisted ventilation in critically ill patients in .I.C.U (need ventilator support.) This can be facilitated by continuous IV infusion of neuromuscular blockers
5. To protect the patients from convulsion during eletroconvulsive therapy.
6. In severe cases of tetanus and status epilepticus.

Adverse effects

-respiratory paralysis. prolonged apnoea are the most common problem (antidote Neostigmine is given to reverse the action very quickly), histamine release –fall in BP.

DEPOLARIZING AGENT (SUCCINYLCHOLINE)

- It is a depolarizing skeletal muscle relaxant

⁚ Mechanism of action :Ref above before

Pharmacological actions

I. Action on skeletal muscle: It produces initial fasciculation and twitching followed by skeletal muscle relaxation. Other actions on skeletal muscle are similar to that of non – depolarizing agents. It produces excellent intubating conditions, viz. relaxed jaw, vocal cord apart, and immobile with no diaphragmatic movement is obtained within 2 min.

II. No Histamine release

III. Autonomic ganglia → slight stimulation of sympathetic ganglia → rise in BP

Clinical uses :

1. It is employed for brief procedures like endotracheal intubation, laryngoscopy, bronchoscopy, esophagoscopy, reduction of fractures, dislocation and to treat laryngospasm.

Adverse effects: ↑ (rise in) BP, tachycardia, hyperkaelemia (common in burns, uraemia and arrhythmia), Prolonged apnoea in patients with atypical pseudocholinesterase, soreness of muscle (due to fasciculation).

DANTROLINE

Mechanism of action : (ref: before)

Clinical uses :

1. In malignant hyperthermia due to general anaesthetic like Halothane

2. Reduce the spasticity in the upper motor neurone disorders like hemiplegis, paraplegia and multiple sclerosis. It reduces the voluntary muscle power also. (Hence centrally acting skeletal muscle relaxants are useful in the above mentioned conditions, since they do not affect the voluntary muscle power)

Adverse effects: muscular weakness, sedation, troublesome diarrhoea.

Advantages of newer neuromuscular blockers over the older ones:

1. No cardiac or vascular side effects
2. No/minimum Histamine release
3. Rapid and short acting – easy reversal

CENTRALLY ACTING SKELETAL MUSCLE RELAXANTS:

They are also called as spasmolytic of skeletal muscle.

DRUGS:

Mephenesin group: Mephenesin, Chlorzoxazone

Diazepam

Baclofen

Tizanidine

Gabapentine

Mechanism of action :

They ↓ (Inhibit) the internuncial neurones in the spinal cord → ↓ (inhibit) the stretch reflex → ↓ (reduce) skeletal muscle spasticity → ↓ (inhibit) pain due to spasticity

They selectively depress spinal and supraspinal polysynaptic reflexes involving in the regulation of muscle tone without affecting the voluntary muscle power.

Diazepam : ↑ (Facilitate) the action of GABA in the synapses of the brain → ↓ (inhibition) of stretch reflux → acts at the level of supraspinal site.

Clinical uses :

1. In upper motor neurone disorders- hemiplegia, paraplegia, multiple sclerosis or any hypertonia of spinal cord injury

2. In acute muscle spasm; Over stretching muscle, sprain, tearing of ligament and tendons, dislocations, fibrositis, bursitis, which cause painful spasm of muscles

3. Anxiety with muscle spasm (Diazepam)

4. Tetanus (IV Diazepam)

5. Orthopaedic manipulations: Under the influence of Diazepam, it is very easy for reduction.

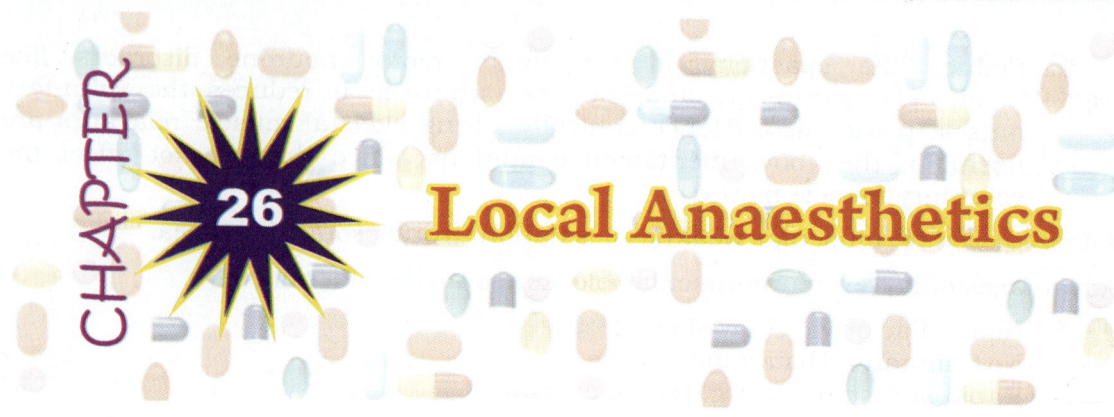

CHAPTER 26

Local Anaesthetics

These drugs produce reversible loss of sensory perceptions, especially pain at the local site of administration of local anaesthetics.

CLASSIFICATION

Injectable anaesthetic

Low potency, short duration

> Procaine
>
> Chloroprocaine

Intermediate potency and duration

> Lidocaine (Lignocaine)
>
> Prilocaine

High Potency, long duration

> Tetracaine (Amethocaine)
>
> Bupivacaine
>
> Ropivacaine
>
> Dibucaine (Cinchocaine)

Surface anaesthetic

Soluble	Insoluble
Cocaine	Benzocaine
Lidocaine	Butylaminobenzoate
Tetracaine	(Butamben)
Benoxinate	Oxethazaine

Mechanism of action : (Fig.32)

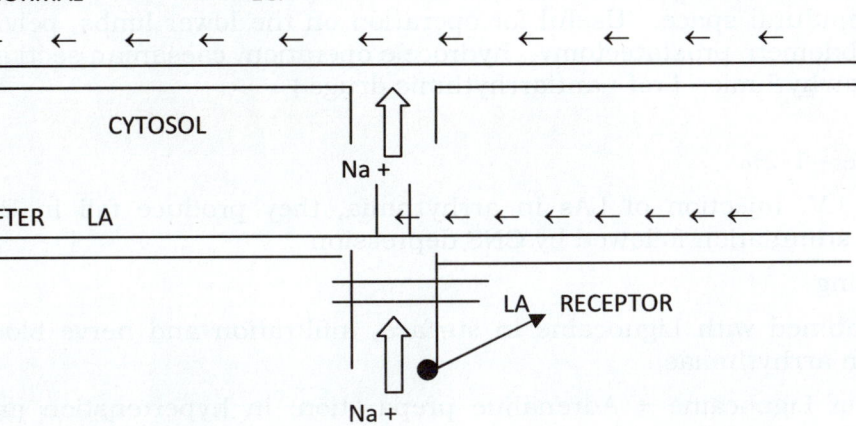

LA – Local Anaesthetic

Fig.32 Conduction of pain impulse through sensory nerves and site of action of LA

Normally if any impulse comes across nerve → Na+ enters through voltage gated Na+ channel → generates and conducts nerve impulse → pain is felt.

After local anaesthetic → LA binds with LA receptor present near the intracellular end of the voltage gated Na+ channel → ↓ (blocks) them → ↓ (prevents) the entry of Na+ through voltage gated Na+ channel → ↓ (blocks) both the generation and conduction of impulses → anaesthesia is produced in the proximal areas of the block

Local actions:
1. Block the sensory and motor nerves
2. Smaller sensory nerves are anaesthetized first
3. LAs fail to provide adequate pain relief in inflammed areas
4. Normally Adrenaline is combined with local anaesthetics : The advantages are i) Prolong the duration of action of LAs. ii) reduces the systemic toxicity iii)reduces the bleeding in the field of surgery and iv) enhances the intensity of anaesthesia

Systemic actions: if LAs are absorbed i)vasodilatation and fall in BP ii) CNS stimulation followed by CNS depression. iii) inhibit the heart- (bradycardia)

Clinical uses : LIGNOCAINE

1. As surface anaesthesia: local application on skin and mucous membrane: to relieve pain in corneal ulcer, corneal surgery, tonometry, stomatitis, sore throat, endoscopies, endotracheal intubation, ulcer, burns, itching, dermatoses etc.,
2. As infiltration anaesthesia: LAs are injected subcutaneously in and around the area to be anaesthetised, for I.V. cannulation, skin surgery, for catheterization, in fissure and painful piles, proctoscopy

3. As nerve block anaesthesia: injection of LAs near the nerve trunk. (lingual nerve block in tooth extraction)
4. As spinal and epidural anaesthesia: LAs are injected into subarachnoid space/epidural space: Useful for operation on the lower limbs, pelvis, lower abdomen, prostatectomy, hydrocele operation, caesarean section
5. As antiarrhythmic: (ref : antiarrhythmic drugs)

Dose of Lignocaine – 1-2%

Adverse effects: I.V. injection of LAs in arrhythmia, they produce fall in BP, bradycardia, CNS stimulation followed by CNS depression

Delay wound healing

Adrenaline is combined with Lignocaine in surface, infiltration and nerve block anaesthesia (not in arrhythmias).

Contraindication of Lignocaine + Adrenaline preparation: in hypertenstion and ischaemic heart diseases.

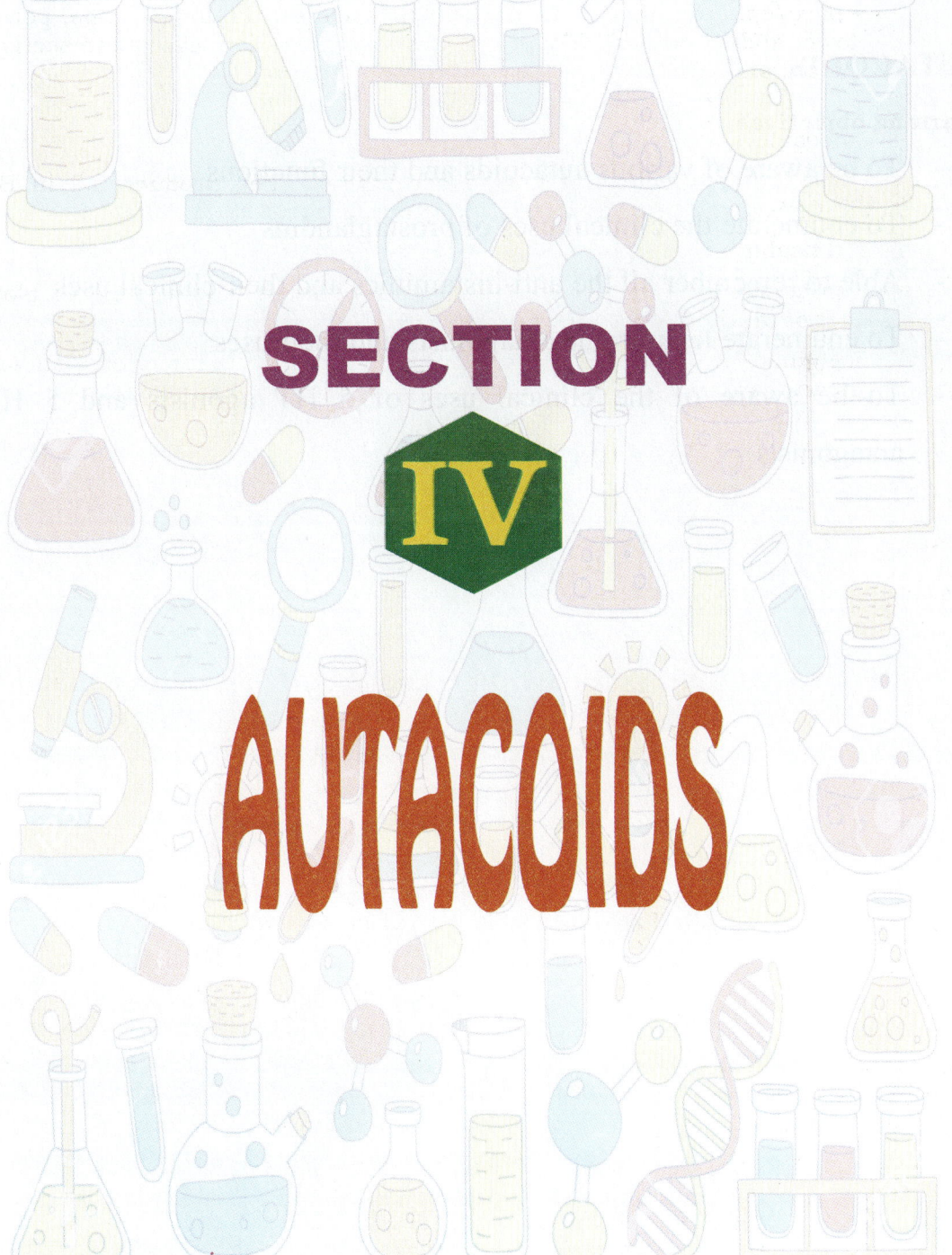

SECTION

IV

AUTACOIDS

AUTACOIDS

Learning objectives

- To be aware of various autacoids and their functions

- To enumerate the clinical uses of prostaglandins

- Able to remember all the anti-histaminics and their clinical uses

- To enumerate leukotriene antagonists and their uses

- To be aware of the clinical uses of 5 HT agonists and 5 HT antagonists

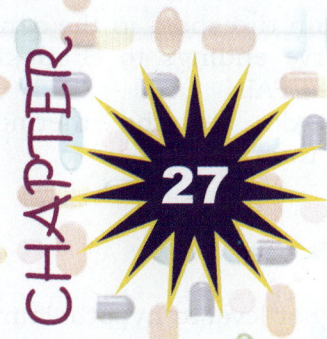

Introduction, Prostaglandins, Leukotriens antagonists

CHAPTER 27

The term 'Autacoid' is derived from Greek word 'auto = self' akose = healing substance/remedy. But most of the autacoids are harmful to the body.

- They are synthesized and released by a wide variety of cells in the body
- They are also called as "local hormones", resemble hormone except that autacoids act locally at the site of release (whereas hormones act throughout the body)
- Autacoids are involved in a number of physiological and mostly pathological processes.

Autacoids are:

1) Histamine

2) 5 HT –5 Hydroxy Tryptamine or Serotonin

3) Prostaglandins

4) Leukotriens

5) Platelet Activating Factor (PAF)

6) Bradykinin

7) Angiotensin

8) Others: Cytokines (interleukins), TNFα, gastrin, Vasoactive Intestinal Peptide (VIP) may be considered as autacoids.

PROSTAGLANDINS (PGs)

- They are synthesized in various cells but not stored → synthesized → released

Synthesis:

Arachidonic Acid

↓ COX (Cyclo-oxygenase)

Prostaglandins (including thromboxane – A_2)

Actions of PGs:

1. Pain producing substances – PGs reduce pain threshold in the sensory nerve. They also sensitize the sensory nerve endings to Bradykinin, Substance – P, pain producing substances → PAIN

2. Fever producing substances. Bacteria/toxin set the thermostat mechanism at higher level in hypothalamus through PGs.

Bacteria, toxins

↓

Increase PGs Synthesis

↓

Set the thermostat mechanism at higher level in hypothalamus

↓

FEVER

3. Inflammatory producing substances :

PGs produce vasodilatation → increase capillary permeability → increase exudation of fluid → and also release the mediators of INFLAMMATION

4. On uterus & cervix – They stimulate uterus → Contraction during pregnancy and also softening of cervix. They cause dysmenorrhoea.

5. On GIT – Inhibit gastric acid production and increase mucus production (useful in peptic ulcer)

6. On Eye –↑ (increase) uveoscleral outflow and partly ↓ (inhibit) synthesis of aqueous humour → ↓ (reduce) IOP (Intra Ocular Pressure) → useful in glaucoma.

7. They maintain patency of ductus arteriosus in foetal life

8. PGs produce vasodilatation → Local injection into cavernous muscle → vasodilatation → Useful in EDF (erectile dysfunction)

Clinical uses of PGs : (Misoprostol)

1. To induce abortion → It is very Effective → Used to terminate the pregnancy (1st and 2nd trimester abortion). Also soften the cervix (easy for inducing abortion).

2. For facilitation of labour (next to Oxytocin or if Oxytocin is C/I)

3. In Post Partum Haemorrhage (PPH). It is alternate to Ergonovine (contraction of uterus → blood vessels are compressed → stop haemorrhage.)

4. In peptic ulcer → for quick healing of ulcers, they are combined with Proton Pump Inhibitor (particularly effective against NSAIDs induced ulcer)

5. In pulmonary hypertension (PGI$_2$) → PGI$_2$ decreases periphery, pulmonary & coronary resistance. It reduces pulmonary hypertention.

6. To keep the ductus arteriosus patent in congenital pulmonary artery stenosis in neonates during surgery.

7. In peripheral vascular diseases. (due to its vasodilatory action – local injection)
8. In glaucoma (it is also 1st line drug). (Refer Glaucoma).
9. In erectile dysfunction. PG is injected locally into carvernous muscle → dilate the blood vessels → erection of penis → treated in impotency also.

PGs – preparations: vaginal tablets, injection, eye drop.

Adverse effects:

Systemic – they are very rarely used. If used systemically → they produce fever, arthralgia, bone pain, inflammation, fall in BP, syncope & flushing etc.,

LEUKOTRIENS (LT)

Zileuton – inhibits leukotriene synthesis

Zafirlukast, Montelukast – Leukotriene Receptor Antagonists – blocks LT Receptors in the bronchial smooth muscles → relieve bronchospasm

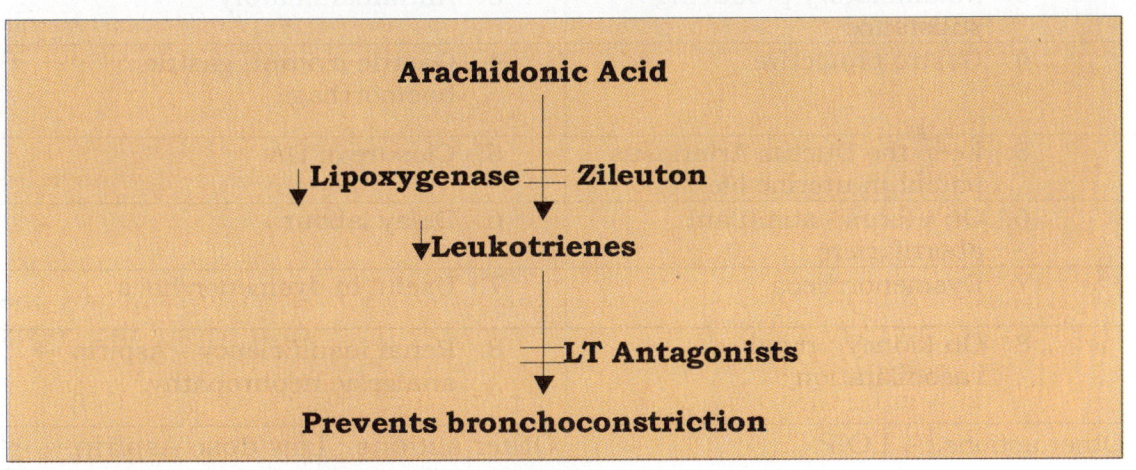

Clinical use:

1. Mainly used as prophylactic in allergic type of asthma as adjuvant with inhaled corticosteroids in poorly responding cases of asthma patients. They also reduce the dose of β_2 agonists.
2. Also useful in allergen induced and NSAIDs induced bronchoconstriction

Dose: Zafirlukast - 10-20 mg/orally /day, Montelukast – 5 – 10 mg/day

Adverse effects: Zileuton is a hepatotoxic (use is restricted), mild GIT upset, headache.

Zafirlukast is an enzyme inhibitor. It increases the toxicity of warfarin (bleeding), whose dose to be reduced, GIT upset, Headache.

NSAIDs

- Nutshell about NSAIDs.
- NSAIDs act by inhibiting PGs synthesis.
- Actions of NSAIDs are opposite to PGs.

Actions of PGs	Actions of NSAIDs (Inhibit PGs Synthesis)
1. Pain producing substance	1. Analgesic
2. Fever producing substance	2. Antipyretic
3. Inflammatory producing substance	3. Antiinflammatory
4. Gastro protective	4. Gastric irritant, gastric haemorrhage
5. Keep the Ductus Arteriosus patent in uterine life	5. Closure of DA
6. On uterus - stimulant abortifacient	6. Delay labour
7. Dysmenorrheoa	7. Useful in dysmenorrhoea
8. On kidney : renal vasodilatation	8. Renal insufficiency – Aspirin → analgesic nephropathy.

Other actions : ↓ I.O.P   Other actions : Low dose Aspirin

Nonsteroidal anti-inflammatory drugs (NSAIDs)

CHAPTER 28

NON STEROIDAL ANTI INFLAMMATORY DRUGS
(Steroidal Antiinflammatory drugs are Glucocorticoids)

    1. They are also referred as 'Non opioid analgesics' (Opioid analgesics are → Morphine, Pethidine).

    2. They are also referred as analgesics, antipyretic and antiinflammatory drugs

Mechanism of action

They ↓ (Inhibit) cyclo oxygenase enzyme →↓ (inhibit) Prostaglandins synthesis → Act as analgesic, antipyretic and antiinflammatory.

CLASSIFICATION OF NSAIDs

I.   Non selective irreversible inhibitors of COX : (inhibit both COX-1 and COX-2)

    1) Aspirin (acetyl salicylic acid), Sulfasalazine & Olsalazine

II.   Non selective reversible inhibitors of COX: (inhibit both COX-1 and COX-2)

    1) Indomethacin

    2) Ibuprofen

    3) Naproxen

    4) Mefenamic Acid

    5) Piroxicam

    6) Ketorolac

    7) Diclofenac & Aceclofenac

    8) Nimesulide

III.   Selective COX – 2 Inhibitors:

    1) Celecoxib

    2) Valdecoxib

IV. COX- 3 Inhibitors or Reversible Inhibitors of Hypothalamic COX – 1:

1) Paracetamol (crocin, Dolo-650)

2) Metamizol (analgin)

V. NSAIDs, which do not inhibit prostaglandin synthesis:

1) Nefopam

Mechanism of action of NSAIDs

Prostaglandin synthesis is increased when there is a tissue injury. There are some important actions of prostaglandins –

- They are mediators of inflammation, sensitizes the pain receptors in sensory nerve ending by reducing the pain threshold.
- They potentiate sensitizing action of (5HT, Substance –P, bradykinin) on pain receptors in the sensory nerve ending.
- Prostaglandins are less potent in producing pain by themselves. But in the presence of other mediators like 5HT, Substance –P, bradykinin, the pain is more intense.
- So, by inhibiting prostaglandin synthesis, pain is effectively relieved.
- Prostaglandins are synthesized from arachidonic acid by the enzyme cyclooxygenase (COX-1 and COX-2)
- COX- enzyme is predominant in GIT (parietal cells) and platelets. COX-2 is predominant in inflammatory producing cells.
- Aspirin inhibits both enzymes and has anti-inflammatory and ulcerogenic activity.
- Selective COX-2 inhibitors are having only anti-inflammatory action and no ulcerogenic action.

Pharmacological actions of Aspirin (Ref : Prostaglandins)

I. **Analgesia:** it is effective analgesic only in relieving integumental pain (pain arising from skin, muscle, joints etc.,). It is not effective in visceral pain (pain due to MI, malignancy and fracture of long bone). It does not produce tolerance or dependence.

II. **Antipyretic action:** It brings only symptomatic relief. The actual cause of the fever is to be evaluated. It does not affect the normal body temperature. It reduces the temperature only at hyperpyrexia. Prostaglandins set the thermostat mechanism at higher level in hypothalamus. Aspirin decreases prostaglandin synthesis and resets the thermostat mechanism at normal level.

III. **Anti-inflammatory action:** Prostaglandins produce vasodilatation, increase capillary permeability, exudation of fluid and cause inflammation. Aspirin produces anti-inflammatory action only in high doses (5-6 times of analgesic dose). There will be also adverse effects more intense. It is very effective in inflammatory pain. The actual cause of inflammation is not removed. The new NSAIDs are preferred for this action. It stabilizes leukocyte lysosomal membrane and prevents the spread of inflammation.

IV.   **On uterus:** prostaglandins are uterine stimulant. The excess contraction (ischemia of myometrium) may be responsible for dysmenorrhoea. Aspirin inhibits prostaglandins synthesis and useful in dysmenorrhoea.

V.   **On ductus arteriosis:** the ductus arteriosis is kept patent by prostaglandins in foetal life. At the time of birth, level of prostaglandins will decline and there is closure of ductus arteriosis. In some infant, the ductus arteriosis does not close. At that time NSAID drugs are given for early closure of ductus arteriosis.

VI.   **On GIT:** Aspirin inhibits prostaglandin synthesis in parietal cells of stomach. So, there is an increased gastric acid secretion and reduced mucous production. There will be gastric irritation, gastric haemorrhage, ulcerogenic effects. So, it is contraindicated in peptic ulcer.

VII.   **On respiration and acid base balance:** Aspirin stimulates respiration – in therapeutic dose by uncoupling of oxidative phosphorylation, produces CO_2, which is washed away by respiratory stimulation. In large doses – due to direct stimulation of respiration lead to respiratory alkalosis and then compensatory respiratory acidosis, lead to metabolic acidosis.

VIII.   **Antiplatelet action:** Antiplatelet action is seen only in low dose. (Ref- antiplatelet drugs). And also long term use of Aspirin produces hypoprothrombinaemia, which is responsible for bleeding.

IX.   **On uric acid level:** Aspirin in low dose decreases the excretion of uric acid and large dose increases uric acid excretion (uricosuric action) but other NSAIDs act as uricosuric agent at all dose levels, preferred in gout.

X.   **On kidney:** It causes analgesic nephropathy characterized by chronic nephritis and renal papillary necrosis. It is due to the inhibition of prostaglandins induced vasodilatation.

XI.   **Reye's syndrome:** it is very rare and at times fatal by the treatment of Aspirin in infants. It is characterized by liver damage and encephalopathy which occur when they are recovering from febrile viral infection. Hence, Paracetamol (not Aspirin) should be preferred in fever of unknown origin in children under 12 years.

Clinical uses of Aspirin

1. As analgesic: In integumental pain like headache, bodyache, arthralgia, toothache, myalgia, etc.,
2. As antipyretic: It is for only symptomatic treatment. The actual cause of fever is not removed. It reduces body temperature only in fever, not in normal body temperature.
3. As anti-inflammatory: It prevents the spread of inflammation. It is very effective in relieving inflammatory pain due to sprain, dislocation, rheumatoid arthritis and gout.
4. In dysmenorrhoea: It relieves pain due to dysmenorrhoea, which is due to excess synthesis of PGs in uterus.

5. For closure of ductus arteriosis: In some infants, the ductus arteriosis remains patent after birth, which is not wanted. NSAIDs are very much useful for the closure of ductus arteriosis.

6. Clinical uses of low dose aspirin (75-150 mg per day)

    i.   In pre-eclampsia (pregnancy induced hypertension): the hypertension in pregnancy is due to excess Thromboxane A_2. Aspirin in low dose specifically inhibits TXA_2.
    ii. In Myocardial Infarction: Due to its antiplatelet action by inhibiting specifically the TXA_2. The treatment is lifelong.
    iii. In colonic and rectal cancer: Aspirin reduces the risk of colonic and rectal cancer. COX-2 enzymes are found to be more concentrated there. So, specific COX–2 inhibitors may produce better effects.
    iv. Familial colonic polyps: May be due excess Thromboxane A_2 level at that site. Aspirin in low dose inhibits the synthesis of Thromboxane A_2 and suppresses polyp's formation.
    v.   In cataract: Aspirin in low dose slows down the cataract progression by unknown mechanism.
    vi. Niacin induced cutaneous flush and pruritus: This is probably is mediated through PGs. Aspirin inhibits PGs synthesis and relieves all the symptoms.
    vii. In alzheimer's disease: Aspirin lowers the risk and retards the onset of alzheimer's disease.

Adverse effects of Aspirin:

Gastric irritation, gastric haemorrhage, vomiting, metabolic acidosis, analgesic nephropathy, Reyes syndrome in children (especially below 12 years), bleeding, tendency in long term use, bronchoconstriction (due to diversion of excess arachidonic acid for the synthesis of LTs, which are powerful broncho-constrictors).

Contraindication:

Pregnancy – it may cause early closure of ductus arteriosis in foetus.

Drug interaction:

1. With warfarin – Aspirin displaces Warfarin from the protein binding site, produces hypoprothrombinemia lead to toxicity of Warfarin (bleeding)
2. Low dose of Aspirin – aggravate gout and reduces the efficacy of uricosuric agents.

Other NSAIDs (Non-selective COX-1, COX–2 inhibitors):

Pharmacological actions:

- Analgesic
- Antipyretic
- Anti-inflammatory
- Uricosuric action
- On GIT
- On Uterus
- On ductus arteriosis

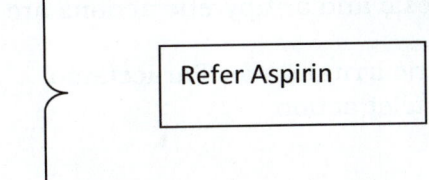

Refer Aspirin

Clinical uses – (Ref: like that of Aspirin except that of low dose of Aspirin) and also used in acute gout.

Adverse effects: gastric irritation, bronchoconstriction.

Dose:

- Aceclofenac sodium – 100 mg tab/BD/daily
- Diclofenac sodium – 50 mg tab/TDS/daily
- Ibuprofen – 200-400 mg tab/TDS/daily
- Indomethacin – 25-50 mg cap/TDS/daily
- Ketoralac – 10 mg tab/TDS/daily
- Mefanemic acid – 250 mg tab/TDS/daily
- Naproxen – 250 mg tab/BD/daily
- Piroxicam – 20 mg/BD/daily

Selective COX–2 inhibitors

- Examples : Rofecoxib, Celecoxib, Valedecoxib
- There is no action at the site of GIT, Platelets
- There is no gastric irritation (gastroprotective)
- There is no platelet inhibitory action, less bleeding tendency
- The main actions are analgesic, antipyretic and anti-inflammatory
- Long term use of COX-2 inhibitors increase Thromboxane A_2 concentration which will increase the cardiac toxicity (Hence some of them are banned).
- They are very much useful in long term treatment of rheumatoid arthritis.

Dose: Celecoxib – 100-200 mg/ BD/daily, Valdecoxib – 10-20 mg / once/daily

Adverse effects: not much, occational oedema, mild hypertension, skin rash.

Paracetamol

- It is also called as acetaminophen
- It is a COX-3 inhibitor or reversible inhibitor of hypothalamus COX-1
- It is one of NSAIDs

Mechanism of Action

- It inhibits COX – 3/COX – 1 in hypothalamus → ↓ (inhibits) PGs synthesis in hypothalamus
- The analgesic and antipyretic actions are due to inhibition of COX-3 in CNS
- Least gastric irritation for Paracetamol
- No antiplatelet action

Clinical uses

1. As analgesic – it is the first choice drug in relieving integumental pain
2. As antipyretic – it is very potent. It is the first choice drug and preferred in children.

Dose: Paracetamol (crocin 500 mg, Dolo-650 mg, Calpol 500 mg, Metacin 500 mg)

Adverse effects:

Mild side effects, well tolerated, Skin rashes.
Acute toxicity can occur mainly in children.

Adverse effects: Well tolerated, nausea occasionally.

Paracetamol poisoning in children: Toxic metabolite of Paracetamol → conjugated and excreted. In children there is a deficiency of glucoronide conjugation of enzyme →↓ (reduced) conjugation capacity → the toxic metabolite of Paracetamol is not conjugated and excreted → ↑ (increase) blood level of toxic metabolite →↑ (increase) the toxicity (liver, kidney).

Antidote: N-Acetyl cysteine conjugates the toxic metabolite and excretes it.

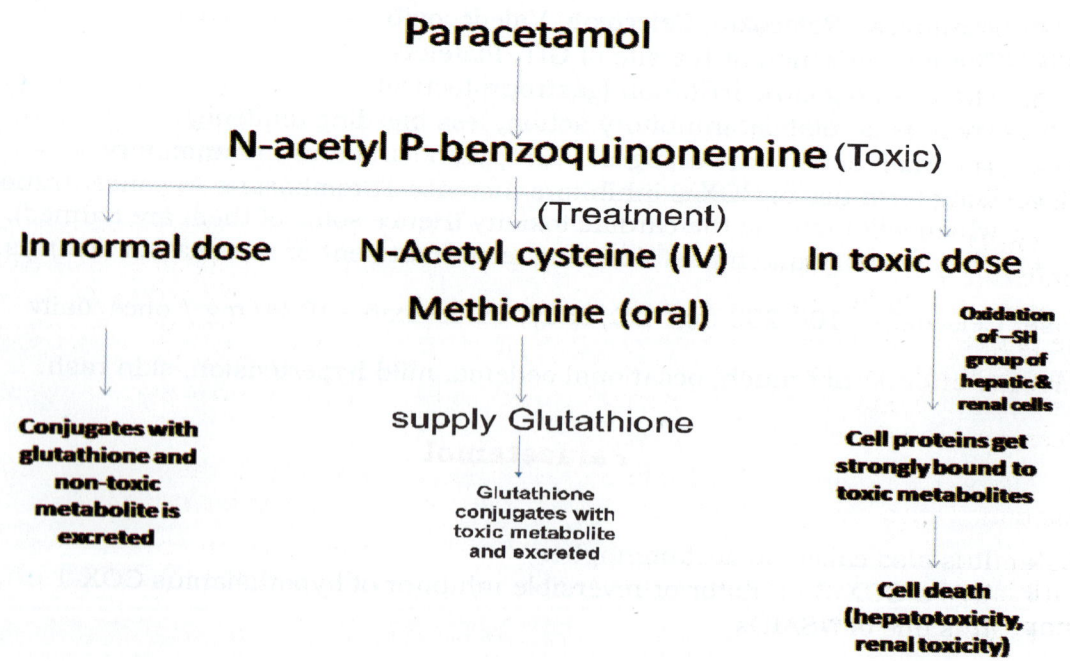

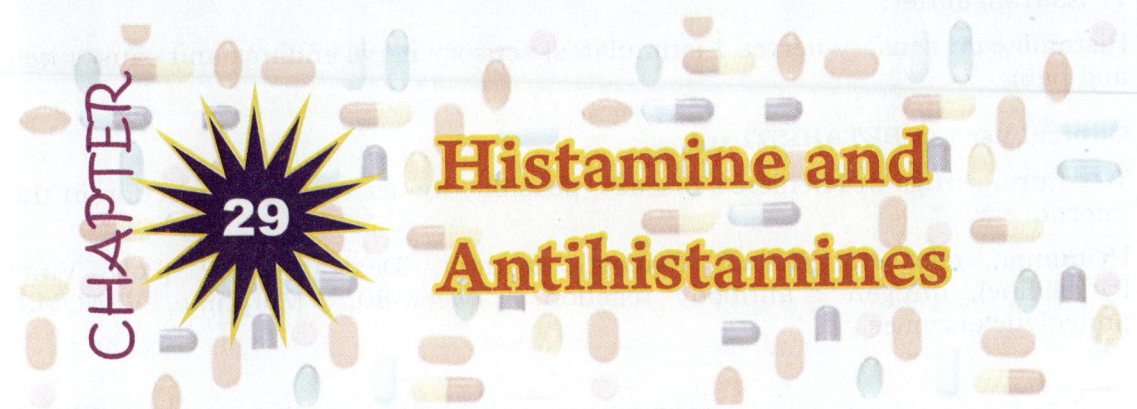

Histamine and Antihistamines

CHAPTER 29

Histamine means, tissue amine.

Histamine is present in the mast cells, venoms and pathological fluids.

HISTAMINE RECEPTORS: H_1 and H_2

H_1 is mainly concerned with allergic manifestations and emetic action.

H_2 is concerned with acid secretion from the parietal cells of stomach.

Actions of Histamine:

1.   On blood vessels: Histamine causes vasodilatation → fall in BP → anaphylactic shock (partly due to Histamine).

2. On smooth muscles: Histamine causes contraction of smooth muscles → diarrhoea and brochoconstriction.

3. On sensory nerve endings: Histamine stimulates the sensory nerve endings → pain and itch.

4. On CNS: Histamine stimulates CNS → Wakefulness: Non mast cells Histamine in RAS (Reticular Activating System) is responsible for wakefulness. Sedation is the most important side effect of Antihistamines. ↑ (stimulates) Chemoreceptor Trigger Zone → vomiting → antihistamines are antiemetic.

5.   On GIT (H_2 receptor): ↑ (stimulates) Gastric acid secretion. Histamine has got dominant physiological role. Histaminocytes (non mast cells, present very close to parietal cells in the stomach) → release Histamine → occupies H_2 receptor in the parietal cells of stomach → ↑ (stimulates) Cyclic AMP → ↑ (stimulates) in turn Proton pump → ↑ (stimulates) gastric acid secretion. Histamine is also released by the stimuli from vagus, cholinergic drugs, gastrin and certain drugs. In peptic ulcer, excess release of Histamine is found.

6.   Allergic phenomenon: The important role of Histsmine is the hypersensitive reaction. Released by antigen: antibody reaction as one of the main mediators.

Histamine causes urticaria, angioedema, bronchospasm and anaphylactic shock. Antihistamines are effective in the above conditions except asthma and anaphylactic shock.

7. As transmitter:

Histamine on sensory nerves ↑ (stimulates) sensory nerve endings and causes itch and pain.

Clinical uses of BETAHISTINE:

To control vertigo in Mieniere's disease, possibly due its vasodilating action in the internal ear.

Histamine releasers: Tissue damage, trauma, Dextran, PVP (Poly Vinyl Pyrrolidine), antigen : antibody reaction, Tween-80, Morphine, VENOMS, proteolytic enzymes.

ANTIHISTAMINES

ANTIHISTAMINES: are drugs which inhibit the actions of Histamine (H_1 receptors) called as Antihistamines or H_1 antagonists. The action of H_2 receptors is inhibited by H_2 antagonists (discussed under Peptic ulcer).

CLASSIFICATION: (on the basis of sedative action)

I. Highly sedative:

1. Diphenhydramine
2. Promethazine

II. Mild and moderately sedative

1. Pheniramine (Avil)
2. Meclizine
3. Buclizine
4. Cyclizine
5. Cinnarizine

III. NON SEDATIVE ANTIHISTAMINE OR SECOND GENERATION ANTIHISTAMINES:

1. Cetrizine
2. Levocetrizine (Levosiz)
3. FEXOFENADINE (Allegra)
4. Ebastine (Ebast)
5. Loratadine
6. Azelastine

IV. H_2 antagonists: (ref: peptic ulcer)

Actions of Antihistamines:

1. On CNS:

Antihistamines produce CNS DEPRESSANT action and SEDATION

ANTIEMETIC (ANTI MOTION SICKNESS) ACTION (Antihistamines inhibit H_1 receptors in semicircular canal in internal ear.

2. Anticholinergic actions are useful IN MOTION SICKNESS

Side effects like dryness of mouth, constipation and urinary retention are due to anticholinergic actions.

3. ANTI ALLERGIC ACTIONS: Many manifestations of Type I hypersensitive reactions (like urticaria, angioedema, dermatitis, conjunctivitis, itching are well controlled) are suppressed by antihistamines.

Clinical uses :

1. IN ALLERGIC DISORDERS: like urticaria, andioedema of lip and eye lid, dermatitis, conjunctivitis, itching etc., They are not effective against cell mediated immune reactions, since Histamine is not involved.

2. They relieve pain and itch due to insect bite, ivy plant poisoning (ivy plant is Histamine releaser on contact).

3. In pruritus: Antihistamines are first choice drugs in idiopathic pruritus.

4. In motion sickness: Promethazine is effective and it taken half an hour before proposed journey by the susceptible individuals.

5. In vertigo (only cinnarizine).

6. In common cold: Antihistamines produce symptomatic relief (by its anticholinergic, antiallergic and sedative action) → ↓ (inhibits rhinorrhoea).

7. In cough: ↓ Antihistamine inhibit cough centre, and its sedative action is also useful in cough.

8. In Parkinsonism: (due to its anticholinergic action) particularly useful in drug induced Parkinsonism. (Promethazine)

9. As sedative and anxiolytic used in children.

Adverse effects: Dryness of mouth, constipation, urinary retention, blurring of vision (all are due to their anticholinergic actions), SEDATION (driving to be avoided, tendency to sleep, motor incordination, impairment of psychomotor performances)

NONSEDATIVE OR SECOND GENERATION ANTIHISTAMINES:

DRUGS:

1. Cetrizine (mild sedative-not used)
2. LEVOCETRIZINE
3. LORATADINE
4. EBASTINE

5. FEXOFENADINE

6. AZELASTINE

Differences between conventional antihistamines and non sedative antihistamine

1. THEY DO NOT CROSS Blood Brain Barrier → No central actions - NO SEDATION, no central anticholinergic USES and no central anticholinergic side effects.

2. Higher H_1 selelctivity.

3 Additional anti allergic mechanism →↓ (inhibit) late phase allergic reactions → ↓(inhibit) LTs and PAF actions → so, potent anti allergic action.

4. These drugs do not impair psychomotor performances (driving, operating machinery → not contraindicated in them, particularly in taxi driver)

5. They do not produce sleepiness and do not potentiate CNS depressants, alcohol etc.,

6. They are mainly useful in allergic disorders.

7. All the drugs are having same action and USES except some pharmacokinetic properties.

Clinical uses

Mainly in allergic disorders

1. In allergic rhinitis.

2. In allergic conjunctivitis.

3. In hay fever, pollinosis (due to pollen grains).

4. To control sneezing and running nose due to allergy.

5. In itching.

6. In urticaria, dermatitis, atopic eczema.

7. In acute allergic reactions due to food and drugs.

Adverse effects: Minimum and well tolerated

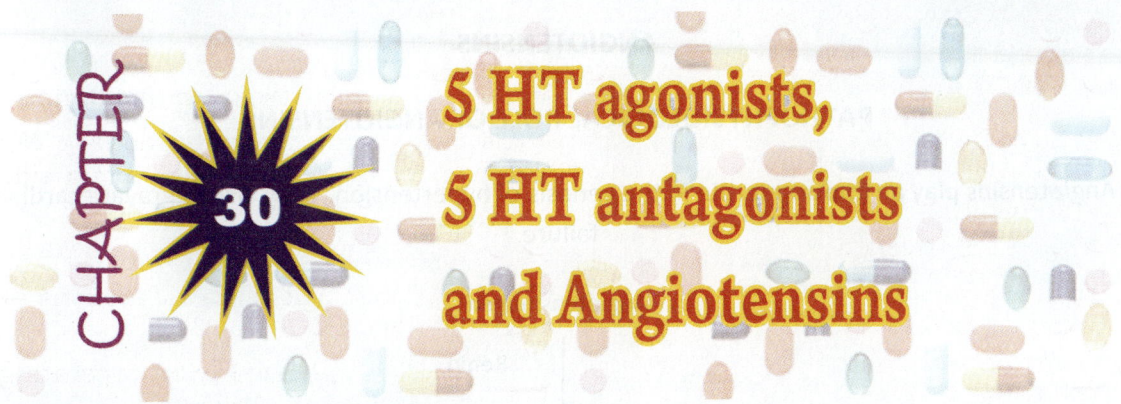

CHAPTER 30

5 HT agonists, 5 HT antagonists and Angiotensins

Clinical uses of 5 HT AGONISTS:

1. SSRI (ref: Antidepressants)

2. Sumatriptan- Selective $5HT_{1B}$ agonist- used in migraine (ref: Migraine)

Clinical uses of 5 HT ANTAGONISTS:

1. Ondansetron: Selective $5 HT_3$ antagonist→ antiemetic (ref: antiemetic).

2. Atypical antipsychotic drugs −↓ (inhibit) reuptake of 5 HT (ref: atypical antipsychotic drugs).

3. Cyproheptadine: In carcinoid syndrome (due to excess 5 HT).

4. Ergotamine: Used in acute attack of migraine.

5. Methysergide: Used as prophylactic in migraine.

ERGOT ALKALOIDS:

Source: From fungus Claviceps purpurea grown on rye plant.

Ergot alkaloids: Ergotamine, Ergonovine (Ergometrine)

Ergotamine: α adrenergic blocking action → vasodilatation. But direct vasoconstrictor action is more potent. Hence useful in migraine.

Ergometrine: direct vasoconstriction, powerful uterine stimulant (hence it is useful in PPH- Post Partum Haemorrhage)

C/I in pregnancy- because they contract all parts of the uterus at a time – foetal asphyxia (unlike Oxytocin, which contracts upper portion and relaxes lower portion).

ANGIOTENSINS

PATHOPHYSIOLOGICAL ROLE OF ANGIOTENSINS

Angiotensins play an important role in the genesis of hypertension. They also aggravate cardiac failure.

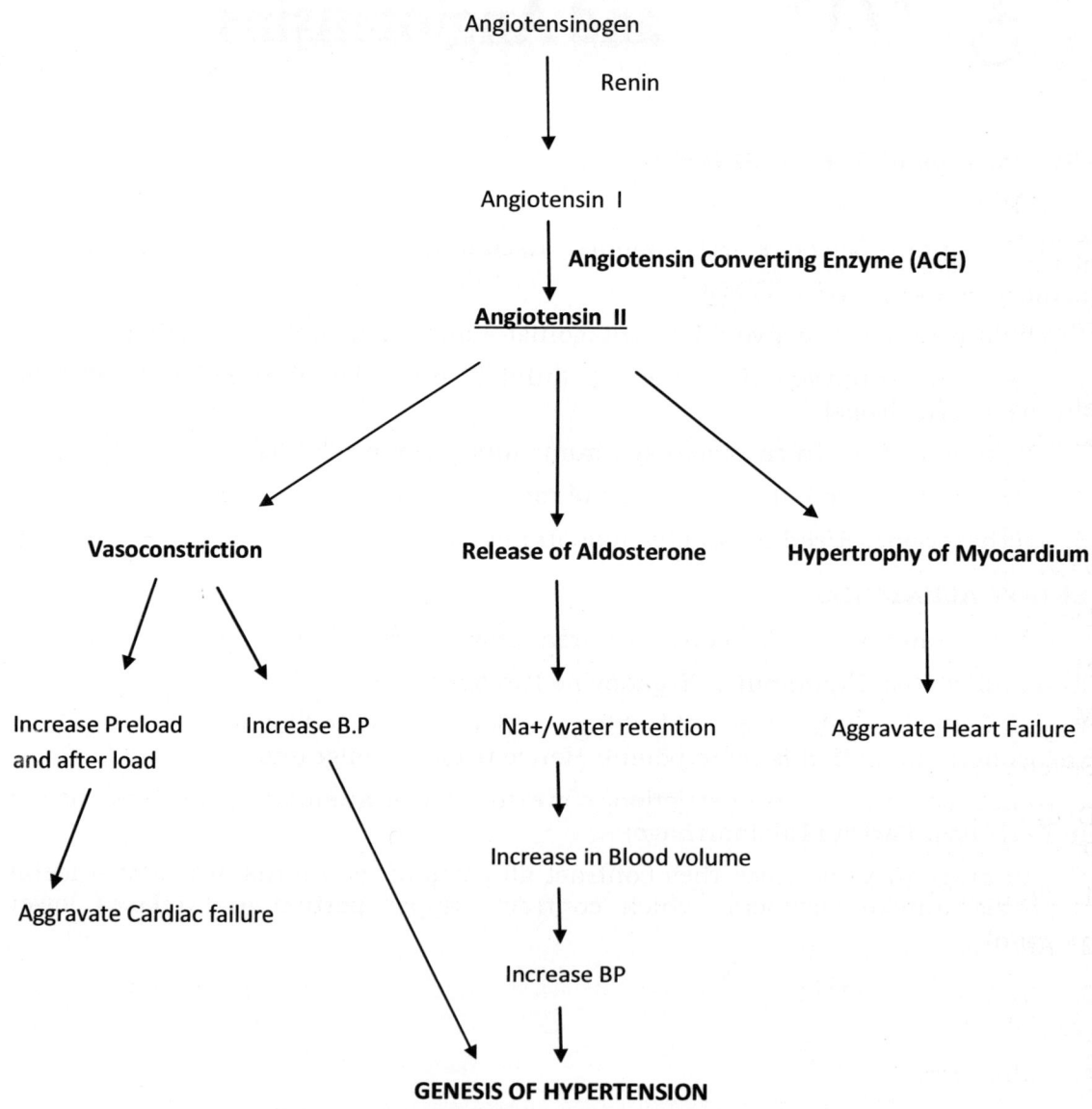

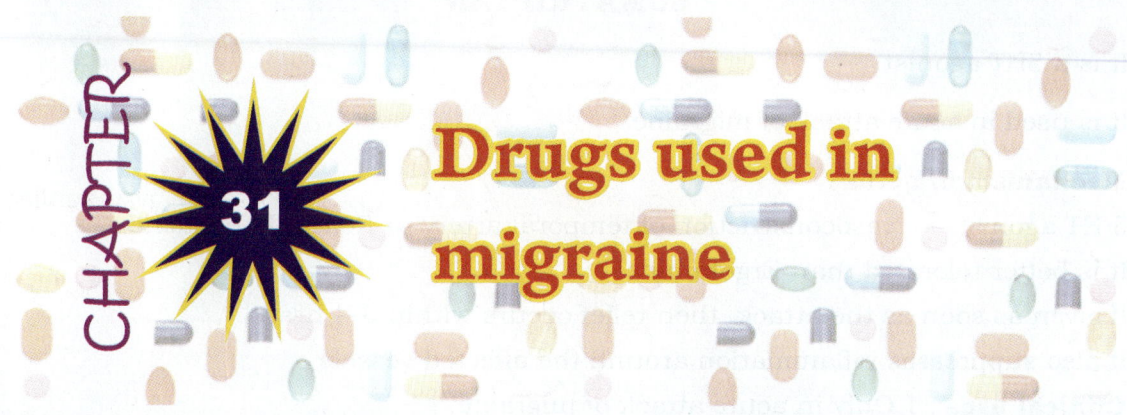

CHAPTER

31

Drugs used in migraine

Migraine, a symptom complex of periodic headache (usually one sided, temporal) often with nausea, vomiting and photophobia, preceded by constriction of the cranial arteries (ischaemia → pain) often with resultant prodromal sensory (ocular) symptoms (aura) and commencing with vasodilatation of temporal arteries that follows → produce headache.

Neurotransmitters theory of migraine: 5 HT plays an important role. The efficacy of the drugs having actions in the serotoninergic (5 HT) system to prevent/ abort/ terminate migraine attacks suggests a pivotal role of 5 HT in this disorders.

The drugs used in acute attack produce vasoconstriction of temporal artery.

The drugs used in prophylaxis produce vasodilatation of cranial artery or vasoconctriction of temporal artery.

Drugs used in acute attack:

Mild: Analgesic/NSAIDs with an antiemetic

Moderate: NSAIDs/Ergotamine/Sumatriptan with an antiemetic

Severe: Ergotamine/Sumatriptan with an antiemetic

Drugs used as prophylactic: Prophylactics are needed, if acute attack occurs once or twice a month.

1. Propranolol

2. Amitriptyline (inhibits reuptake of 5 HT)

3. Flunarizine and other calcium channel blockers (produce vasodilatation of cranial arteries)

4. Valproic acid

5. Methysergide (5 HT antagonist)

SUMATRIPTAN

It is a 5HT agonist.

It is used in acute attack of migraine.

Mechanism of action

5 HT agonist → vasoconstriction of temporal artery → Relief of headache

It is better tolerated than Ergotamine.

If given as soon as the attack, then relief occurs within 3-4 hrs.

It also suppresses inflammation around the affected vessels

Clinical uses : 1.Only in acute attack of migraine.

Adverse effects: mild, dizziness, weakness, infrequent but serious coronary vasoconstriction

C/I. in ischaemic heart diseases

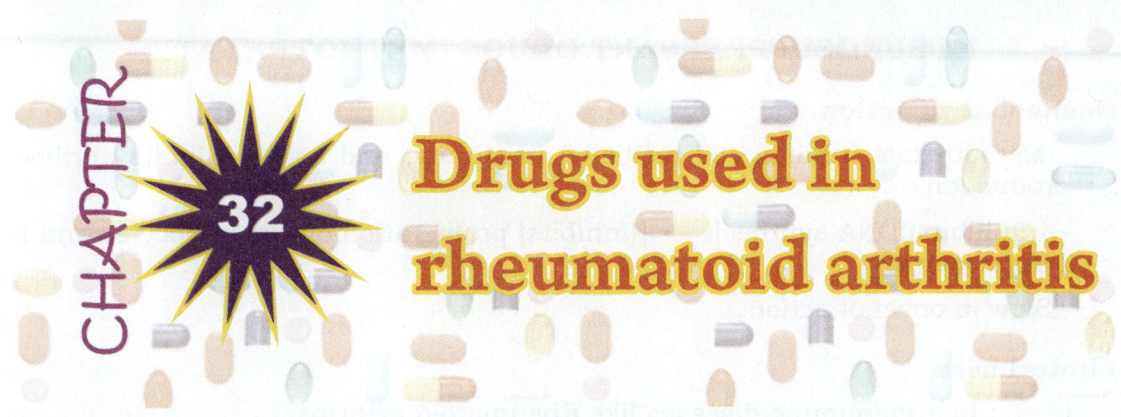

CHAPTER 32

Drugs used in rheumatoid arthritis

Rheumatoid arthritis is an autoimmune disease, a chronic systemic disease primarily of the joints, usually polyarticular, marked by inflammatory changes in the synovial membrane and destruction of articular cartilage and erode bones. In later stage, deformity develops

Main symptoms: stiffness in the joints, joint swelling, inflammatory pain, restricted joint mobility. Later stage joint deformity, very difficult in joint mobility.

First NSAIDs are tried. Then oral / intra articular Glucocorticoids are tried. If glucocorticoids are contraindicated/long term toxicity, then the last chance is by DMARDs (Disease Modifying Anti Rheumatic Drugs). If that fails, the only option is knee replacement.

The DMARDs can suppress the rheumatoid process and bring about remission, by specific anti-inflammatory action.

DISEASE MODIFYING ANTIRHEUMATIC DRUGS (DMARDs)

The goals of the treatment in rheumatoid arthritis are:

1. Ameliorate pain, swelling and joint stiffness.

2. Prevent articular damage and bony erosion.

3. Prevent joint deformity and preserve the joint function.

DMARDs are acting slowly. But less toxic for long term use.

1. Immunosuppressants: Methotrexate

2. Salfasalazine

3. Hydroxy chloroquine

4. Gold compounds

5. d- Penicillamine

6. Biologic response modifier:TNF- α inhibitors i) Infliximab ii) Adalimumab

7. Adjuvant drug: Glucocorticoids

IMMUNOSUPPRESSANT DRUGS (METHOTREXATE)

Mechanism of action

- Methotrexate inhibits cell mediated immunity, and also ↓ inhibits antibody production

- ↓ (inhibits) DNA synthesis → ↓(inhibits) proliferation of T-lymphocytes and B-Lymphocytes.

- Slow in onset of action.

Clinical uses

i.   In autoimmune diseases like Rheumatoid arthritis
ii. To prevent graft rejection in organ transplantation

Adverse effects: (ref: general toxicity of anti cancer drugs)

C/I in pregnancy.

SALFASALAZINE

- It is a DMARD
- It is also useful in ulcerative colitis
- **Mechanism of action** Salfasalazine is converted to 6 Amino Salicylic Acid, which is an anti-inflammatory.
- It is useful in rheumatoid arthritis and ulcerative colitis.
- It is second line drug for milder cases of Rheumatoid arthritis.

HYDROXY CHLOROQUINE

- It is an anti-inflammatory drug
- It ↓(inhibits) B-lymphocytes →↓(inhibits) antibody production- useful in autoimmune diseases. (Rheumatoid arthritis)
- **Adverse effects**: Retinal damage (long term use), greying of hair, irritable bowel syndrome, myopathy.

BIOLOGIC RESPONSE MODIFIERS

- They are monoclonal antibodies. (Refer Monoclonal antibody)
- They bind with cytokines and inhibit them. It affords sustained relief in Rheumatoid Arthritis.
- There are also useful in Inflammatory Bowel Disease, psoriasis.

ADJUVANT- GLUCOCORTICOIDS

- They are potent immunosuppressant and anti-inflammatory.
- Both actions are useful in Rheumatoid Arthritis.
- They produced symptomatic relief.
- They do not reduce progression (do not arrest the rheumatoid process).
- Precautions: (ref:glucocorticoids)

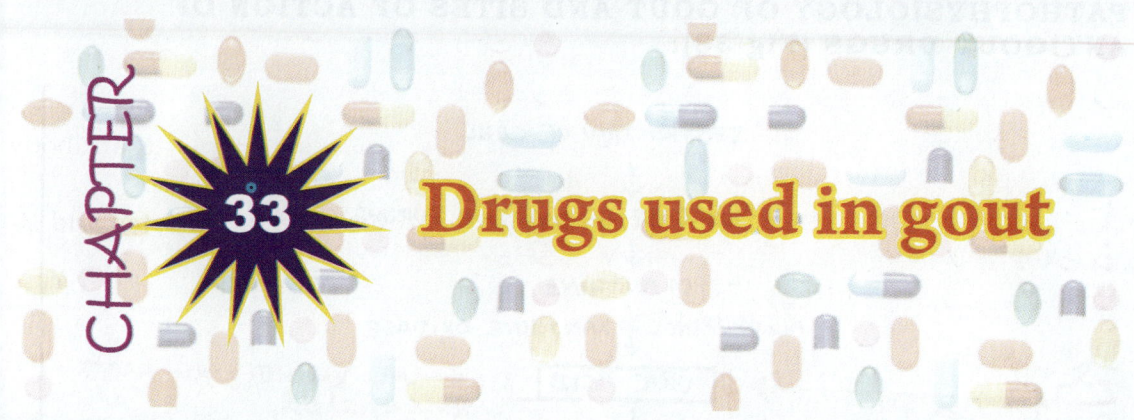

Drugs used in gout

CHAPTER 33

Gout is a disorder of purine and pyrimidine metabolism characterized by hyperuricemia (normal blood uric acid is 1-4 mg/dl) and typhi (chalk like stone) deposited in the soft tissues of kidney, ears, cartilage of smaller joints. If it is not treated in time lead to joint immobility, swelling and pain in the form of acute attack.

The uric acid is a waste product from the purine and pyrimidine metabolism. There will be hyperuricaemia in over producers or under excretors of uric acid. Hyperuricaemia in acidic medium gets precipitated into urate crystals in the joints → irritate the cartilage → form inflammation surrounding the joints → causes swelling and pain → slow destruction of joint tissues.

If untreated in time, it will lead to swelling, joint immobility and pain, which will be represented as acute attack. Inflammation due to release of chemotactic factors → infiltration of granulocytes into the joints → phagocytosis of urate crystals with the release of glycoprotein (free radical) → destroys more joints and release of lysosome enzyme with more precipitation of urate crystals (acute attack). The vicious cycle is going on with all the precipitating factors if it is not treated.

CHRONIC GOUT:

Hyperuricaemia forms subcutaneous tophi in the pinna of external ear, eye lid and around joints. The tophi will also affect synovial, articular damage → joint deformities, pain, stiffness in the joints which persist in between the attack.

The uricosuric agents and the drugs which inhibit the synthesis of uric acid are useful.

PATHOPHYSIOLOGY OF GOUT AND SITES OF ACTION OF ANTIGOUT DRUGS (Fig 33):

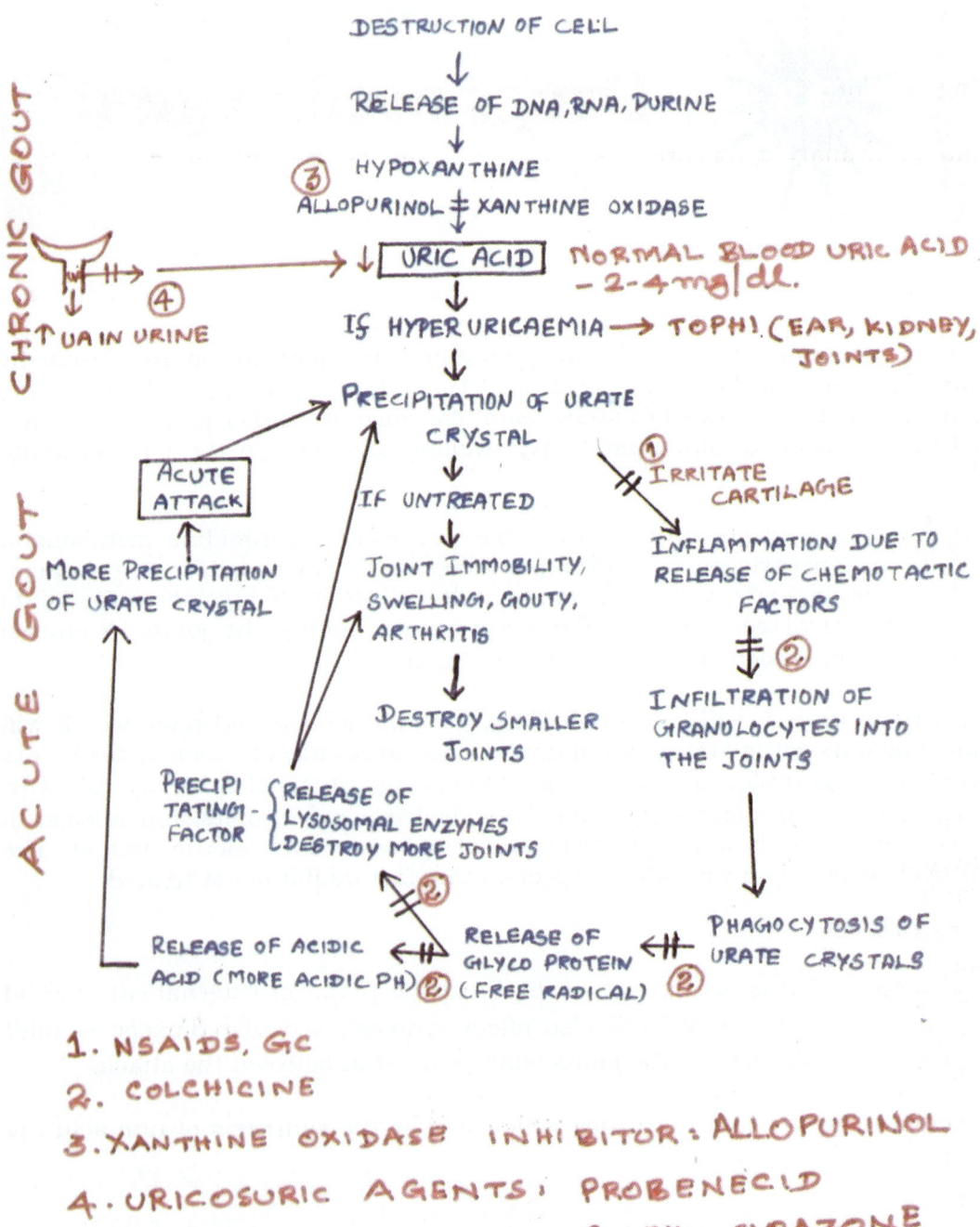

DESTRUCTION OF CELL
↓
RELEASE OF DNA, RNA, PURINE
↓
③ HYPOXANTHINE
ALLOPURINOL ⊥ XANTHINE OXIDASE
↓
↓ URIC ACID   NORMAL BLOOD URIC ACID — 2-4 mg/dL.
↓
IF HYPERURICAEMIA → TOPHI (EAR, KIDNEY, JOINTS)
↓
PRECIPITATION OF URATE CRYSTAL

CHRONIC GOUT

④ ↑UA IN URINE

ACUTE GOUT

ACUTE ATTACK

MORE PRECIPITATION OF URATE CRYSTAL

IF UNTREATED
↓
JOINT IMMOBILITY, SWELLING, GOUTY, ARTHRITIS
↓
DESTROY SMALLER JOINTS

① IRRITATE CARTILAGE
↓
INFLAMMATION DUE TO RELEASE OF CHEMOTACTIC FACTORS
⊥ ②
INFILTRATION OF GRANULOCYTES INTO THE JOINTS
↓
PHAGOCYTOSIS OF URATE CRYSTALS

PRECIPI- TATING- FACTOR { RELEASE OF LYSOSOMAL ENZYMES DESTROY MORE JOINTS

RELEASE OF ACIDIC ACID (MORE ACIDIC PH) ② ← ⊥ ② RELEASE OF GLYCO PROTEIN (FREE RADICAL) ←⊥ ②

1. NSAIDS, GC
2. COLCHICINE
3. XANTHINE OXIDASE INHIBITOR: ALLOPURINOL
4. URICOSURIC AGENTS: PROBENECID
        SULPHINPYRAZONE

ACUTE GOUT:

It is due to painful arthritic attack of sudden onset. The common joint affected is the first metatorsophalangeal joint (podagra-gouty pain in the great toe). Other sites that may be affected later are knee joint, elbow joint, ankle joint, wrist joint and fingers joints. This severe arthritic pain progressively worsen

Patients of primary hyperuricemia- 1.either over producers (the drugs which inhibit the synthesis of uric acid is useful in this condition- ALLOPURINOL 2. Or due to under excretors (the drugs which increase the excretion of uric acid (uricosuric agents) are useful in this condition-PROBENECID AND SULFINPYRAZONE.

In secondary hyperuricemia, (which may occur during the course of some diseases like leukemias, lymphomas and during anticancer drugs treatment destroy cancer cells and release purine and pyrimidine bases, which are then converted into uric acid).

Gout is a metabolic disorder characterized by hyperuricemia (normal plasma urate is 1-4 mg/dl). The urate crystals are precipitated and deposited in the joints, S.C tissues (tophi-chalk like stone under the skin in pinna, eye lids, nose, around joints and other places). Smaller joints are affected and unilateral.

Uric acid is the degradation product of purine metabolism.

Secondary hyperucricemia occurs in Leukemia and other cancers, when treated with anti cancer drugs, where large number of cells are destroyed and uric acid is synthesized in excess.

Drug induced- Frusemide, Thiazides, Pyrazinamide etc., by inhibiting the secretion of uric acid, increase the plasma uric acid level → hyperuricemia.

Symptoms are mainly due to the deposition of urate crystals in the joints → pain, stiffness in the joints and arthritis.

I. DRUGS FOR ACUTE GOUT: sudden onset of severe inflammation in a smaller joints (commonest is the metatarso-phalangeal joint of great toe) due to the precipitation of urate crystals in the joints space → pain.

1. Colchicine

2. NSAIDs

3. Glucocorticoids

II. DRUGS FOR CHRONIC GOUT:

1. Uricosuric agents: i) Probenecid ii) Sulfinpyrazone

2. Uric acid synthesis inhibitors: i) Allopurinol

COLCHICINE

- It is an alkaloid obtained from colchicum autumnale.
- It is not analgesic or anti-inflammatory action (it is effective anti-inflammatory only in urate crystals induced inflammation)
- It does not inhibit the synthesis of uric acid.
- It does not increase the excretion of uric acid.
- It is useful only in acute attack. In chronic gout it is toxic.

Mechanism of action: (Ref : fig 33)

- It inhibits only the gouty inflammatory response
  1. It inhibits fibrillar protein tubulin and disappearance of micro tubule in the granulocytes and by preventing the migration of granulocytes into the inflamed joints.
  2. It Inhibits the release of glycoprotein → decreases the acidity → further decreases the urate crystals formation → and by inhibiting the release of lysosomal enzymes → prevent the destruction of joint tissues further.
  3. It interrupts the vicious cycle and relieves the acute attack and pain.

Clinical uses:

1. Only in acute gout.

Dose: 0.5mg/day

Adverse effects:

DIARRHOEA, abdominal pain, peripheral neuritis , haematuria, oliguria.

GLUCOCORTICOIDS

- Intra articuclar injection of Glucocorticoids are useful in acute attack (oral NSAIDs are preferred).

NSAIDs

- They are commonly used in acute attack, and they are less toxic.
- They are analgesic and anti-inflammatory

Mechanism of action (Fig.33)

- NSAIDs → ↓ (Inhibit) PGs synthesis → anti-inflammatory and analgesic → very much useful in acute attack of gout.

- onset of action is also quick.

DRUGS USED IN CHRONIC GOUT: i) Uricosuric agents ii) Drugs inhibit uirc acid synthesis

When pain and stiffness persist in joints between attacks, gout becomes chronic.

- Hyperuricemia, tophi are present.

URICOSURIC AGENTS: Those drugs which increase the excretion of uric acid.

PROBENECID

- Useful only in chronic gout.
- Since it is not anti-inflammatory, not suitable for acute attack.

Mechanism of action (Fig.33 / 34)

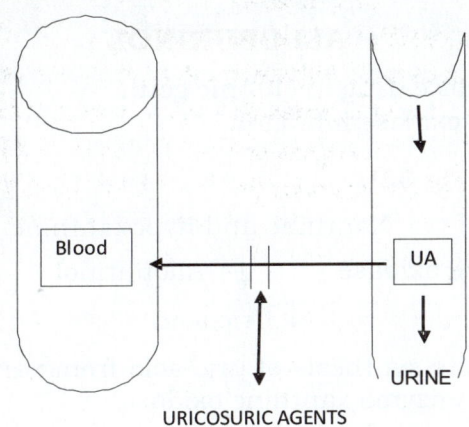

URICOSURIC AGENTS

Fig. 34 Excreation of Uric Acid (UA)

- Probenecid ↓ (inhibits) the tubular reabsorption of uric acid in the renal tubule → ↑ (increases) excretion of uric acid in the urine → reduces plasma uric acid level.

- Also, it competitively ↓ (inhibits) the secretion of Ampicillin and Amoxicillin → ↑ (increases) the concentration of those drugs in the plasma. Higher concentration of Ampicillin and Amoxicillin is needed in the treatment of gonorrhoea. The high concentration of Ampicillin in the plasma cannot be achieved for the treatment of gonorrhoea by giving high oral dose, since it produces intolerable diarrhoea. So, Ampicillin (in normal therapeutic dose) is combined with Probenecid only for the treatment of gonorrhoea.

Clinical uses : 1. In chronic gout

3. To prolong/increase the plasma concentration of Ampicillin.

Adverse effects: May cause uric acid stone, when excess uric acid is excreted in the urine. When uric acid is mobilised from the joints, urate crystals are affected, which may cause pain (NSAID is given), allergic dermatitis, GIT upset, dyspepsia

Dose : Probanecid 250 – 500 mg.

SULFINPYRAZONE

-It is used in chronic gout.

-Mechanism of action similar to that of Probenecid.

 Adverse effects: similar to that of Probenecid.

 Dose : 200 mg.

 Clinical uses: similar to that of Probenecid.

DRUG WHICH INHIBIT URIC ACID SYNTHESIS:

ALLOPURINOL

- -   It is the first choice drug in chronic gout.
- -   It is a xanthine oxidase inhibitor.

Mechanism of action (Fig.33)

Xanthine and hypoxanthine

xanthine oxidase   ⫢ Allopurinol

↓ Uric acid

- •   Allopurinol inhibits synthesis of uric acid from xanthine and hypoxanthine by inhibiting the enzyme xanthine oxidase.

Adverse effects : aggravate acute gout, GIT upset, hypersensitivity reaction, cataract formation due to deposition of Allopurinol on lens

Dose of Allopurinol : 100 mg./OD

Clinical Uses :

1. Only in chronic gout (not useful in acute attack)
   - • It is useful in UA excretion exceeds 1.0 g./day
   - • It is useful, if uricosuric agents are contraindicated.
2. In hyperuricemia due to anticancer drugs treatment.

It is also used in Kala azar as an adjuvant with Sodium stibogluconate.

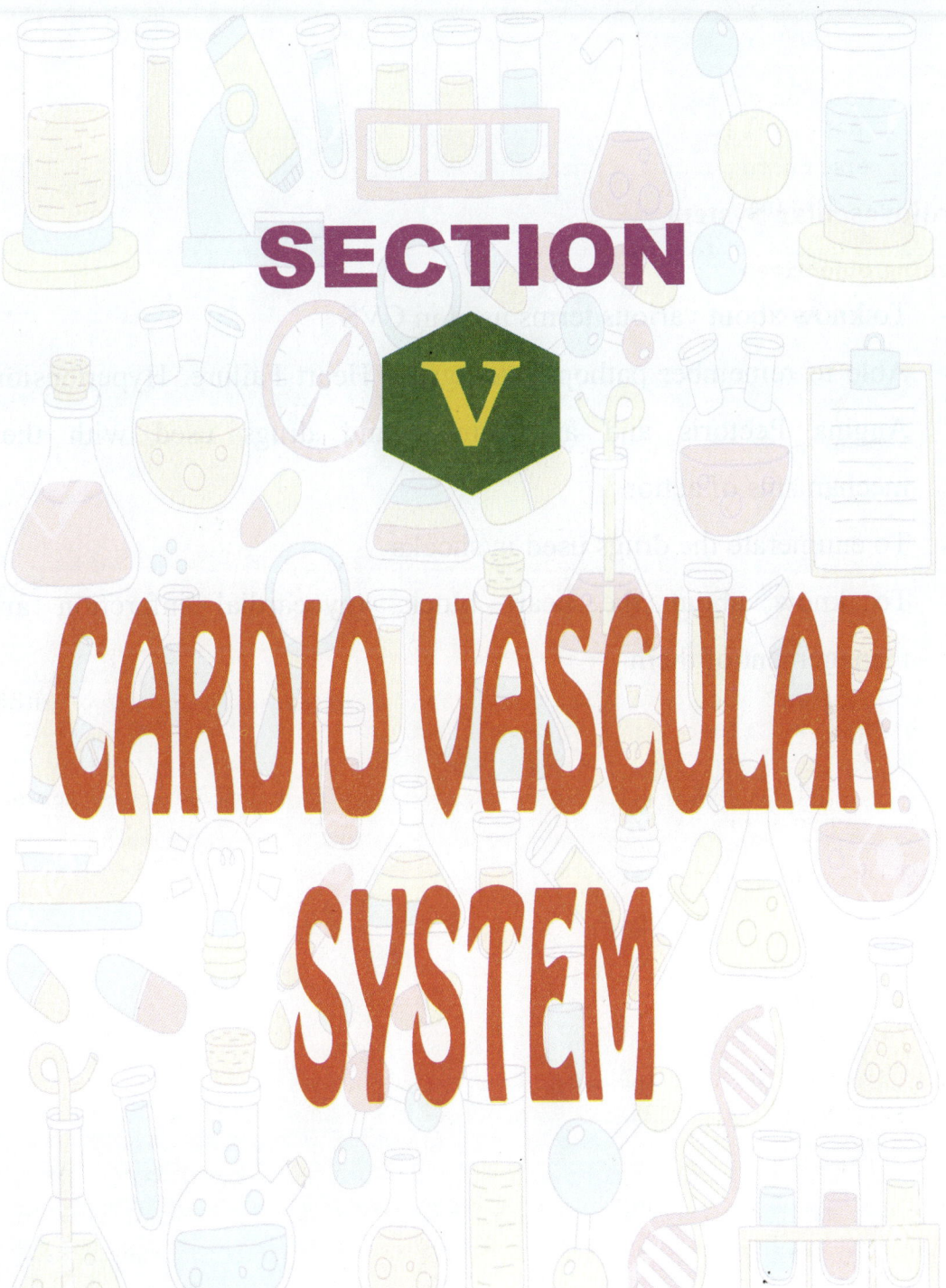

SECTION
V

CARDIO VASCULAR SYSTEM

Cardiovascular System

Learning objectives

- To know about various terms used in CVS
- Able to remember pathophysiology of Heart Failure, Hypertension, Angina Pectoris and arrhythmias and drugs used with their mechanisms of action
- To enumerate the drugs used in shocks
- To know about the heart block, myocardial infarction and management of them

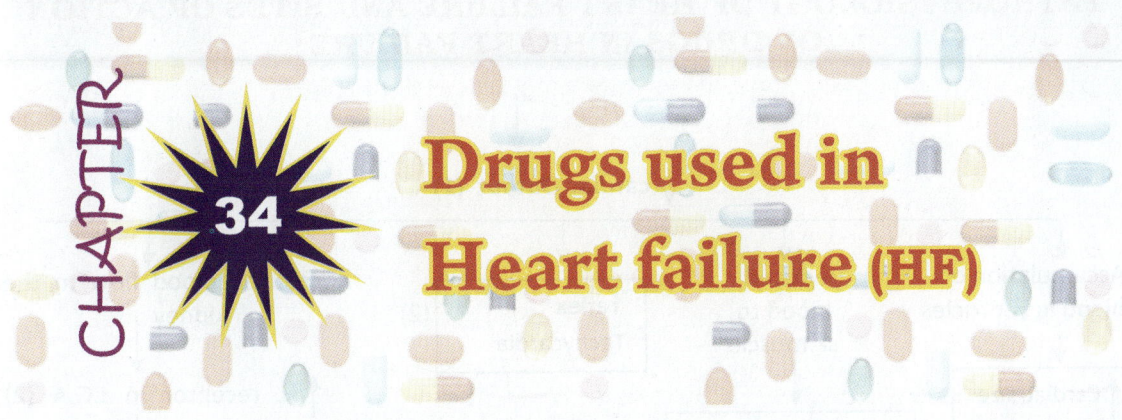

Drugs used in Heart failure (HF)

CHAPTER 34

HF means, the inability of ventricles to pump out sufficient blood to meet the demand.

HF is of mainly two types:

1. High Output Failure – In these conditions the C.O.P (Cardiac Output) is increased, but even then it could not meet the oxygen demand of the tissues. Example: Anaemia, thyrotoxicosis, beri beri etc. In these conditions, the specific treatment will be useful.

2. Low Output Failure - In which there is a reduced cardiac output may not be sufficient to meet the demands of tissues. This is called Heart Failure. We will discuss the drugs used in this condition under "Heart Failure".

CAUSES OF HEART FAILURE (LOW OUTPUT FAILURE)

1. Valvular Diseases
2. Hypertension
3. Arrhythmias

These are the common causes of heart failure

SYMPTOMS

1. Dyspnea (pulmonary Oedema)
2. Fatigue
3. Reflex tachycardia, which in turn aggravate H.F
4. Oedema
5. Increased After load which in turn aggravate H.F
6. Increase blood volume ⟶ increase B.P

PATHOPHYSIOLOGY OF HEART FAILURE AND SITES OF ACTION OF DRUGS IN HEART FAILURE

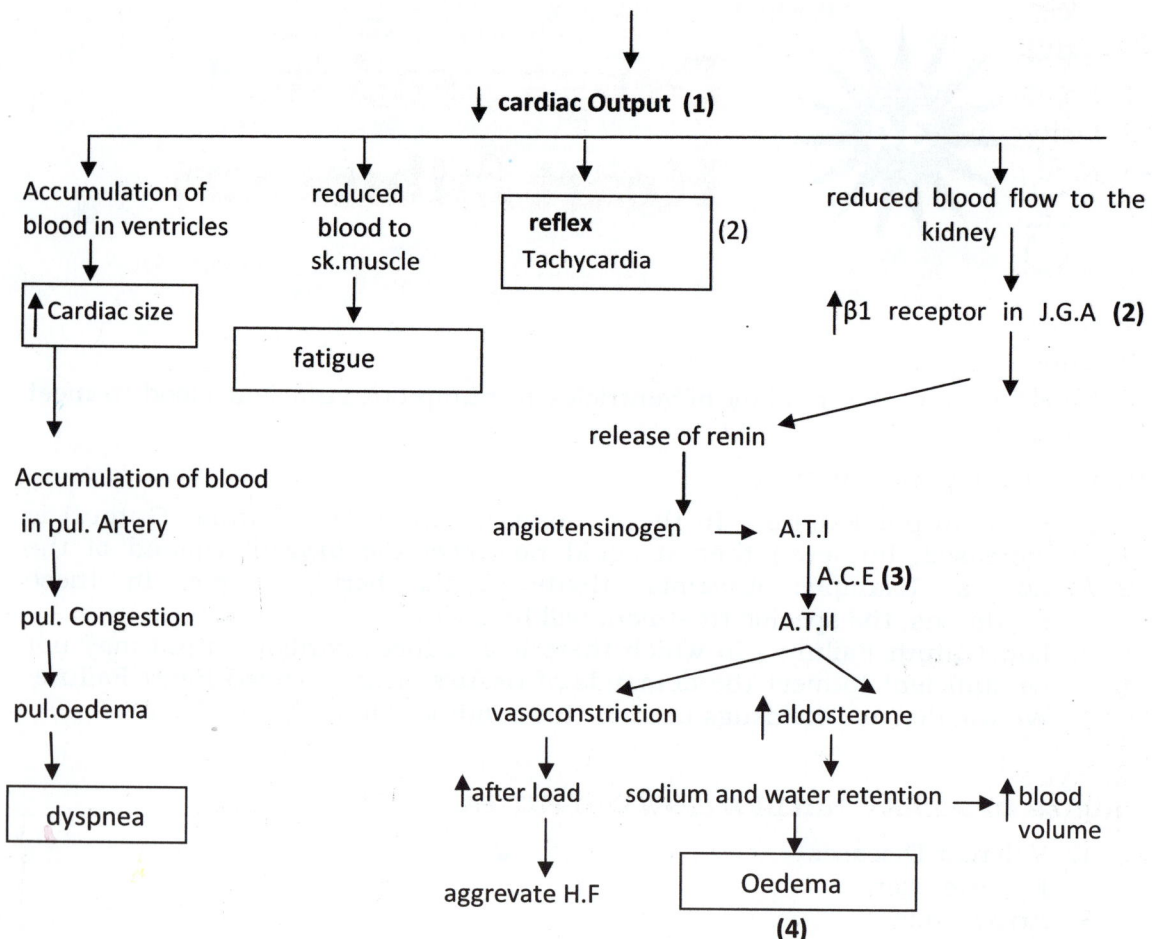

(1) digoxin & Amrinone

(2) β - adrenergic blockers

(3) ACE inhibitors and ARB (Angiotensin Receptor Blockers)

(4) Diuretic

DRUGS USED IN HEART FAILURE

I. Digoxin (Cardiac Glycoside)

II. Angiotensin Converting Enzyme(ACE) Inhibitors

1. Enalapril
2. Lisinopril
3. Ramipril

III. Angiotensin Receptor Blockers (AT$_1$ – Receptor Blocker)

1. Losartan
2. Candesartan
3. Valsartan

IV. β-adrenergic blockers

1. Metoprolol
2. Atenolol

V. Diuretics

1. Frusemide
2. Hydrochlorothiazides
3. K$^+$ retaining diuretics (are contraindicated with ACE inhibitors).

VI. Amrinone

VII.GTN (Glyceryl trinitrate)

DIGOXIN

It is a cardiac glycoside

Earlier digoxin was the first choice in H.F. But due to its narrow margin of safety and better drugs are being available, digoxin is no longer the first choice (except some specific condition like H.F associated with atrial arrhythmias).

Mechanism of action: in heart failure (Fig.35)

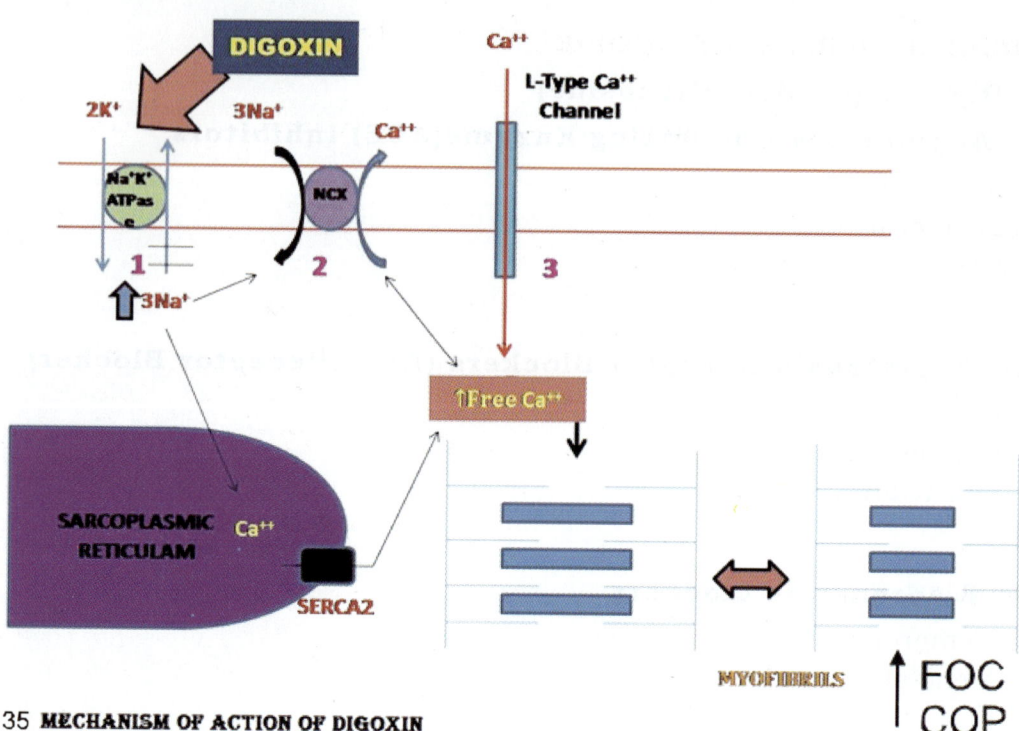

FIG:35 **MECHANISM OF ACTION OF DIGOXIN**

Digoxin (1) inhibits the enzyme sodium potassium ATPase (sodium pump, which helps in efflux of sodium) situated on the cell membrane of cardiac muscle → Prevents the efflux of sodium → increases the concentration of sodium intracellularly, which inturn exchanged with calcium (2) which enters in to the cell. The increased intracellular sodium will release ca++ in the sarcoplasm in to free ca++. Ca++ (3) also enters through L-Type Calcium channels and increases the concentration of free calcium. Now the increased free ca++ ion concentration increases the actin-myosin fibres → increases the force of contraction →increases the cardiac work.

1. Inhibits Na$^+$ K$^+$ ATPase (Sodium pump)
2. Increases intracellular active calcium
3. That calcium stimulates actin-myosin fiber
4. Increases the FOC and hence C.O.P
5. Reverses all the symptoms of H.F

ACTIONS OF DIGOXIN:

I.   CARDIAC ACTIONS:
1. Refractory Periods: Digoxin increases Refractory period in A.V node (A,V. block), reduces Refractory period in atrium and ventricles ⟶ flutter and fibrillation occur
2. Inhibits heart ⟶ bradycardia

II.   EXTRA CARDIAC ACTIONS:
   • Stimulates Chemoreceptor Trigger Zone ⟶ vomiting
   • Diuretic action, only in H.F (not in normal individual)

III.   On E.C.G. Prolong PR interval (slow down AV conduction) and shortening of QT interval (shortening of ventricular systole)

Clinical uses :

1. In H.F - last choice (if other drugs fail)
2. In Atrial flutter and atrial fibrillation (refer antiarrhythmic drugs)

Adverse effects:

There is no cardiac side effects when used in atrial flutter and fibrillation. The only side effect is vomiting.

When it is used for H.F, the cardiac side effects are atrial flutter, atrial fibrillation, and ventricular arrhythmias, AV block and vomiting.

A.C.E.I (ANGIOTENSIN CONVERTING ENZYME INHIBITORS) IN H.F:

These drugs inhibit the enzyme A.C.E, which is released in H.F and hence the symptoms.

And secondly, they inhibit Aldosterone release → inhibit the sodium and water retention → reduce blood volume and oedema, which are common symptoms of H.F.

And thirdly, they produce vasodilatation and reduce the Peripheral Resistance → decreases afterload → increase the efficiency of ventricles, increase cardiac output and relieve all the symptoms of Heart Failure.

And fourthly, they produce venodilatation → reduce preload → increase the efficiency of ventricles → increase COP → relieve all the symptoms of HF.

ARB (Angiotensin Receptor Blockers) in HF :

They block AT_1 receptors and produce all the above actions of ACE inhibitors without inhibiting ACE.

There is no adverse effect of cough.

BETA ADRENERGIC BLOCKERS:

1. They inhibit the Heart. The reflex tachycardia which aggravate HF is antagonised
2. They reduce renin secretion (β blockers inhibit $β_1$ receptors in Juxta Glomorular Apparatus). The consequences of renin action is prevented by β adrenergic blockers and reverse all the symptoms of HF.

DIURETICS

They inhibit the Sodium and water retention and oedema. Also they reduce the blood volume which are the common symptoms of HF. Example: Frusemide

The Aldosterome antagonist should not be combined with A.C.E inhibitors/ARB since both the drugs produce hyperkaelemia which lead to muscle weakness.

AMRINONE:

1. Non-glycoside and non-sympathomimetic inotropic drug

Mechanism of action of Amrinone:

1. It inhibits the enzyme phosphodiesterase → inhibits the degradation of AMP from c-AMP → accumulation of c-AMP → increased cardiac contractility and vasodilatation (called as ' INODILATOR')

Clinical uses:

1. In heart failure due to its inodilator action (given as IV infusion). But limited use only.

TREATMENT OF HEART FAILURE

Heart failure is the inability of the ventricles to pump out the blood efficiently to meet the demands of the tissues.
The signs and symptoms of Heart failure

- Dyspnea
- Fatigue
- Renal congestion
- Reflex tachycardia
- Increase in cardiac size

Aim is to prevent the progression of the disease and prolong the survival time.
As discussed before, Digoxin is no longer considered as the drug of choice in Heart Failure, because of its narrow margin of safety. Better and less toxic drugs available now. The first line drugs for all types of HF are ACE inhibitors / Angiotensin Receptor Blocker with Frusemide.
If needed, β-adrenergic blocker is added, because they afford survival benefit. Beta adrenergic blocker is used with caution in depressed heart. At the beginning of the treatment there is a reduced cardiac output (C.O.P.) due to cardiac inhibition. Later cardiac efficiency is increased by blocking aggravating factors like sympathetic over activity to the heart, the increased renin secretion and the consequences symptoms.
The β-adrenergic blockers should be started with low dose and slowly increased.
The β-adrenergic blocker should not be withdrawn suddenly.
If the above treatment is failed to respond, digoxin can be tried. The digoxin is also preferred in Heart Failure with atrial flutter and fibrillation.

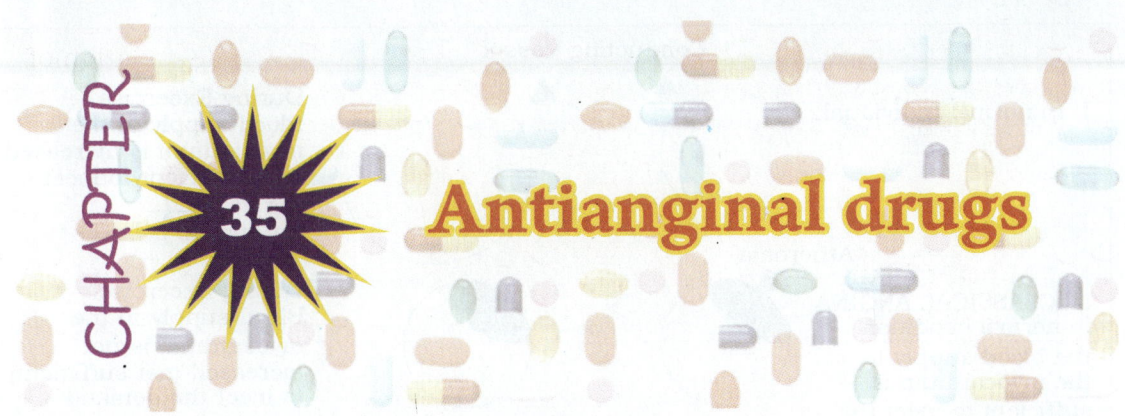

Antianginal drugs

Angina Pectoris is an ischaemic pain syndrome characterised by retrosternal pain that radiates to chest, left shoulder, upper arm and neck. This is due to imbalance between oxygen supply and oxygen demand in a portion of myocardium.

In normal individual oxygen supply ══════ oxygen demand
(depends on coronary blood supply) (depends on HR, FOC, systolic wall tension, preload and afterload)

In angina pectoris, there is reduced (↓) oxygen supply increased (↑) oxygen demand or both in myocardium

TYPES OF ANGINA PECTORIS (Fig.36)

1. Classical angina (Angina at effort) : is due to obstruction by atheroma (atherosclerotic plaque) in the coronary vessels. If the individual takes rest → anginal pain is relieved → otherwise drug is to be given. It occurs only during exercise, coitus, any hard work etc.,
2. Prinzmetal's angina (Angina at rest) : is due to sudden vasospasm. Anginal attack occurs even at rest. Rest will not relieve anginal pain. Drug is to be taken.
3. Unstable angina (pre infarct stage): is due to both atheroma and vasospasm. Many drugs are to be given.

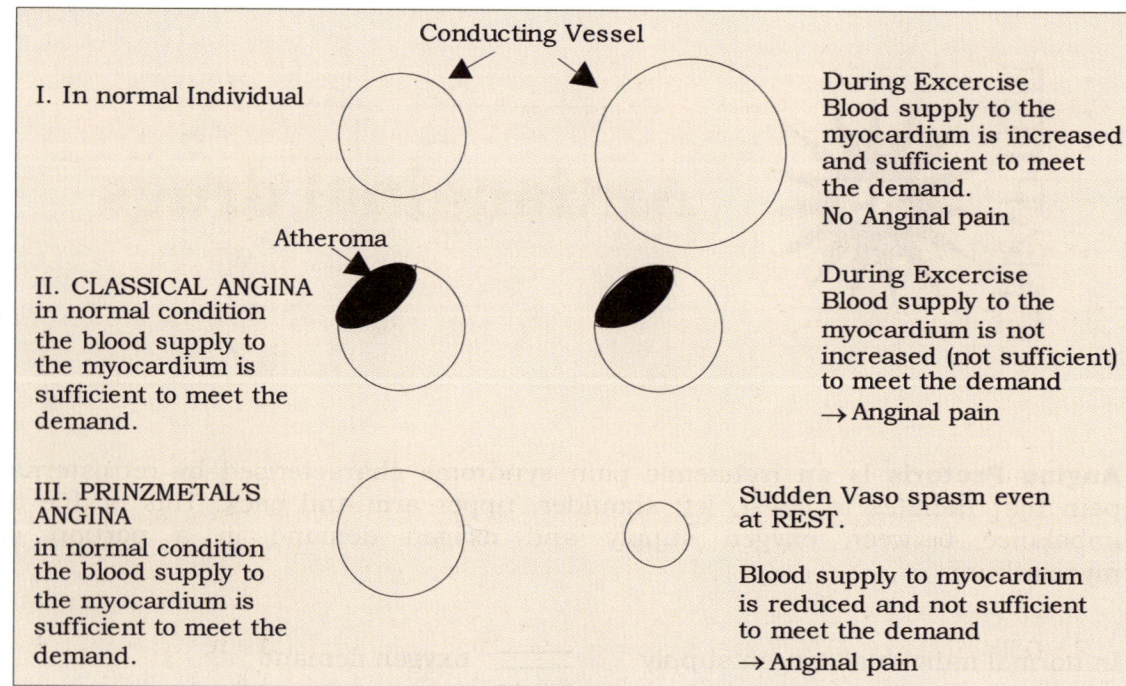

Fig. 36 Types of Angina Pectoris

The treatment should be either to increase the oxygen supply (by coronary vasodilatation) or reduce the oxygen demand of the myocardium. There is no effective drug available to increase the oxygen supply (because the drugs cannot dilate further in atherosclerotic vessel). All the available drugs used in angina pectoris mainly reduce the oxygen demand and relieve anginal pain.

CLASSIFICATION OF ANTIANGINAL DRUGS:

I . NITRATES

1. Short/fast acting : Glyceryl trinitrate (nitro glycerine)
2. Long/slow acting : Isosorbide dinitrate (Sorbitrate), Isosorbide Mononitrate, Erythrital tetranitrate, Pentaerythritol tetranitrate

II. BETA ADRENERGIC BLOCKERS

Propranolol, Atenolol, Metoprolol

III. CALCIUM CHANNEL BLOCKERS

Verapamil, Diltiazem, Nifedipine, Amlodipine, Felodipine etc.,

IV. POTASSIUM CHANNEL OPENERS: Nicorandil

GLYCERYL TRINITRATE (GTN) / NITROGLYCERINE

- It is not effective orally (due to high 1st pass metabolism of the drug)
- It is given by Sublingual administration in acute attack
- It is a powerful antianginal drug

Mechanism of action

- GTN → formation of free radical Nitric oxide (NO) → Decreases tone of blood vessels → VASODILATATION (mainly **veins**)
- Also increases the formation of EDRF (Endothelial Derived Relaxing Factor) → relaxation of smooth muscles including blood vessels → Vasodilatation (mainly veins)

Pharmacological action:

1. **GTN** reduces **PRELOAD** (due to **Venodilatation**) GTN causes venodilatation → pooling of blood in the periphery → (reduces) venous return → reduces venous filling pressure → reduces preload → decreases the work load on the heart → reduces oxygen consumption → increases the efficiency of myocardium → relieves anginal pain
2. **GTN** reduces **AFTERLOAD** (due to **Arteriolar Dilatation**) GTN causes dilatation of Arterioles → reduces the peripheral vascular resistence → decreases the afterlaod → decreases the myocardial consumption of oxygen → improves efficiency of myocardium → relieves anginal pain.
3. Mild coronary vasodilator (secondary effect)
4. Divert the blood from non ischaemic area to ischaemic area
5. On other smooth muscles
   i. G.I.T – Relaxation of gastro intestinal smooth muscle → constipation
   ii. Bronchus – bronchodilatation
   iii. Relaxation of biliary and oesophageal spasm

Clinical uses :

1. In angina pectoris : The nitrates commonly used is GTN. It is used in acute attack in all types of angina pectoris. GTN is administered sublingually. The pain is relieved within 2-5 minutes. It is used as and when required. It is short acting (30 min). To prevent night attack, long acting Nitrates (oral) or GTN transdermal patch is used and also as prophylactic whenever is needed.

2. In HF & LVF : GTN (IV infusion) produce veno-dilatation and arteriolar dilatation, reduces preload and afterload. GTN improves the efficiency of the ventricles and increases the force of contraction and reverses all the symptoms of HF. In the long-term, survival benefit has been obtained with ACE inhibitors/ARB.

3. In biliary colic, oesophageal spasm. Sublingual GTN is given, the pain is relieved within 3-5 mts.
4. In cyanide poisoning (Sodium Nitrite 3%/IV)

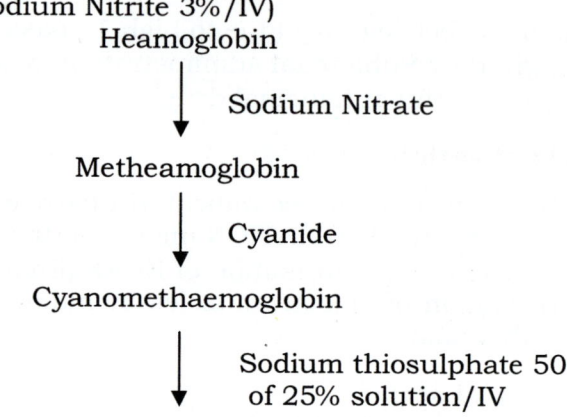

Heamoglobin

↓ Sodium Nitrate

Metheamoglobin

↓ Cyanide

Cyanomethaemoglobin

↓ Sodium thiosulphate 50 ml of 25% solution/IV

Methaemoglobin + Sodium thiocyanate
(easily excreted)

GTN → Metheamoglobinemia + Cyanide → Cynometheamoglobinemia + Sodium thiosulphate (intravenous) → Sodium thiocynate + Metheamoglobinemia → Sodium thiocynate is non toxic → excreted
5. In Myocardial Infarction (IV)
6. In hypertensive emergency (IV GTN) – GTN reduces both preload and afterload

Adverse effects: Headache, flushing, tolerance, fall in BP

OTHER DRUGS USED IN ANGINA PECTORIS

I. Beta Adrenergic Blockers
   • They are useful only in classical angina where it decrease workload on heart and decrease FOC reduce HR, reduce COP, reduce the oxygen consumption (reduce oxygen demand) and relieve anginal pain.
   • They are not coronary vasodilator. On the contrary they are coronary vasoconstrictor. They aggravate Prinzmetal's angina and hence contra indicated in prinzmetal's angina.
   • **Other USES** (refer Beta Adrenergic blockers)
II. Calcium Channel Blockers

Mechanism of action :

   • Calcium → opens Calcium channel → entry of Ca^{++} into smooth muscles and heart → contraction of smooth muscles including blood vessels → vasoconstriction and cardiac stimulation
   • Calcium channel blockers block the calcium channel → prevent the entry of Ca^{++} into the smooth muscles, heart → relaxation of smooth muscles and inhibition of heart

- On G.I.T → relaxation of gastro intestinal smooth muscles and so constipation
- On Bronchus → bronchodilatation
- On Blood vessels → they produce coronary vasodilatation and arteriolar dilatation → reduce after load (useful in hypertension)
- They slightly reduce the oxygen demand by decreasing the heart rate, force of contraction and cardiac output → useful in angina pectoris
- On uterus : Relaxation of uterus → useful to delay labour in threatened abortion
- Other actions on Heart : inhibit the heart → useful in cardiac arrhythmias

Clinical uses of Calcium channel blockers

1. In Hypertention → Arteolar dilatation → fall in diastolic pressure → fall in BP. They are useful in ACEI resistant cases.
2. In Heart failure: They reduce the cardiac output, heart rate reduce the work load on the heart, reduce oxygen consumption, reduce after load
3. In cardiac arrhythmias → they decrease automaticity and prolong refractory period of myocardium
4. In angina pectoris : They are useful in reducing frequency and severity of classical and prinzmetal's angina. They reduce oxygen consumption, cardiac output, heart rate and reduce oxygen demand. So they are useful in angina pectoris. There is also slight coronary vasodilatation and hence they are useful in prinzmetal angina.
5. They are useful to delay labour in threatened abortion.

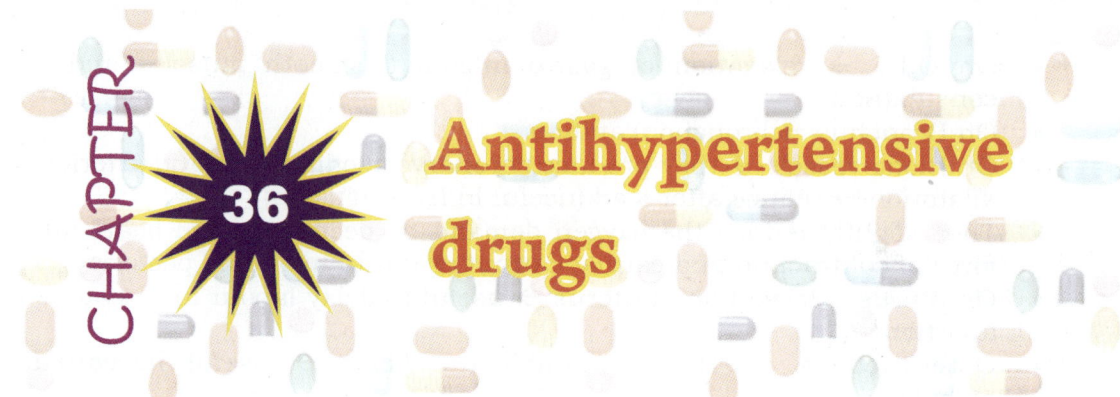

CHAPTER 36

Antihypertensive drugs

Antihypertensive drugs are those drugs which are used only in primary/essential (cause is not known) hypertension.

Hypertension is a cardio vascular disorder characterised by the diastolic BP is more than 90mmHg.

- Normal BP is denoted as 120 (Systolic Pressure)/ 80 (Diastolic Pressure)
- Systolic pressure is proportional to C.O.P
- Diastolic pressure is proportional to Peripheral vascular Resistance (arteriolar constriction).
- Clinical manifestations and complications of hypertension are mainly due to constriction of arterioles (increased diastolic Pressure)
- W.H.O recommendation – the hypertension is divided on the basis of diastolic pressure into

Normal	= 120/80
Mild	= D.B.P 90 to 99 mmHg
Moderate	= D.B.P 100 to 109 mm Hg
Severe	= D.B.P 110 to 119 mm Hg
Very severe	= D.B.P > 120 mm Hg

- If systolic B.P is above 140 mmHg and diastolic B.P of below 90 mmHg is termed as Isolated Systolic Hypertension
- In the early stage many patient missed the diagnosis since they feel the symptoms are mild like sweating, dizziness. Most of the patients come to the doctor when there are complications. If it was found earlier atleast the complications would have been prevented. That is why any person goes to the doctor for any ailment they take B.P to ensure that there is no hypertension. Many have been identified as Hypertensive when they go to the doctors for some other ailments.

CLINICAL MANIFESTATIONS AND COMPLICATIONS:

Hypertension, if untreated leads to a variety of cardiac, cardiovascular and renal complications with shortened life expectancy because of continued arteriolar constriction, reduced blood flow to all the tissues and organs.

- Heart failure (is due to reduced blood flow to myocardium)
- Reduced blood flow through the kidney → stimulate beta$_1$ receptors in Juxta Glomerular Apparatus → release renin → converts angiotensinogen to angiotensin I → by ACE → angiotensin II → vasoconstriction (increase B.P), release aldosterone (sodium and water retention), increase blood volume → increase B.P
- Reduced blood flow to the skeletal muscle → fatigue
- Reduced blood flow to the brain → dizziness
- Reduced blood flow to the kidney → reduced GFR → renal failure
- Increased in diastolic pressure due to arterioles constriction → rupture, thrombosis, haemorrhage in brain (stroke), myocardial infarction (heart attack)

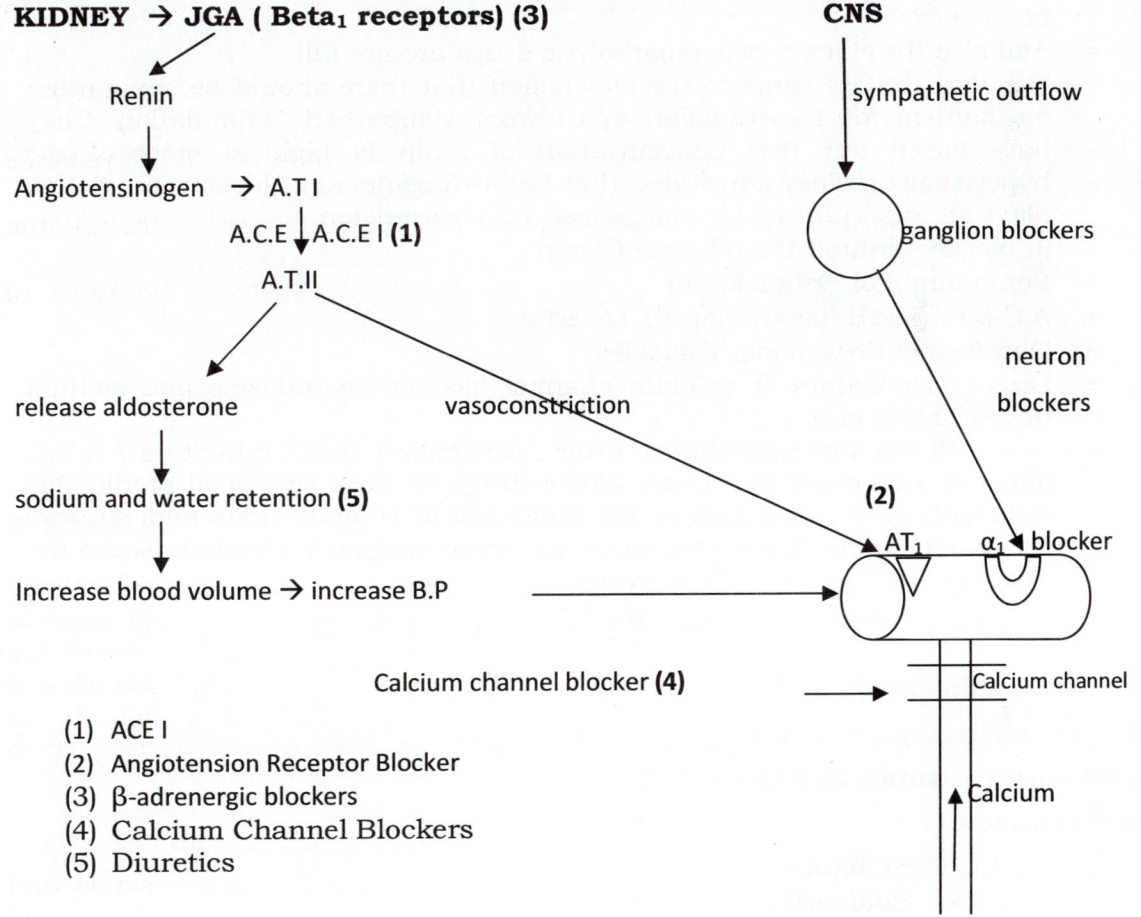

KIDNEY → JGA (Beta$_1$ receptors) (3)

Renin

Angiotensinogen → A.T I

A.C.E ↓ A.C.E I **(1)**

A.T.II

release aldosterone   vasoconstriction

sodium and water retention **(5)**

Increase blood volume → increase B.P

Calcium channel blocker **(4)**

CNS

sympathetic outflow

ganglion blockers

neuron

blockers

(2)

AT$_1$ α$_1$ blocker

Calcium channel

Calcium

(1) ACE I
(2) Angiotension Receptor Blocker
(3) β-adrenergic blockers
(4) Calcium Channel Blockers
(5) Diuretics

ETIOLOGY OF ESSENTIAL HYPERTENSION

The blood vessels (arterioles) are supplied only by sympathetic nerves. It was thought, due to some reason that the sympathetic system is stimulated → increase the Noradrenaline release from sympathetic nerve ending → Noradrenaline will occupy alpha$_1$ receptors on the blood vessels → arteriolar constriction → increase diastolic blood pressure → genesis of hypertension.

So, the sympathetic blockers were tried on that basis.

- Central sympatholytic (clonindine, α methyl dopa)
- Sympathetic ganglion Blockers → hexamethonium
- Adrenergic neuron blockers → bretylium → act on post ganglionic fiber of the sympathetic nerve by inhibiting synthesis and release of Noradrenaline
- α adrenergic blockers → block α$_1$ receptors in the arterioles → arteriolar dialatation (reduce the diastolic B.P)
- But unfortunately 2 important side effects that affect the quality of life by the sympatholytic antihypertensive drugs are postural hypotension and impotency.
- And also the efficacy of sympatholytic drugs are not full
- The Researchers came to the conclusion that there should be some other mechanism for hypertension apart from sympathetic stimulation. They have found out that concentration of renin is high in most of the hypertensives. They concluded that Renin-Angiotensin-Aldosterone system plays an important role in the genesis of hypertension.
- β$_1$ blockers inhibit the release of renin
- Renin inhibitor → (Aliskiren)
- A.C.E.I / A.R.B like Enalapril/ Losartan
- Diuretics → Frusemide, Thiazides
- Direct vasodilators → calcium channel blocker, hydralazine and sodium nitroprusside etc.,

All the above mentioned drugs, particularly A.C.E inhibitors / A.R.B alone or with other anti hypertensive drugs produce very good predictable reduction in B.P and reduce the incidence of complications and improve the quality of life on long term use. So, these drugs completely replaced the drugs acting via sympathetic system.

CLASSIFICATION OF ANTIHYPERTENSIVE DRUGS (ABCD)

A → A.C.E inhibitors/ A.R.B

B → Beta adrenergic blockers

C→ Calcium Channel Blockers

D → Diuretics

I.   A.C.E Inhibitors:
- Enalapril
- Lisinopril
- Ramipril

II.   AT₁ Receptor Blocker: (ARB)
- Losartan
- Candesartan
- Telmisartan

III.   Beta Adrenergic Blockers:
- Atenelol
- Metoprolol
- Esmolol

IV.   Beta and Alpha Adrenergic Blockers: used in Pheochromocytoma
- Labetolol
- Carvedelol

V.   Calcium Channel Blockers:
- Amlodipine, Felodipine
- Nifedipine

VI.   Diuretics:
- Frusemide & Thiazides (with Potassium retaining diuretics)

VII.   Hypertension in pregnancy – α methyldopa, Hydralazine

VIII.   In hypertensive emergency – Sodium nitroprusside (I.V) & G.T.N (I.V)

IX.   Renin inhibitor : Aliskiren

A.C.E Inhibitors (Angiotensin converting enzyme inhibitor)

- They are the first line antihypertensive drugs

Mechanism of action

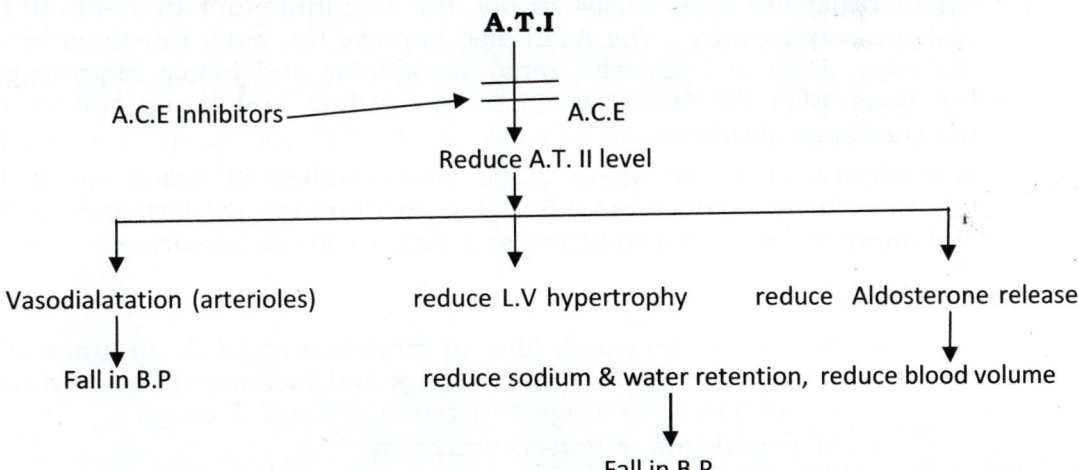

Clinical uses of A.C.E INHIBITORS/ A.R.B

1. In hypertension : They are first line drugs in all grades of Hypertension. Most of the patients respond to monotherapy. In others they are combined with β-adrenergic blockers, calcium channel blockers, diuretics. They are

best suited in hypertension with Diabetes mellitus, Diabetic nephropathy, HF, Myocardial infarction. There is no postural hypotension, no brocho-constriction, no rebound hypertension, no hyperuricemia, no hyperlipidemia, prevents K^+ loss due to Frusemide & thiazide diuretics, no reduced sexual performance

- Quality of life is little affected.
- They reduce the (complications) cardiovascular morbidity and increase the life expectancy.

2. In H.F – Now, they are the first line drugs (since digoxin is having narrow margin of safety) in non associated hypertensive patients. They are usually given with diuretics. They reduce preload → reduce peripheral resistance → reduce outflow pressure and also reduce aftreload. Reduce Aldosterone secretion → reduce sodium & water retention → reduce blood volume → reduce oedema and workload on the heart, reduce pulmonary arterial pressure → reduce pulmonary oedema → reduce dyspnea → prolong survival time.

3. In M.I. They are administered to all patients within 24 hours of onset of symptoms→ slow the progression of H.F → slow down pregression of M.I. They reduce the recurrent M.I. More benefits will be obtained if the patients are hypertensive and diabetic.

4. Diabetic Nephropathy: Long term use of ACE inhibitors prevent renal damage in diabetes mellitus. Albuminuria (an index of nephropathy) is significantly reduced. The creatinine clearance is also increased, when compare to the treatment before. All Diabetic nephropathy patients, whether they are hypertensive or not, the ACE inhibitors are given. In non-diabetic nephropathy : The ACEI also improve the renal functions in non-diabetics. They are powerful renal vasodilator and hence improve renal functions. After the ACEI treatment, they reduce proteinuria and increase the creatinine clearance.

5. Scleroderma crisis → where A.T.II concentration is found to be high (increase BP and reduce renal function) ACEI inhibit the formation of AT-II and improve the above conditions and they are life saving drugs.

Adverse effects:

- Persistent dry cough (due to inhibition of A.C.E. in lungs which degrade bradykinin in the lungs and increase the concentration of bradykinin in lungs→ irritation of lungs → cough
- Hyperkalemia → muscle weakness
- Muscle cramps
- Altered taste sensation
- Pregnancy → they are contraindicated

Dose

- Enalapril → 5 to 20 mg once daily

- Ramipril → 5 to 20 mg once daily
- Lisinopril → 5 to 20 mg once daily

ANGIOTENSIN RECEPTOR BLOCKER (ARB)

Mechanism of action They inhibit AT_1 receptor in the blood vessel → vasodilatation → fall in B.P. They do not inhibit A.C.E.

All actions are similar to A.C.E inhibitors

Clinical uses similar to A.C.E inhibitiors

Adverse effects: similar to A.C.E inhibitors except cough.

β ADRENERGIC BLOCKERS (Cardio selective β 1 receptor Blockers are preferred)

Mechanism of action in HYPERTENSION

- They inhibit central sympathetic outflow
- They inhibit Renin release → fall in B.P (Mechanism : Ref β-adrerergic blocker)
- They reduce C.O.P → useful in isolated systolic hypertension
- Sudden withdrawal of β adrenergic blockers is to be avoided, otherwise there will be rebound hypertensive crisis
- Other clinical uses and adverse effects (refer β adrenergic blockers under A.N.S)

CALCIUM CHANNEL BLOCKERS

- They are also first line antihypertensive drugs.

Mechanism of action

- blood vessels are having calcium channels which are activated by Ca^{++} → entry of Ca^{++} into the blood vessel → vasoconstriction and contraction of smooth muscles. Calcium channel blockers block the calcium channels and block the entry of Ca^{++} into the blood vessels and the smooth muscles → vasodilatation, relaxation of smooth muscles and inhibition of heart.

Clinical uses

1. in hypertension (particularly in low renin patients in whom A.C.E inhibitors do not produce the expected result).
2. In cardiac arrhythmias (Ref : antiarrhythmic drugs)
3. In angina pectoris (mainly as prophylactic) in both classical and prinzmetal anginas
4. In biliary colic
5. To delay labour in pre term delivery

DIURETICS

Mechanism of action

- They reduce Na+/water retention
- They reduce blood volume → fall in B.P
- Thiazides have got additional direct vasodilatation action also and hence they are preferred in hypertension.

Clinical uses (refer diuretics)

Adverse effects: (refer diuretics)

ANTIHYPERTENSIVE PREFERENCES

- First line drug is A.C.E. inhibitors/ ARB with or without other antihypertensive drugs
- If they are not effective (in few individuals who are suspected to have low renin status) calcium channel blockers are preferred
- The antihypertensive drug is started with low dose and slowly increased till the desired effect is achieved
- As far as possible keep the systolic B.P less than 140 mm Hg and diastolic B.P less than 90mm Hg
- Beta blockers are to be avoided in bronchial asthma and diabetes mellitus with antidiabetic agent (insulin)
- Hypertension with H.F → A.C.E inhibitors/ ARB, diuretics
- Hypertension with classical angina → beta adrenergic blockers (not in Prinzmetal's angina, in which they are contraindicated)
- Hypertension with mitral valve prolapse syndrome → beta adrenergic bockers
- Hypertension with L.V hypertrophy → A.C.E inhibitors / ARB
- Hypertension with peripheral vascular disease → calcium channel blockers
- Hypertension with renal failure → A.C.E inhibitors/ ARB
- Hypertension with diabetes mellitus → A.C.E inhibitors/ ARB, calcium channel blockers
- Hypertension with thyrotoxicosis → beta adrenergic blockers

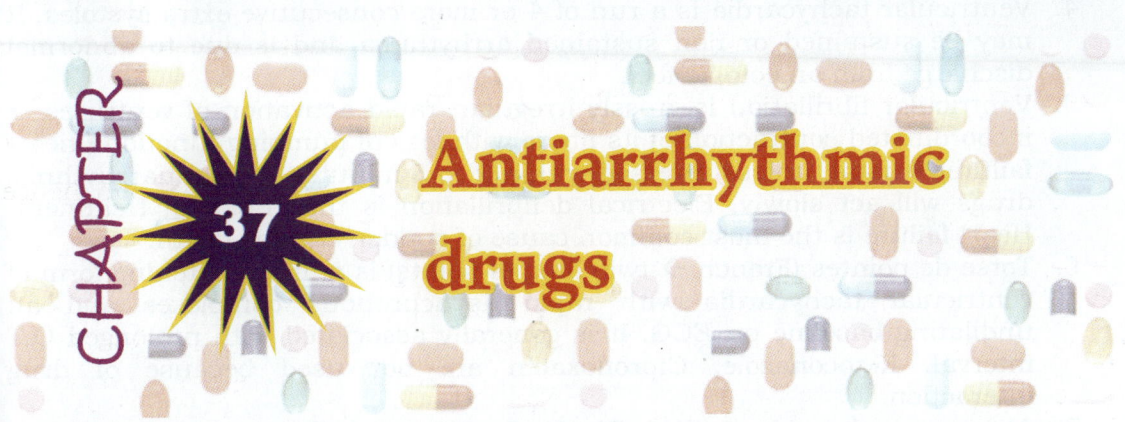

Antiarrhythmic drugs

CHAPTER 37

Arrhythmia means abnormal rhythm of heart.

If the heart beat is higher, then it is referred as "Tachyarrhythmia".

Here we discuss the drugs used in tachyarrhythmia mainly.

If the heart beat is slow then it is referred as "Bradyarrhythmia".

Normally impulses are generated in S.A node (Pace Maker) in the absence of external stimuli unlike skeletal muscle, which contract only after receiving external stimuli. That is called as intrinsic generation of impulses (Automaticity).

Arrhythmia results from abnormal generation of impulses (abnormal Pace Makers activity / abnormal Automaticity) or increased conduction of impulses (reduced refractory period) at many number of sites in the heart.

Common Arrhythmias are as follows:

Here we refer arrhythmias means only Tachyarrhythmias.

Common Tachyarrhythmias are as follows:

1. Paroxysmal Supra Ventricular Tachycardia (PSVT) is a sudden onset episodes of atrial tachycardia (rate is between 150 and 200 per minute) with 1:1 atrioventricular conduction.

2. Atrial flutter – Atria beat at a rate of 200 to 350 per minute and there is a physiological 2:1 or 4:1 or higher AV block (because AV node cannot transmit impulses faster than 200 per minute) → C.O.P is reduced due to ineffective beats.

3. Atrial fibrillation – Atrial fibers are activated asynchronously at a rate of 300 to 550 per minute (due to many abnormal foci → increases automaticity → and also electo physiological inhomogenecity at atrial fibers) associated with grossly irregular and often fast (100 to 150 per minute) ventricular response. Atria remains dilated and quiver like a bag of worms → HF

4. Ventricular tachycardia is a run of 4 or more consecutive extra systoles. It may be sustained or non sustained arrhythmia and is due to abnormal discharge from an ectopic foci.

5. Ventricular fibrillation is grossly irregular, rapid activation of ventricles → incoordinated contraction of its fibers with loss of pumping function (heart failure) → fatal, unless reversed within 2 to 5 minutes. The antiarrhythmic drugs will act slowly. Electrical defibrillation is the choice of treatment. Heart failure is the most common cause of sudden cardiac death.

6. Torse de pointes (French → twitching of points) is a life threatening form of ventricular tachycardia with rapid asynchronous complexes and an undilating baseline on ECG. It is generally associated with prolonged Q.T interval. Ketoconazole, Ciprofloxacin are not used because of drug interaction.

7. Atrioventricular block (AV Block) is due to depression of impulse conduction through AV node and Bundles of His, mostly due to vagal influence or Ischaemia.

CAUSES OF ARRHYTHMIAS

I . PATHOLOGICAL

- Ischaemia
- Acute myocardial infarction
- Electrolytes and pH imbalance
- Mechanical injury to myocardium
- Neurogenic

II. DRUG INDUCED:

- Digoxin
- General anaesthetics
- Terfenadine
- Astemizole
- Erythromycin (higher dose)
- Cisapride

} with microsomal enzyme inhibitors

CLINICAL MANIFESTATIONS:

- Palpitation
- Breathlessness at rest or on exertion
- Coronary insufficiency (H.F, angina)
- Cerebral insufficiency (syncope, dizziness, vertigo)

COMMONLY USED ANTIARRHYTHMIC DRUGS

1. Lignocaine – ventricular tachycardia
2. Adenosine – PSVT, ventricular tachycardias
3. Beta adrenergic blockers – atrial flutters, atrial fibrillation, prevent arrhythmias due to acute myocardial infarction.

4. Calcium channel blockers – to produce AV Block and protect ventricles from atrial flutters and fibrillations.

5. Digoxin – Atrial flutter, atrial fibrillation (particularly associated with Heart Failure)

I.   Abnormal automaticity:

S A Node generates impulses at faster rate than the other Pace Maker cells exhibiting automaticity. This SA Node normally sets the pace of contraction for the myocardium.

However, if cardiac sites other than the SA Node show enhanced automaticity, they may generate abnormal impulses and arrhythmias may arise.

Abnormal automaticity may also result in myocardial injury or electrolyte imbalance.

II.   Effect of drugs in automaticity:

Most of the antiarrhythmic drugs suppress automaticity by blocking either Sodium or Calcium channels. More effective on ectopic pace makers than on the normal cells.

III.   Abnormal impulse conduction:

Mainly due to the reduced refractory period → results in abnormal excess impulse conduction.

IV.   Effects of drugs on abnormal conduction:

Antiarrhythmic drugs increase refractory period or prevent re entry by slowing the impulse conduction.

ACTION POTENTIALS OF CARDIAC MUSCLES (ELECTROPHYSIOLOGY OF CARDIAC RHYTHM)

I.   Impulse generation

Electrophysiologically, there are two types of myocardial fibers.

1) Non automatic fibers: (Fig.37)

These are the ordinary working myocardial fibers. They cannot generate their own impulse. But they can conduct impulse coming from SA node. When stimulated, they depolarize rapidly generate impulse by fast moving Na^+ channel (phase '0') reaches +30mv, and then short repolarization (phase-1), due to efflux of K+. Then it is followed by a Steady state called plateau phase of slow repolarization – (phase-2), due to slow Ca+ entry. followed by fast repolarization (Phase-3) due to fast efflux of K+ and then reaches resting membrane potential and stable (-90 mv) – phase-4, waiting for the next impulse to come.

From the beginning of phase '0' to the end of phase'3' (or beginning of Phase-4) – equal to one heart beat. The number of heart beats per minute is increased in arrhythmias(due to increased automaticity or increased conduction velocity)

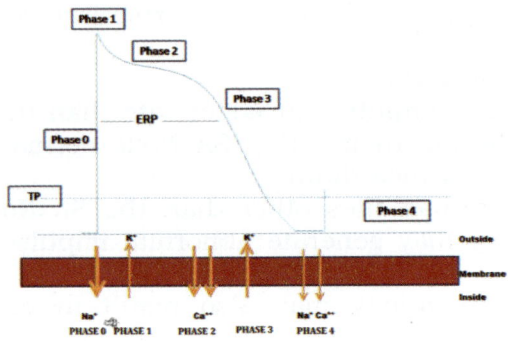

TP - Threshold Potential
ERP - Effective Refractory Period
→ thick arrow indicates prominent movement of electrolytes
Phase 0 - Fast Na⁺ entry through Na⁺ channel (Na⁺ channel blocker → will act as anti-arrhythmic)
Phase 1 - Na⁺ channel closes, K⁺ channel opens → outward movement of K⁺ - rapid repolarisation
Phase 2 - Plateau phase → due to slow entry of Ca⁺⁺ mainly at SA node and AV node. Slow repolarization
Phase 3 - outward movement of K⁺ → prolong repolarization (prolong repolarization → K⁺ channel blockers) - refractory period & Automaticity.
Phase 4 - Na⁺ and Ca⁺⁺ entry → slow diastolic depolarization
Phase 0 to Phase 4 → one heart beat. If heart beat is increased will lead to arrhythmia Antiarrhythmiac

Fig.37 Action potential of Nonautomatic fiber

Automaticity = The capacity of a cell to initiate an impulse without an external stimuli. The automaticity is increased in arrhythmias.
2) Automatic fibers (SA node, AV node, Purkinje fiber) (Fig.38A/38B)

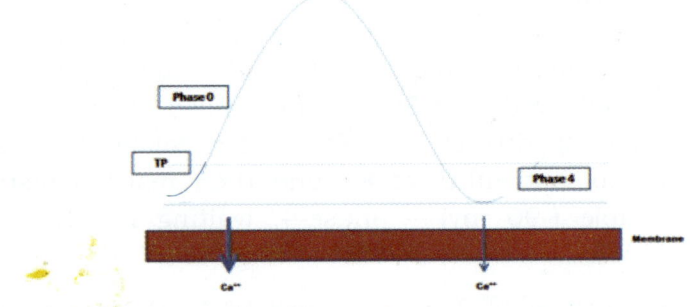

TP - Threshold Potential

Fig.38A Action potential of automatic fiber

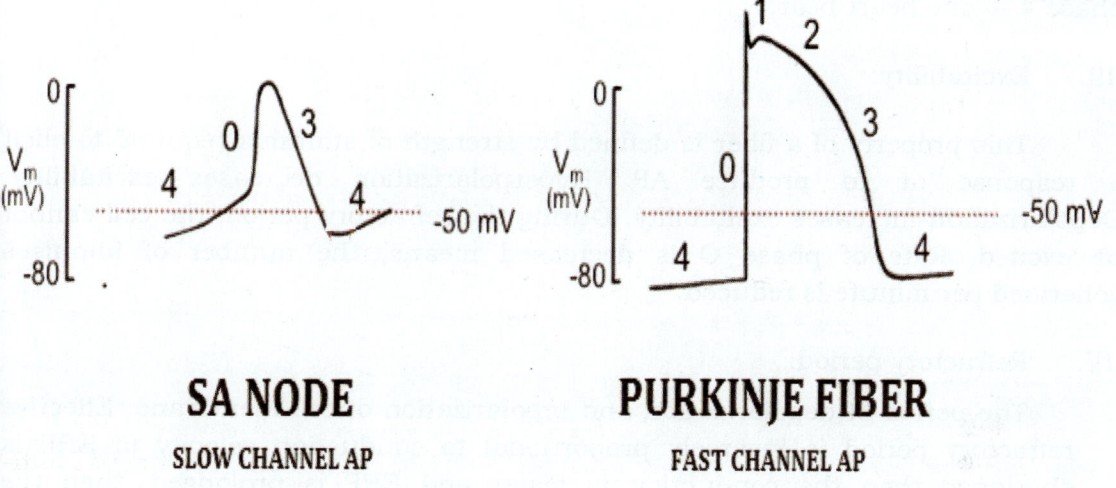

Fig.38B Action potential of automatic fiber

Automatic fibers are capable of generating impulse without any external stimuli.

The characteristic features of these fibers are that they produce phase-4 slow diastolic depolarization, that is after depolarization to the maximum value, the membrane potential decays spontaneously. Spontaneous depolarization occurs till it reaches the threshold value and then suddenly it will lead to fast depolarization (Spontaneous = without any external stimulus). SA node is the fastest in generating impulse, and it is called as 'pace maker' and propagate impulse to the rest of the heart.

SA node → atrium → AV node → Bundle of His → Ventricle → Contraction. But other fibers are called as 'latent pace makers'. In SA/AV node the action potential develops slowly. In this phase 0,1,2,3 are not distinguishable. There is prominent phase-4.

II.   Conduction:

A drug (Anti-arrhythmic drug) which reduces the slope of '0' phase shifts the action potential curve to the right and impedes conduction. AV node has very low conduction velocity. Purkinje fibers have high conduction velocity – 4000mm/sec to 20 m/sec. From the beginning of phase '0' to the beginning of phase 4 → one heart beat.

III.   Excitability:

This property of a fiber is defined by strength of stimulus required to elicit a response or to produce AP. Hyperpolarization decreases excitability. Depolarization increases excitability. During the refractory period, the cell cannot be excited. Rate of phase O is decreased means, the number of impulses generated per minute is reduced.

IV.   Refractory period:

The period of depolarization and repolarization of cell membrane. Effective refractory period is inversely proportional to conduction velocity (if ERP is shortened then the conduction is faster and ERP is prolonged, then the conduction is slowed down. Antiarrhythmic drugs prolong the ERP.

Relative Refractory Period + Absolute Refractory Period = Effective Refractory Period (Fig.44).   The Absolute Refractory Period = The period in which the muscle fiber cannot respond to a second stimulus (From phase'0' to mid Phase '3'. The Relative Refractory Period = The period in which the muscle can respond only to a stronger stimulus (from mid phase – 3 to end of phase - 3).

ERP – Depicts a minimum interval between two prolonged responses (fig: From the beginning of phase '0' to the end of phase '3'. From beginning of phase '0' to the end of phase '3' is equal to one heart beat/one impulse.

Rate of phase '0' depolarization is increased in arrhythmias (No. of impulses increased/minute or HR is increased/minute.) In arrhythmias the heart beat is more than 200/min) due to increased automaticity.

Normal heart beat 80/min.

Antiarrhythmic drugs decrease rate of phase '0' depolarization (i.e. the

HR/minute is decreased. i.e. decrease / suppress Automaticity.

Automatic fibers – SA node (Highest rate/min) followed by AV node (slow channel AP) The phases 0,1,2,3 are not distinguishable and purkinje fiber (fast channel AP) with prominent phases.

Non automatic fibers – atrium, ventricle, bundle of His

```
                                      One – Non – automatic fiber
Cardiac action potential ── 3 ──────  Two – Automatic - Slow AP
                                      Three – Automatic – Fast AP
```

V.   Autonomic influences on cardiac muscles

PS (ACh)	S (Adr)
1.Automaticity: SA node –Decreased-Bradycardia	Increased -↑HR (Tachycardia)
2.Ectopic-Ventricles –↓ decreased conduction velocity	↑increased conduction velocity

CLASSIFICATION OF ANTIARRHYTHMIC DRUGS:

Class – I Fast sodium channel blockers

1) LIGNOCAINE
2) Quinidine
3) Procainamide.

Class – II β – adrenergic blockers

1) Propranolol
2) Metoprolol
3) Atenolol
4) Esmolol

Class – III Potassium channel blockers

1) Amiodarone

Class – IV Calcium channel blockers

1) Diltiazem
2) Verapamil

Others

1) Digoxin
2) Adenosine

THE Mechanism of Action OF ANTIARRHYTHMIC DRUGS:

The anti arrhythmic drugs may act by any one or more of the following:

I. **Suppression of enhanced automaticity of pace maker and non pace maker cells:**

1) By decreasing the slope of phase'0' depolarization (Shift phase'0' towards right) (impede conduction) & decrease automaticity. (Fig.39)

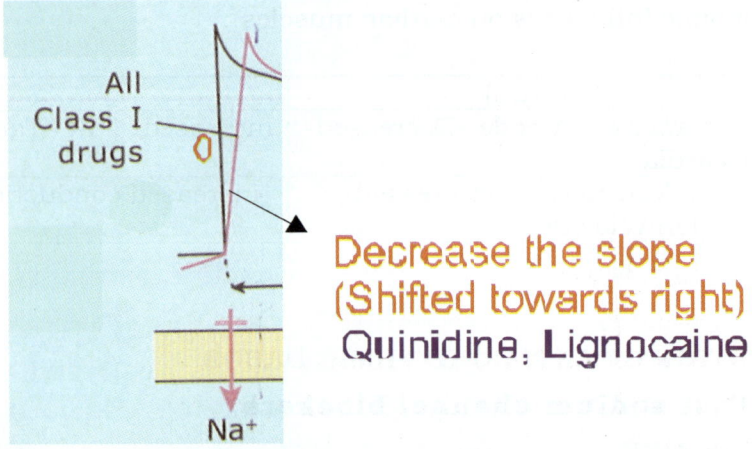

Fig.39 Decrease the slope of phase '0'

2) By decreasing the rate of phase '0' depolarization (the number of impulses generated per minute is reduced. (decrease automaticity.) (Fig.40)

All class I drugs

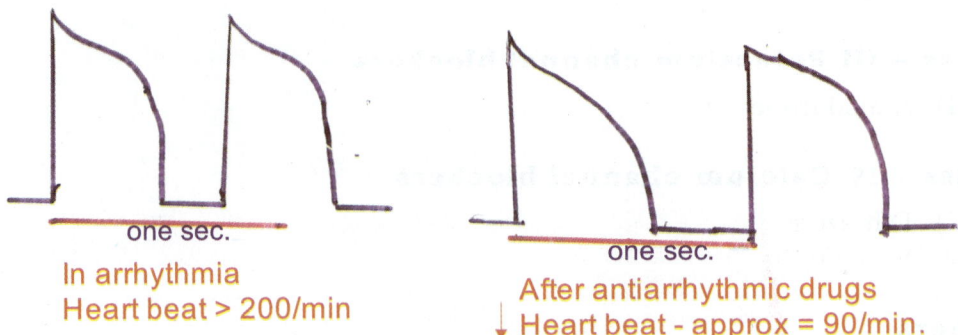

Fig.40 Decrease rate of Phase '0' depolarization

3) Increasing the threshold potential, delay in generating impulses (↓ automaticity) (Fig.41)

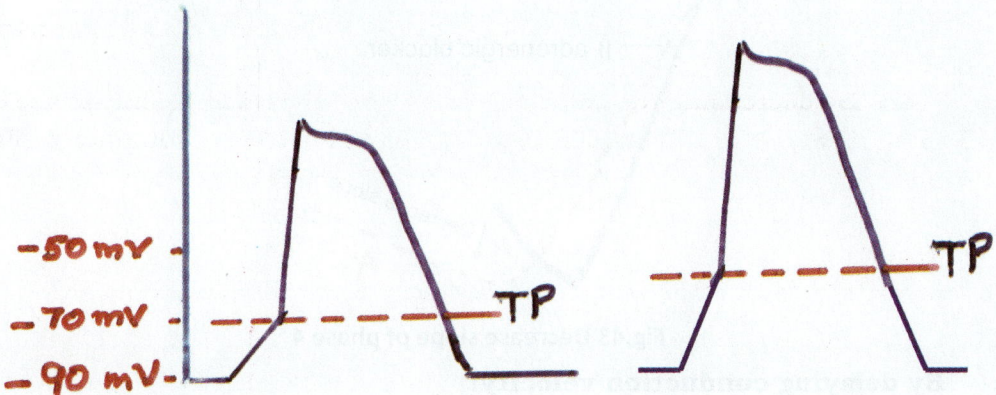

−50 mV

−70 mV

−90 mV

T.P. Threshold potential

Fig.41 Showing increase in Threshold potential by antiarrhythmic drug

4) Prolong phase 4 – diastolic depolarization - decrease automaticity (Fig.42)

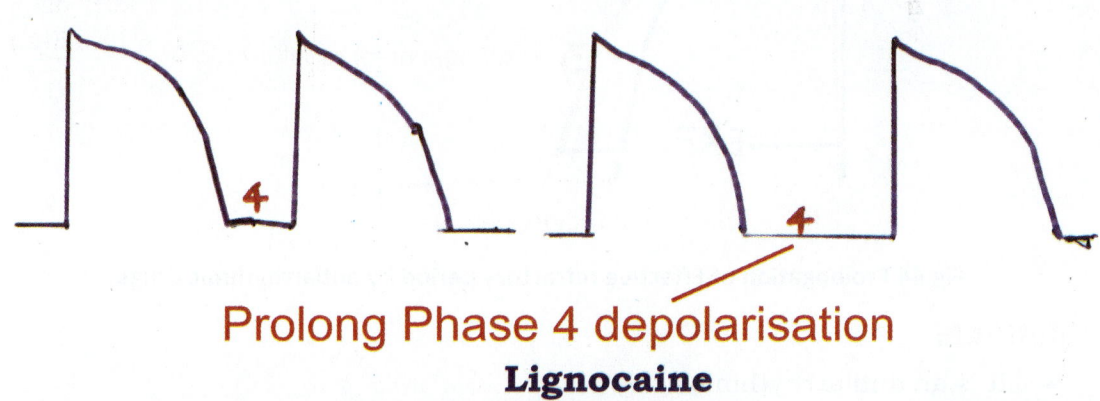

Prolong Phase 4 depolarisation

Lignocaine

Fig.42 Prolong phase 4 depolarisation

5) In automatic fibers

Phase 4 depolarization, AP is shifted to the right, or depress the phase '4' depolarization (Slope of phase – 4 is decreased. (↓ Automaticity) (Fig.43)

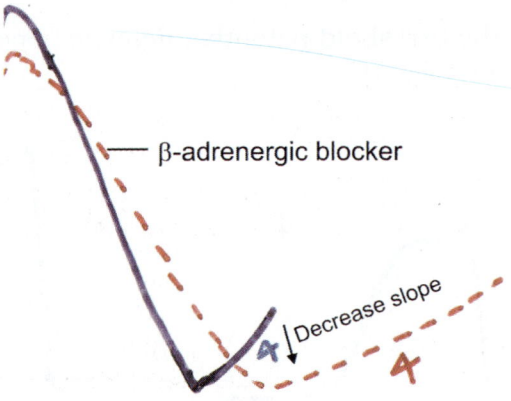

Fig.43 Decrease slope of phase 4

II. By delaying conduction velocity:
1) By prolonging the refractory period (Fig.44)
2) By prolonging the repolarization phase. Antiarrhythmic drugs prolong the refractory period. Both prolong the refractory period and inhibit the conduction velocity. The number of impulses conducted per minute is decreased. (Fig.44)

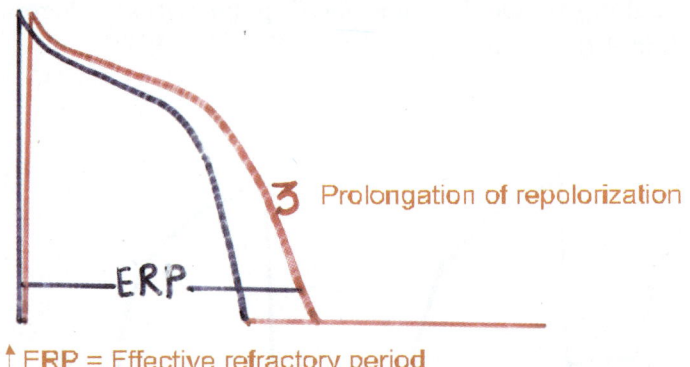

Fig.44 Prolongation of Effective refractory period by antiarrhythmic drugs

QUINIDINE:
- It is an anti arrhythmic drug.
- It is pro arythmogenic in nature, hence not preferred.

Mechanism of action:
1) It decreases the slope of phase '0'. It impedes conduction.
2) It decreases the rate of phase '0'. The number of impulses generated per minute is decreased (decreases Automaticity)
3) It increases ERP, and decreases the conduction velocity.

4) It prolongs phase '3' repolarization, prolongs the ERP → reduces conduction velocity.
5) It also decreases the slope of phase '4' depolarization (AP is shifted towards right) in pace maker cells other than SA node.
Procainamide same as quinidine. Both are rarely used except in Wolf Parkinson White syndrome and last chance in ventricular tachycardia.

LIGNOCAINE

- It is an antiarrhythmic drug.
- It is a blocker of fast Na^+ channel. It inhibits influx of Na^+.
- It is also an important local anaesthetic.

Mechanism of action as antiarrhythmic: (Fig.45)

- Decrease the slope of phase '0' – slow down conduction.
- Decrease the rate of phase '0' - decreases automaticity.
- Prolong phase 4 diastolic depolarization. The number of impulses generated per minute is reduced (decreases Automaticity).

3 Important characteristics of lignocaine as antiarrhythmic:

1) It shortens the refractory period by shortening the phase '3' repolarization. So, it does not have much effect on conduction velocity.
2) It is more effective on arithmogenic cells (rapidly firing cells) than in the normal cells.
3) It is effective only in ventricles (useful only in ventricular arrhythmias).

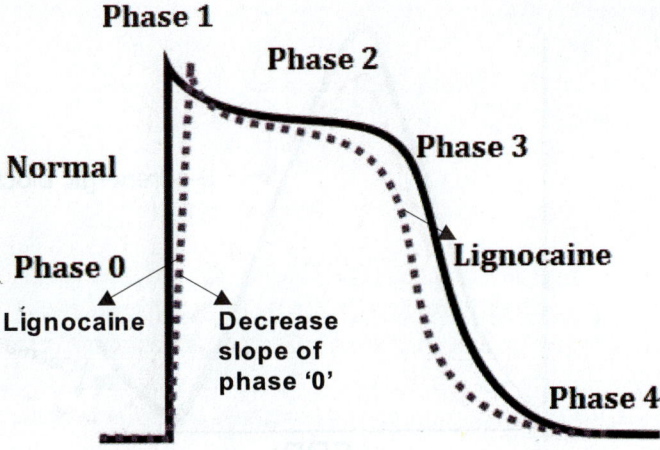

Fig.45 Shows shortening of phase 3 repolorisation and decrease slope of phase '0' depolarization by lignocaine

Clinical uses:

1) In ventricular arrhythmias, a) In arrhythmia following MI, during cardiac surgery, in digitalis toxity.
2) As local anesthetics (Ref: local anesthetics)

Dose:

Lignocaine (Without adrenaline) 50-100mg/IV bolus followed by 20-40mg/every min.

Adverse effects:

Drowsiness, nausea, paresthesis, blurred vision, nystagmus, HYPOTENSION

β – ADRENERGIC BLOCKING AGENTS:

* Cardio selective drugs are preferred.

Mechanism of action: (Fig.46A/46B)

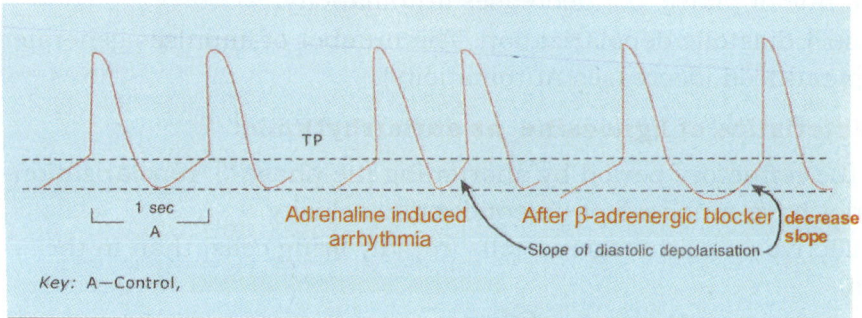

Fig.46A

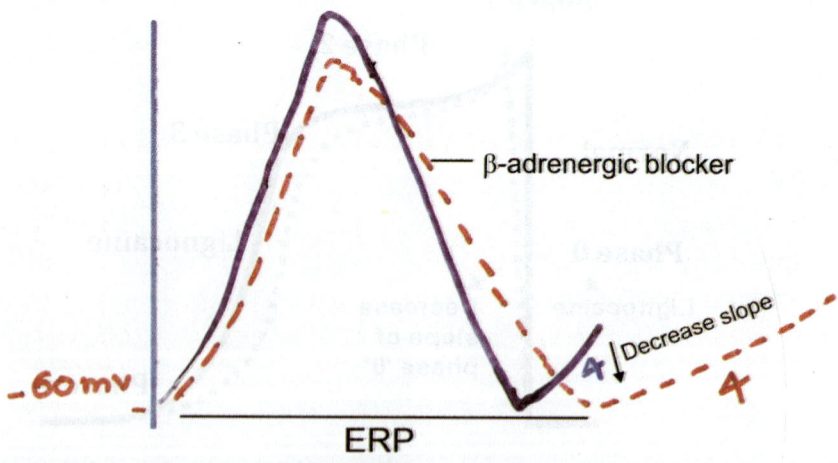

Fig.46B

Fig.46 A & B Mechanism of action of β-adrenergic blockers

- Mainly useful in adrenergic mediated arrhythmias (Halothane induced, digitalis induced and hyperthyroidism induced), pheochromocytoma etc.,
- Adrenaline increases the automaticity in atrium, ventricle, SA node and AV node.
- Toxic dose of adrenaline will cause ventricular fibrillation.
- β-adrenergic blockers competitively inhibit the adrenergically stimulated β_1 receptors in the heart.
- They depress phase-4 diastolic depolarization (decrease the slope of phase 4 depolarization) and decrease the automaticity in SA node, purkinje fiber, other ectopic foci and non automatic fibers (prolong phase 4 – depolarization). They inhibit SA node.
- ERP is prolonged at AV node, Hence decrease AV conduction (Prolongation of PR interval) both the above factors will lead to decreased heart rate per minute.

Clinical uses:

1) In supraventricular arrhythmias (atrial flutter, atrial fibrillation, PSVT). In relative PSVT and in other conditions, they protect ventricles by AV conduction block.
2) To treat arrhythmias induced by adrenergic drugs and sympathetic over activity (Halothane + adrenaline, hyperthyroidism, digitalis induced etc.,)
3) Inappropriate sinus tachycardia in emotion, anxiety etc.,

Other uses/ Adv. Effects/doses – Ref: β – adrenergic blockers under ANS.

AMIODARONE

- It is an antiarrhythmic and exerts multiple actions.
- It produces all actions of antiarrhythmic drugs. (lignocaine like → more effective on arithmogenic tissues, slight β – adrenergic blocking action, also calcium channel blocking action and direct action) → decrease HR, decreases Automaticity in the pace maker cells. (Fig.47)
- The main action is, prolongation of phase '3' repolarization. (Prolong refractory period)

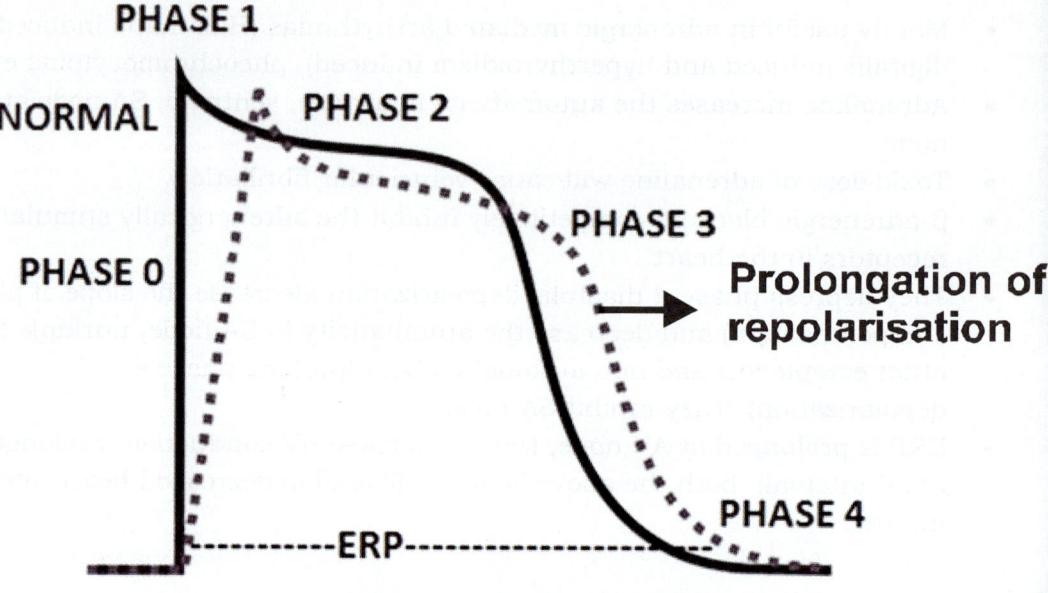

Fig.47 Mechanism of action of Amiodarone

- Decrease the rate of phase '0' depolarization (decreases automaticity). The number of impulses generated /HR/per minute are reduced.

Clinical Uses:

1) In PSVT (atrial flutter, atrial fibrillation)
2) In ventricular tachycardia: reduces HR, protect ventricles, decreases automaticity in ventricles, particularly in resistant and recurrent ventricular tachycardias.
3) Useful in WPW syndrome.

CALCIUM CHANNEL BLOCKERS (CCBs)

- Verapamil and diltiazem are more effective (stronger action on cardiac muscle)

Mechanism of action: (Fig.48)

- They are mainly effective in blocking the action of Ca^{++}, wherever it acts, by blocking L type calcium channel.

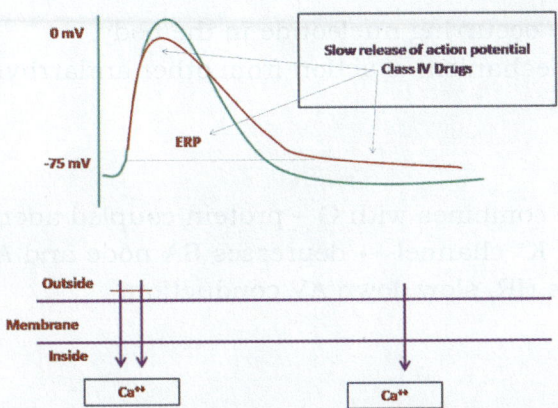

Fig.48 Slow rise of action potential by CCB

- They block Ca^{++} channel mainly at SA node and AV node, where Ca^{++} plays important role.
- They decrease the slope of phase 4 – depolarization at SA node and AV node - decreases automaticity and slow down the conduction also.
- They decrease in inward Ca^{++} current also, which occurs during upstroke, i.e. phase '0' of AP →slow rise of AP → slow in generating and conducting impulses → reduce HR, decrease automaticity.
- ERP is prolonged in AV node. PR interval is prolonged → slow down AV conduction.

Clinical Uses:
1) They are first line drugs in PSVT
2) Rapidly control ventricular response to atrial arrhythmias by AV block (protect ventricle).

Other uses (Ref : before)

Dose Verapamil – 100-120mg/3/daily/oral
      Diltiazem – 30-90mg/3/daily/oral
In emergency – Verapamil – 5-10mg/1V infusion
         Diltiazem – 10-15mg/1V infusion

Adverse effects:
- Peripheral ankle oedema.
- Constipation (due to relaxation of GIT muscle) C/I - in LVF, AV block, should be avoided with β – adrenergic blockers (aggravate bradycardia), with digoxin, reduce the efficacy of digoxin)

ADENOSINE

- It is naturally occurring nucleotide in the body.
- It differs in mechanism of action from other antiarrhythmic drug.

Mechanism of action:

Adenosine → combines with G – protein coupled adenosine receptors → activates ACh sensitive K^+ channel → depresses SA node and AV node and atrial conduction → decreases HR, slow down AV conduction.

Clinical uses:

1) In PSVT: It is very effective in terminating the attack (If CCB fails) very quickly. Some clinicians find adenosine is better than CCBs.

Adverse effects:

Bronchospasm (precipitate asthma), shortness of breath, metallic taste, nausea

Dose – 6 to 12 mg/IV infusion.

DIGOXIN

- It is cardiotonic drug of cardiac glycoside
- Previously it is used in heart failure, but now it is preferred only in atrial flutter and atrial fibrillation associated with Heart Failure or not.

Mechanism of action in Atrial Flutter and Atrial Fibrillation:

- Digoxin prolongs refractory period at AV node → slow down conduction through AV Node → and protects the ventricles
- Flutter is converted into fibrillation due to its reduction in refractory period of the atrial muscles → flutter is converted to fibrillation → now the digoxin is withdrawn suddenly → the fibrillation → becomes flutter → becomes normal rhythm. This is hypothesis, when the cause (digoxin) of recently formed fibrillation is withdrawn → fibrillation → flutter → normal rhythm. The same action will also be applicable to its use in atrial fibrillation. This may be due to rebound inhibition of cardiac rhythm after withdrawal.

Adverse effects:

- Vomiting (stimulation of CTZ)

CHOICE OF DRUGS:

Arrhythmias	First Choice	Alternative
Atrial flutter and fibrillation	• Beta adrenergic blockers • Amiodarone	Digoxin
Ventricular tachycardia	• Lignocaine • Amiodarone	NIL
Ventricular fibrillation	Defibrillator	NIL
PSVT	• Beta adrenergic blocker • CCB • Adenosine	Digoxin
Nodal arrhythmia (sinus tachycardia)	• CCB	
Atrial flutter and fibrillation associated with heart failure	• Digoxin	

Courtesy :

1. Fig.39, 46A Principles of Pharmacology 2nd edition – by HL. Sharma and KK. Sharma

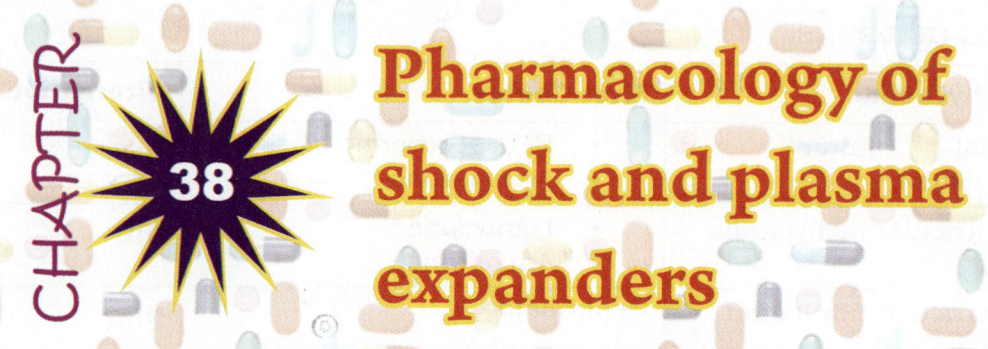

CHAPTER 38

Pharmacology of shock and plasma expanders

PHARMACOLOGY OF SHOCK

Shock (circulatory failure) is due to reduced oxygen supply to the tissues. Shock results in regional hypoxia and subsequent lactic acidosis leading to end organs damage and failure. In shock, symptoms due to reflux sympathetic overactivity are seen like pallor, sweating, cold extremities, tachycardia and fall in B.P.

TYPES OF SHOCKS

1. Anaphylactic shock
2. Cardiogenic shock
3. Hypovolemic shock
4. Septic shock
5. Neurogenic shock

1. **Anaphylatic shock** occurs due to hypersensitive reaction (in susceptible individuals only)

   Antigen – antibody reaction takes place on the mast cells → release of Histamine, Slow Reacting Substance-A, Platelet Activating Factor, Kininins, Leuko Triens etc., → all mediators produce powerful bronchoconstriction & vasodilatation (hypotension). Adrenaline 1:1000 dilution / 1-2 ml/IM is the only drug will reverse both actions simultaneously

   Next alternate drug is Glucocorticoids like Dexamethasone (IV)

2. **Cardiogenic shock:** resulting from severe Heart Failure due to Mycardial Infarction, valvular dysfunction.

   -Fluid replacement, Dopamine or Dobutamine low dose, which increases urine flow and increases Cardiac Output.

3. **Hypovolemic shock:** occurs due to severe haemorrhage and severe burns

   Treatment is by

   - fluid replacement

   - plasma expander is given till suitable blood is available

- Dopamine (in low dose 2-5 µgm/kg/min/IV) increases blood flow to the kidney, increases glomerular filtration rate, increases urine flow → prevents renel failure.

4. Septic shock: is due to release of toxin (exotoxin) from G-ve bacteria.

- infection is to be treated.

- respiratory support is to be initiated.

- fluid replacement

-Dopamine/Dobutamine- in low dose- to maintain proper urinary output.

5. Neurogenic shock: caused by traumatic spinal cord, during epidural anaesthesia.

Treatment is like that of hypovolemic shock.

PLASMA EXPANDERS

Ideally, human plasma, whole blood or reconstituted albumin are preferred in hypovolemic shock. Due to nonavailability of them during emergency forced the clinicians to use plasma expanders temporarily till the suitable blood is available.

- Plasma expanders are synthetic colloids with high molecular weight exerting osmotic pressure comparable to plasma. Ideal plasma expanders do not interfere with blood grouping and should have equal molecular weight like that of plasma .

DRUGS:

- Dextran 70, Dextran 40
- Hetastarch
- Polyvinyl Pyrrolidine
- Human albumin

Clinical uses :

1. They are used as substitute for plasma in conditions like severe burns, hypovolemia and septic shock (not useful in other types of shock)
2. As temporary measure to substitute for blood loss till the same can be arranged

DRAWBACKS:

- no oxygen carrying capacity
- contraindication in anaemia, HF, renal insufficiency, and pulmonary oedema

CHAPTER

39

Drugs used in heart block, Myocardial infarction (heart attack)

DRUGS USED IN HEART BLOCK (AV BLOCK)

1. Atropine: Effective mainly cholinergic drugs or vagal induced AV block (digitalis toxicity and in some cases of MI). Atropine is given 0.6 mg -1.2 mg /IM. Atropine shortens AV node ERP (Effective Refractory Period), bundle of His refractory period and increases conduction velocity in bundle of His.

2. Sympathomimetic drug : (Adrenaline)

It may overcome partial heart block by shortening ERP and improving AV conduction velocity of conducting tissues. It may be used in complete (3rd degree) heart block to maintain a sufficient idio-ventricular rate (by increasing the automaticity of ventricular pace makers), till external pacemaker can be implanted.

MANAGEMENT OF MYOCARDIAL INFARCTION (HEART ATTACK)

Myocardial Infarction (MI) results from prolonged myocardial ischaemia, precipitated in most cases by an occlusive coronary thrombus at the site of pre-existing plaque. Unsable angina, if untreated will lead to preinfarct stage.

MI is the commonest cause of death as a result of 1. pump failure of the ventricle 2. ventricular arrhythmias, which at times become unmanageable. About 25% of cases die even before hospitalisation. Prevention of irreversible ischaemic changes, following MI, by drugs and other supportive measures constitute some important aims of the therapy.

The following is the generalised drug schedule for the treatment of MI:

1. Opioid analgesics: Morphine (4-8 mg) or Pethidine (50 mg) is given intravenously. In most of the cases, pain will lead to shock and death. First, the pain is to be relieved by giving opioid analgesic and then the patient has to be taken to the hospital.

2. Thrombolytic drugs: They lyse the already formed thrombus. They are the most important drug in the treatment of MI. Thrombolytic therapy reduce mortality and limit infarct size in patients with acute MI. The greatest benefit occurs if treatment is initiated within the first 3 to 4 hrs. (golden hours) after the onset of chest pain. 50 to 60% reduction in the mortality can be achieved. The benefits decline rapidly thereafter. Alteplase is preferred, since it is thrombus specific and there is no hypersensitive reactions to Alteplase. It is obtained through DNA recombinant technology. It is given by slow IV infusion. It is a plasminogen activator.

3. Antiplatelet drugs: Low dose Aspirin (Ecosprin) (75 mg -350 mg/once daily) or Clopidogrel (75 mg/ daily/orally) are used as antiplatelet drugs. They prevent further spread of thrombus. They do not dissolve already formed thrombus. Life long treatment is needed.

4. For pump failure: ACE inhibitor with Frusemide is the most effective treatment. They improve the pumping function of the ventricle. Dobutamine / Dopamine are also given for increasing pumping actions of heart.

5. Ventricular arrhythmia is common. → Lignocaine (IV) is given.

6. Anticoagulants Low Molecular Weight (LMW) Heparin / S.C. Little benefit is achieved.

7. If sinus bradycardia-Atropine is given.

8. Calcium Channel Blocker (CCB) (Diltiazem) can be given to prevent reinfarction and ischaemia.

9. Oxygen administration, if dyspnea occurs.

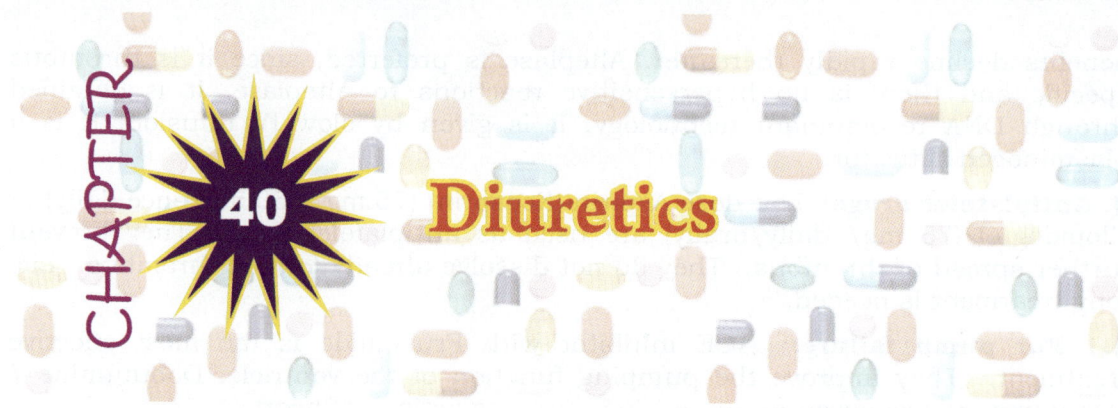

CHAPTER 40 — Diuretics

- Diuretics (clinically used) increase urine flow with net loss of Na+ and water in urine
- Alcohol is also diuretic – but it is not useful clinically, since it produces only "watery dieresis" (no excretion of Na+ along with water)
- The clinically used diuretic are mainly useful in treating oedema (accumulation of Na+ and water in the interstitial tissues).
- Reabsorption of Na+ : (Fig.49) A maximum of 65-70% Na+ is reabsorped from the proximal tubule. But no drug is available to inhibit reabsorption of Na+ at this site. Diuretics inhibit the reabsorption of sodium from the renal tubule and excreted along with equal amount of water and increase urine volume. Next maximum reabsorption of Na+ (25%) takes place at thick ascending limb of loop of Henle. Drugs (Frusemide) which inhibit reabsorption of Na+ at this site will act as high efficacious diuretic. The drugs which inhibit Na+ reabsorption at distal tubule (5%) will act as medium efficacious diuretic. The drug which inhibit sodium reabsorption (1-2%) from the collecting drug will act as low efficacious diuretic.

CLASSIFICATION OF DIURETICS

I.   Higy effecacy diuretics (loop diuretic, since the site of action is ascending limb of loop of Henle). They are also called as high ceiling diuretics (after a single dose, maximum 10L of urine is excreted)
      1) FRUSEMIDE

II.   Medium efficacy diuretics
      1) THIAZIDES – i) Hydrochlorothiazide
                           ii) Benzthiazide
      2) Thiazides like drugs = Chlorthalidone, Indapamide

III. Weak diuretics/ adjuvant diuretics
      1) K+ sparing diuretics (given along with Frusemide and Thiazides to prevent hypokalemia produced by them)
          i)   Aldosterone antagonist→Spironolactone
          ii)   Triamterene
          iii)   Amiloride
      2) Osmotic diuretics: Mannitol, Glycerol

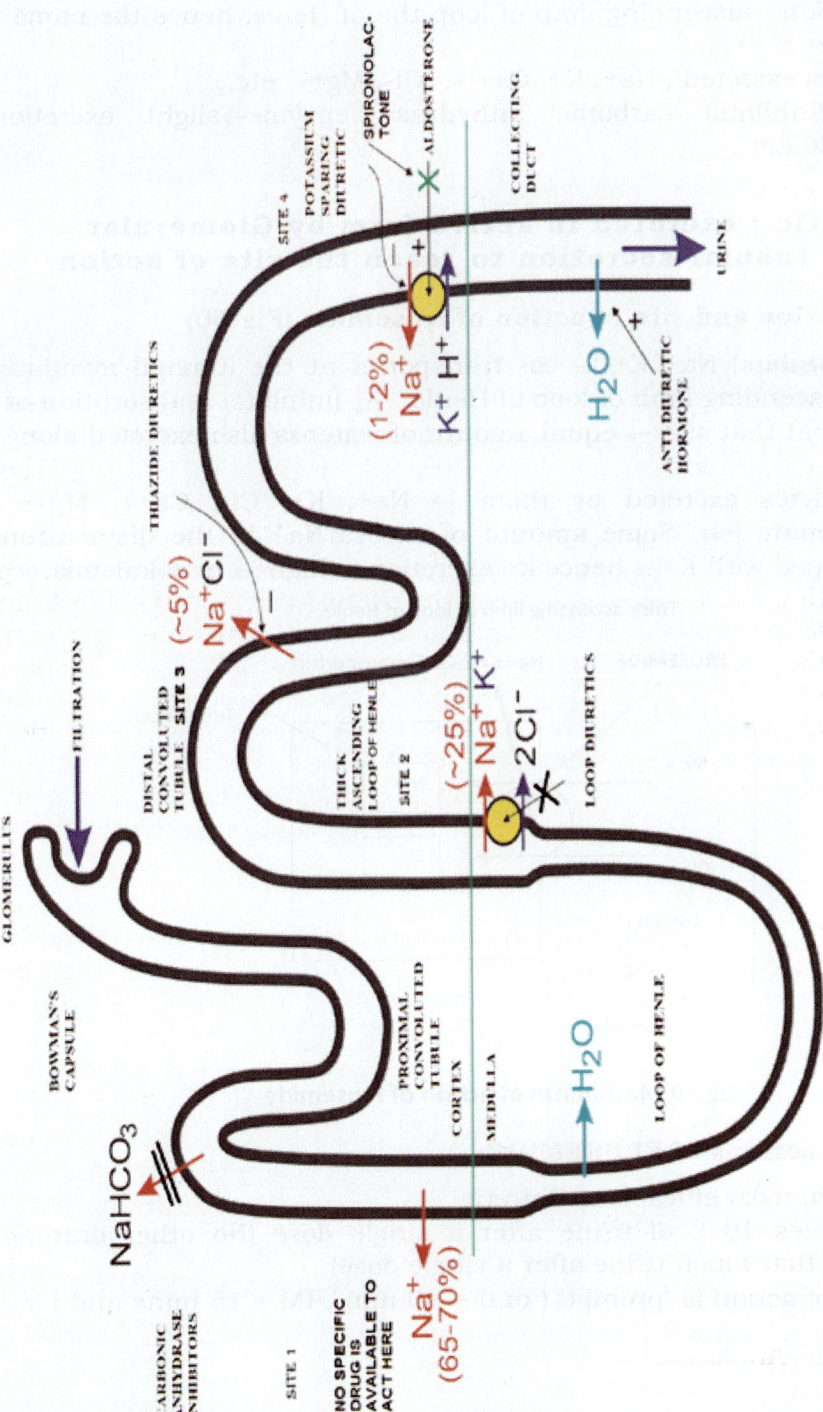

Fig.49 Urine formation and Sodium reabsorption from the urinary tubule

Site 1 - Proximal convoluted tubule → 65 - 70% of Na+ reabsorption akes place. No drug is available to inhibit the Na+ reabsorption at this site.
Site 2 - Thick ascending limb of loop of henle → 25% of Na+ reabsorption takes place loop diuretic act at this site.
         Maximum reabsorption of Na+ takes place next to proximal convoluted tubule. The drugs acting here are very potent (High ceiling Diuretics).
Site 3 - Proximal part of Distal tubule → Approximately 5% of Na+ is reabsorbed. Thiazides act here (Medium efficacy Diuretic).
Site 4 - Distal part of the distal tubule and collecting duct. Pottassium retaining Diuretics act here. Only 1-2% of Na+ is reabsorbed (weak Diuretics).
Anti-Diuretic hormone increases the reabsorption of water in the collecting duct.

FRUSEMIDE (Lasix)

- The most efficacious diuretic
- Site of action →ascending limb of loop the of Henle, hence the name "loop diuretic"
- Electrolytes excreted , Na+, K+, Ca+ +, Cl-, Mg++ etc.,
- Also ↓ (inhibits) carbonic anhydrase enzyme→slight excretion of bicarbonate ion

Pharmacokinetic : excreted in active form by Glomerular Filtration and tubular secretion to reach the site of action

Mechanism of action and site of action of frusemide (Fig.50)

- It ↓ (inhibits) Na+ K+Cl- co- transporter at the luminal membrane of thick ascending limb of loop of Henle →↓ (inhibits) reabsorption of Na+, K+, Cl- at that site → equal amount of water is also excreted along with Na+.
- Electrolytes excreted by them → Na+, K+, Cl-, Ca++, Mg++ with bicarbonate ion. Some amount of excess Na+ in the distal tubule → exchanged with K+→ hence k+ excretion is high → hypokalemia.

Thick ascending limb of loop of Henle

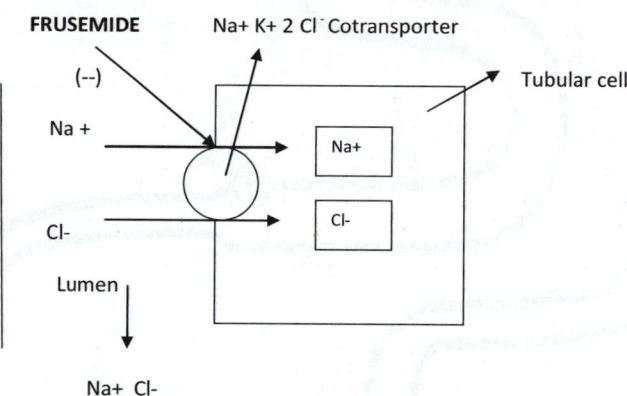

Fig.50 Mechanism of action of Frusemide

Pharmacological actions of FRUSEMIDE:

1) Diuretic action, most efficacious diuretic
   - It excretes 10 L of urine after a single dose (No other diuretic will excrete that much urine after a single dose)
   - Onset of action is 'prompt' (oral = 30 min , IM = 15 mins and I.V = 2-3 mins.)

2) On blood vessals:
  - After I.V administration of frusemide → venodilatation (before diuretic action begins) →↓(reduces) LV filling pressure → relieves pulmonary oedema & dyspnoea.

Clinical uses of FRUSEMIDE :

Dose – 20-40 mg / oral (preferably in the early morning), otherwise it disturbs the night sleep.

1) In oedema – cardiae, hepatic, renal and cerebral oedemas irrespective of the causes of oedema.
2) In acute LVF / pulmonary oedema following M.I (myocardial infarction). It reduces LV filling pressure and relives pulmonary oedema and dyspnea.
3) To make the urine alkaline as in FAD (forced alkaline dieresis) in case of certain drugs poisoning.
4) In hypertension – Thiazides are preferred. But in the presence of HF, renel insufficiency → Frusemide is better.
5) It is given along with blood transfusion in severe anaemia to prevent vascular overload.

Adverse effects:

1) Hypokalemia (prevented by giving along with k^+ retaining diuretic).
2) Acute saline depletion (dehydration).
3) Hearing loss (other ototoxic drugs like gentamicin is to be avoided)
4) Avoided in pregnancy. It decreases blood volume → compromises placental circulation → miscarriage
5) Hyperuricemia – aggravate gout
6) Hyperglycemia → aggravate Diabetes Mellitus
7) Hyperlipidemia (caution in atherosclerosis)
8) Hypercalcemia
9) Mg^{++} depletion
10) Mental disturbances, hepatic coma

THIAZIDES

- They are medium efficacy diuretics.
- They ↓ (inhibit) Na^+ Cl^- symporter.
- It is not metabolized → reach the site of action in active form (by GF & tubular secretion)

Early Distal Tubule

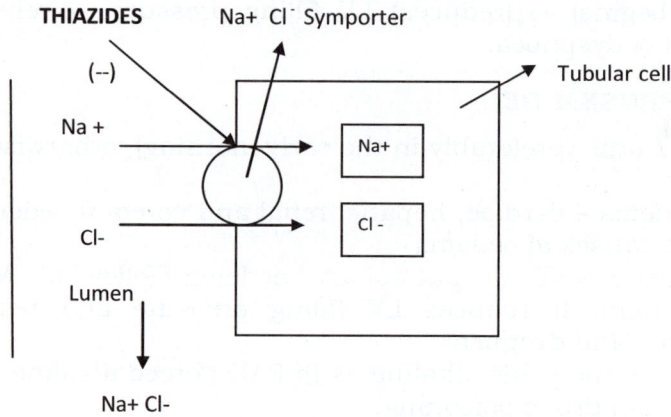

Fig.51 Mechanism of action of Thiazides

Pharmacological actions of THIAZIDES:

1) Diuretic action: mediun efficacy diuretics (useful as maintenance therapy due to their less side effects on long term use).
2) Antidiuretic action – paradoxical action → ↓ they inhibit GFR (not useful in renal failure) but useful action in diabetes insipidus.
3) In hypertension – normally preferred due to their direct vasodilating effect apart from diuretic effect → ↓ (reduce) BP and is more potent when compare to Frusemide and other diuretics.

Adverse effects: (similar to Frusemide - metabolic adverse effects only.)
1) Hypokalemia
2) Hyperlipidemia
3) Hyperuricemia (decrease Uric acid excretion)

Clinical uses of THIAZIDES:

1) In oedema (mild), as maintenance therapy.
2) In hypertension as adjuvant & in 'systolic' hypertension.
3) In diabetes insipidus (both in neurgenic & nephrognic)
4) In hypercalciuria & renal ca++ stone (reduce the excretion of ca++)
Dose – Hydrochlorothiazide -25 – 100mg / daily

K+ sparing / retaining diuretics:

I.   Aldosterone antagonist – Spironolactone
II. Directly acting : Amiloride,Triameterene

SPIRONOLACTONE :

- It is an aldosterone antagonist.
- It is a weak diuretic.
- It is a K+ retaining diuretic.

Mechanism of action :

Aldosterone → stimulates mineralocorticoid receptors → stimulates AIP (Aldosterone induced protein) → retention of Na+ and excretion of K+. Spironolactone → is converted into active metabolite, canrenone → combines with mineralocorticoid receptors at Distal Tubule & Collecting Duct and blocks → inhibits AIP → ↓ (inhibits) the action of Aldosterone → increases excretion of Na+ / water & retention of K+.

Clinical uses :

1) In hyperaldosteronism.
2) In cardiac oedema, H.F & REFRACTORY OEDEMA.
3) To counteract the K+ loss due to Frusemide/ Thiazides.

Adverse effects:

1) Hyperkalemia (should not be given with ACEI / ARB, when used in hypertension & in H.F) → weakness
2) Hirsutism, gynaecomastia, impotence & menstrual irregularities (androgenic action)
3) Peptic ulcer – aggravated

AMILORIDE / TRIAMTERENE

- They are K+ retaining diuretics
- They act directly

Mechanism of action :

- It is similar to spironolactone, but directly acting at Distal tubule & Collecting Duct by inhibiting Na+K+ ATP ase & Na+ channel → excretion of Na+ / water and retention of k+

Clinical uses :

1) Similar to Spironolactone (except in hyperaldosteronism)
2) In Li induced Diabetes Insipidus – Amiloride is preferred

Adverse effects :

Muscle cramp, headache, increase blood urea level

OSMOTIC DIURETIC (MANNITOL)

- It is very weak diuretic
- It promotes G.F.R

Mechanism of action :

- It is pharmacologically inert, not metabolized
- Excreted By Glomerular Filtration
- Large volume is to be given by I.V route → increases osmolarity of plasma and tubular fluid → inhibits reabsorption of Na+ / water in kidney → Na+ / water are excreted
- It also draws water (with Na+) from C.S.F to maintain the osmolarity → useful in cerebral oedema.
- In the ciliary process → it inhibits synthesis of aqueous humour - reduces I.O.P

Clinical uses :

1) In Increased intracranial pressure (head – injury & stroke) and in acute cerebral oedema
2) In acute congestive glaucoma - ↓ I.O.P (after I.V. administration)
3) As forced diuresis - ↑ (increases) GFR → useful in drugs poisoning. (phenobarbitone poisoning)

Adverse effects: (Not useful in chronic oedema)
Nausea, vomiting, headache

- C/I – Heart Failure (due to volume over load → aggravate Heart Failure) and Acute Left Ventricular Failure
- Cerebal haemorrhage (Intra cranial pressure is reduced)

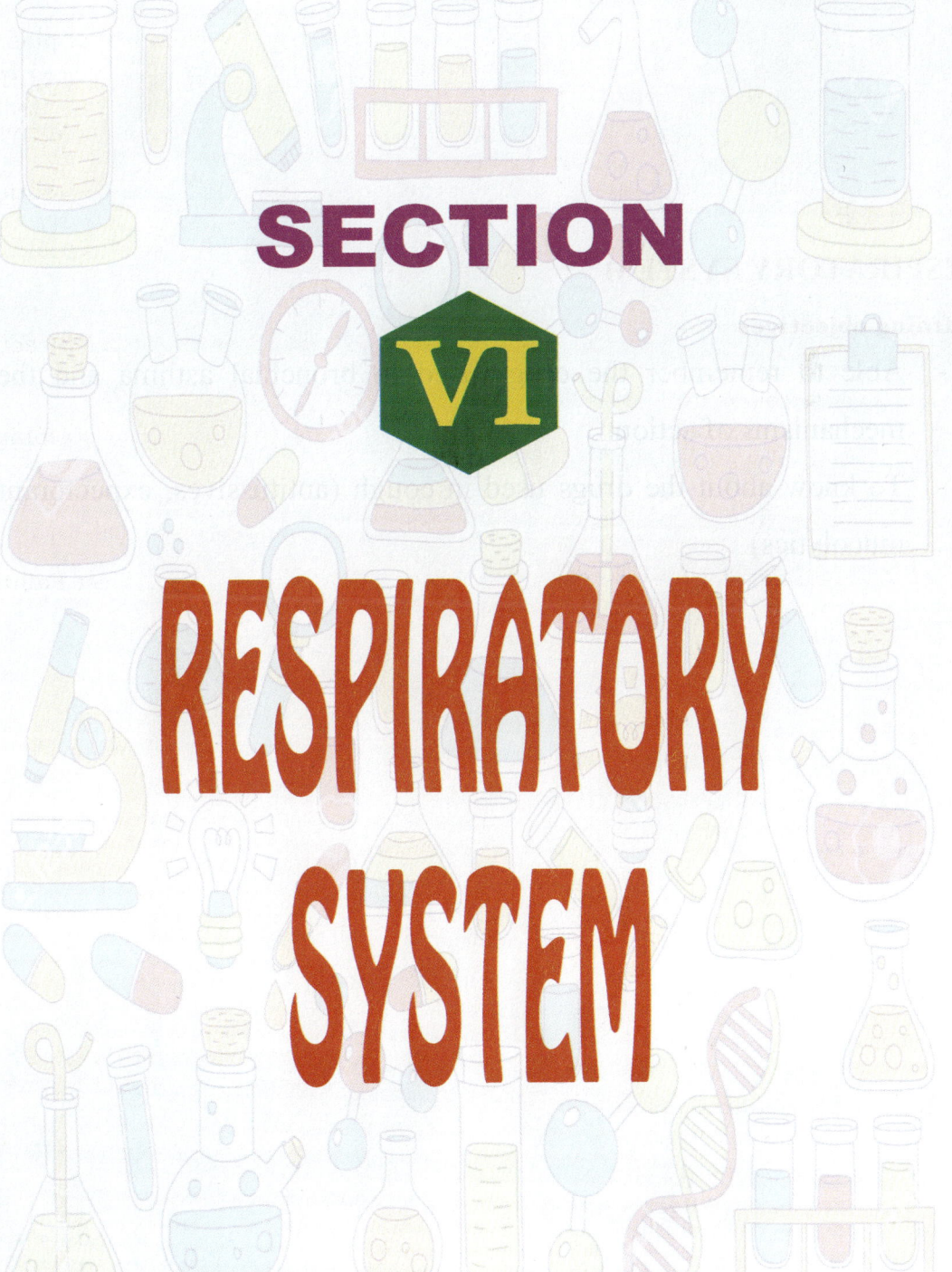

SECTION

VI

RESPIRATORY
SYSTEM

RESPIRATORY SYSTEM

Learning objectives

- Able to remember the drugs used in bronchial asthma and their mechanisms of action
- To know about the drugs used in cough (antitussives, expectorants, mucolytics)

CHAPTER 41

Drugs used in bronchial asthma, Chronic obstructive pulmonary disease(COPD)

DRUGS USED IN BRONCHIAL ASTHMA:

Two important characteristic features in pathology of asthma are 1.INFLAMMATION OF THE RESPIRATORY MUCOUS MEMBRANE (MAY BE DUE TO ALLERGY). 2. HYPER-RESPONSIVENESS OF AIRWAY TUBE (BRONCHOCONATRICTION) TO THE EXTERNAL STIMULI. THE INFLAMMATION IS ALSO PARTLY RESPONSIBLE FOR HYPER- RESPONSIVENESS.

INFLAMMATION+BRONCHOCONSTRICTION → WHEEZE, DYSPNEA → AND PARTLY RESPONSIBLE FOR COUGH.

AIM OF THE TREATMENT IS: 1. Remove inflammation or prevent inflammation and brochoconstriction. 2. Bronchodilators.

The term asthma is derived from Greek word meaning "difficulty in breathing". In the early phase (acute) response, besides smooth muscle spasm, there is excessive secretion of mucus that may clog the bronchi and bronchioles and worsen the attack.

In late (chronic) phase, inflammation continues with oedema and necrosis (death) of bronchial epithelial cells.

- Forced expiratory volume per second (FEV_1) is significantly reduced.
- Asthma may be extrinsic (when exposed to allergens like pollen, house dust mite). It is episodic less prone to develop into status asthmatics.
- Intrinsic – Secondary to a chronic or recurrent condition. It occurs mainly after the age of 40 yrs, has no identifiable external precipitating factor or immunological basis for asthmatic attack. It is perennial and more prone to develop into status asthmatics (Ref below).
  - Many patients may have both intrinsic and extrinsic asthma.

PATHOPHYSIOLOGY OF ASTHMA AND NEURO-HUMORAL CONTROL OF AIRWAYS:

- Antigen (Pollens) in sensitive individual → induces production of antibodies → Circulating in the blood. If the antigen sensitizes the same individual (exposed to antigen for the second time) → Antigen + Circulating antibodies reaction takes place on mast cells of lung → degranulation of mast cells → release of mediators like Histamine, LTs, SRS-A (Slow Reacting Substance of Anaphylaxis), PGs (Early phase) and PAF, cytokines (in later stage) →All are powerful bronchoconstrictors and pro-inflammatory (later stage) (fig:52) → Asthma attack with bronchoconstriction, hyper-reactivity of bronchial muscles, mucus secretion, epithelial damage produces symptoms of wheezing, dyspnea and occasionally cough.

- Neurohumoral control: Balanced by both PS & S system and also by adenosine.

- PS system causes bronchoconstriction & symp. system causes bronchodilation. It is found that PS tone is stronger than sympathetic tone (which is sparse) in bronchial muscles. But β_2 receptors are plenty. Iprotropium is more potent in COPD, where there is more parasympathetic tone to bronchial muscles. But in asthma, β_2 agonists are more potent, since β_2 receptors are plenty.

CLASSIFICATION OF DRUGS USED IN BRONCHIAL ASTHMA

I. Bronchodilators:

1. β_2 AGONISTS: SALBUTAMOL, Terbutaline, Salmeterol

2. Xanthine alkanoids: AMINOPHYLLINE,

3. Anticholinergic drugs: Ipratropium bromide

4. Adrenergic drugs: Ephedrin

II. Drugs that prevent bronchoconstriction:

1. Glucocorticoids; INHALATION: i). Beclomethasone ii). Fluticasone iii). Budesonide iv) Systemic: Hydrocortisone, Prednisolone

2. Leukotriene antagonists: i) Zafirlukast   ii) Montelukast

3. Mast cell stabilizers: i) Cromolyn sodium ii) Nedocromil

4. Anti IgE antibodies : i) Omalizumab

Fig.52 PATHOPHYSIOLOGY OF BRONCHIAL ASTHMA AND SITES OF ACTION OF DRUGS

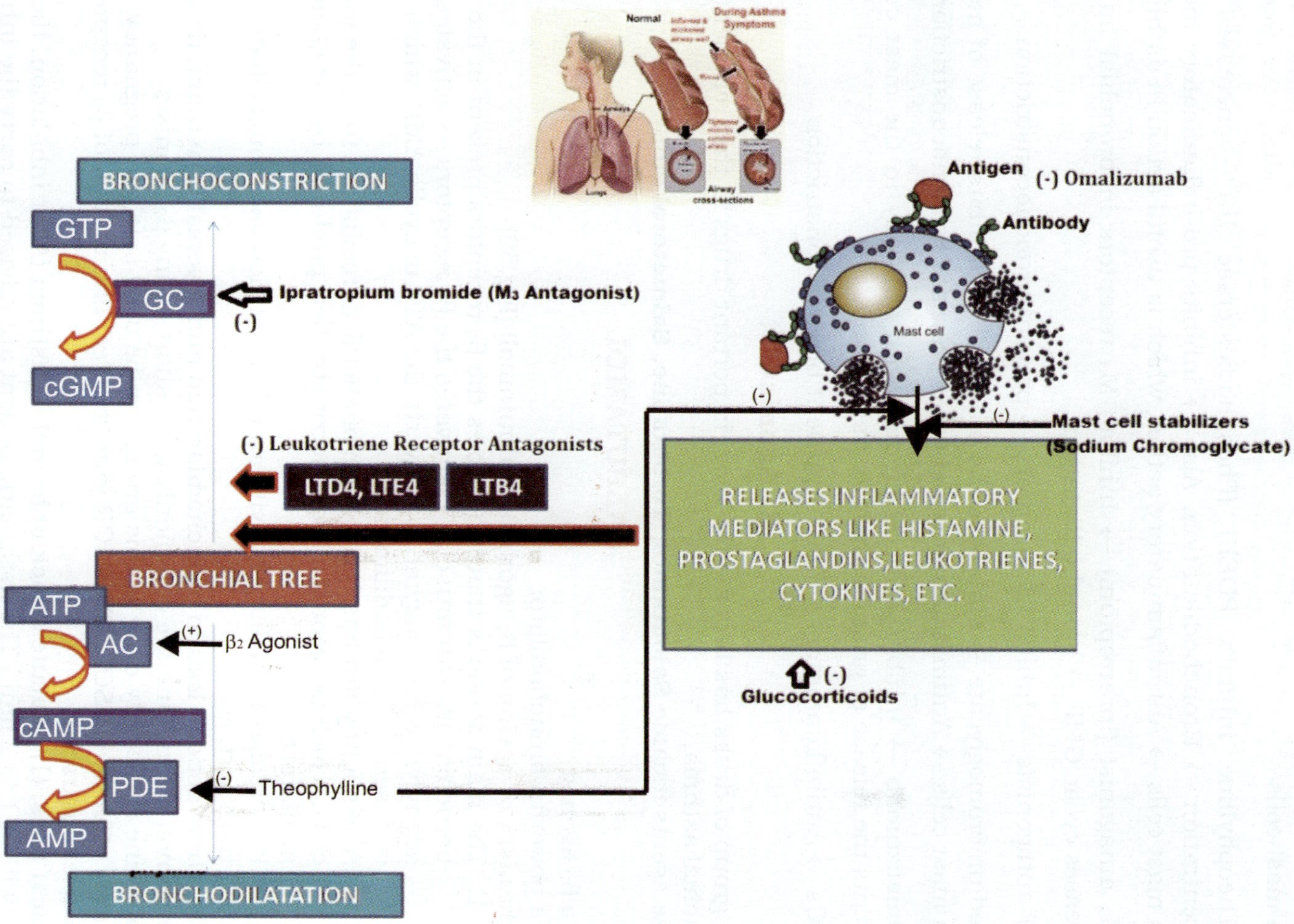

1. β_2 agonists → stimulate β_2 receptors in bronchial muscles → stimulate adenylyl cyclase → increase c-AMP → produces bronchodilatation. Also inhibit mediators from mast cells

2. Theophylline inhibits PDEIII (Phosphodiesterase III) → increases c-AMP concentration → Bronchodilatation. Also → inhibits pro-inflammatory mediators from mast cells → Antiinflammatory action, which is useful action in asthma

3. M_3 antagonist (Ipratropium) → Inhibits M_3 receptors in bronchial muscle → decreases cyclic GMP → bronchodilatation

4. LT antagonists → Inhibit LT receptors → prevent bronchoconstriction.

5. Sodiumcromoglycate → stabilises the mast cell → inhibits release of mediators from mast cells → Antiinflammatory action → prevents bronchoconstriction.

6. Omalizumab → inhibits antigen binding with antibody in the mast cells and prevents the release of proinflammatory mediators.

7. GCs → Antiinflammatory action → prevent bronchoconstriction.

β_2 Agonists

This group of drugs has become the most important drugs in the treatment of bronchial asthma.
These agents include **Salbutamol, Terbutaline, Salmeterol** etc.,

SALBUTAMOL

It is a β_2 agonist
It is a powerful bronchodilator
Mechanism of action of β_2 agonists (Salbutamol) (Fig.52)
1. The main action is that it occupies the β_2 receptors present in the airway bronchial smooth muscles →activates the β_2 receptors → activates adenylyl cyclase enzyme → converts the ATP to cyclic AMP, which is released → bronchodilatation.
2. Also slightly inhibits the release of chemical mediators from the mast cells, which prevent the bronchoconstriction produced by the chemical mediators.
3. It increases the ciliary activity and thereby increases mucociliary transport.
All the above actions lead to bronchodilatation and reversal of asthamatic attack.
Salbutamol, terbutaline are commonly used short acting β_2 agonists.
Terbutaline is the only drug in this group can be used safely in pregnancy.
Adverse effects: MUSCLE TREMOR (due to direct stimulation of β_2 receptors in the skeletal muscles)
Clinical uses: (1) In acute attack of bronchial asthma (After inhalation, there is relief within 1 to 2 min.) The asthmatic patient are advised to carry the inhaler with them. They can use as and when required. (2) In COPD (Chronic Obstructive Pulmonary Disease)

Dose and administration: Metered Dose Inhaler. MDI per puff, 100 mcg of the drug is delivered through inhaler. Nebulizer is also used.

Other uses : As uterine relaxant to delay labour in threatened abortion.

XANTHINE ALKALOIDS

They are bronchodilators and CNS stimulants. Source: Tea leaves, cocoa, coffee seeds

Xanthine alkaloids are caffeine, theophylline (Aminophylline), theobromine.

Mechanism of action: (Fig.52)

- Release of Ca^{++} from sarcoplasmic reticulum, especially in skeletal muscles and cardiac muscles.
- Inhibit PDE (Phospho Di Esterase) III enzyme →increase concentration of cyclic AMP →Relaxation of smooth muscles →Bronchodilatation, stimulate gastric acid secretion, stimulate heart.
- On mast cells: They decrease the release of Histamine and other proinflammatory mediators → Antiinflammatory action (useful in bronchial asthma)

Pharmacological actions

1) On CNS: CNS stimulant → Xanthine alkaloids allay fatigue, insomnia, thinking becomes clearer. That is why the individuals take coffee or tea when they feel dull.
2) On Kidney: Mild diuretic action
3) On GIT: They produce vomiting (Due to stimulation of Chemo receptor trigger zone and gastric irritation)
4) On Skeletal muscle: Enhance contractile power of skeletal muscles → enhanced diaphragmatic contraction (useful in dyspnea)

Clinical uses :

1) In bronchial asthma (in acute attack and in status asthmaticus)
2) In COPD (Chronic Obstructive Pulmonary Disease)
3) In dyspnea (dyspnea in heart failure and bronchial asthma)
4) Apnoea in premature infants.

Dose : Aminophylline – 100 to 200 mg/oral, 25 to 50 mg/IV

Adverse effects:

1) Insomia, tachycardia, gastric irritation, vomiting.

IPRATROPIUM BROMIDE

- It is an anticholinergic drug.
- It is quarternary ammonium compound, hence less absorption through bronchial mucosa (where muscarinic receptors are present to act) and hence less systemic anticholinergic side effects.
- It does not cross BBB & there is no CNS adverse effect.

Mechanism of action: (Fig.52)

- Iprotropium occupies M_3 receptor in bronchial muscles → inhibits M_3 receptor → reduce cGMP level → prevents bronchoconstriction of ACh→ bronchodilatation.
- Less effective than β_2 agonist in bronchial asthma.
- Ipratropium blocks bronchoconstriction due to ACh in the larger airway.
- But in COPD, Ipratropium is better, since parasympathetic tone is stronger in bronchial muscles.
- Combination with β_2 agonist is available, which produces better effect and longer duration of action.

    Duolin inhalation   —— Salbutamol 100 µg + Ipratropium 20 µg

Clinical Use:

1) In bronchial asthma (better effect with salbutamol) 20 µg / metered dose or with salbutamol.
2) In COPD – Better effect than salbutamol.

Adverse effects:

Mild dryness of mouth after inhalation (may be due to its anticholinergic action).

Dose : Metered Inhaler dose – 25 µg/puff, 1-2 puff / thrice daily)

BECLOMETHASONE

- It is an antiinflammatory
- It is not a bronchodilator
- It prevents bronchoconstriction due to allergy

Mechanism of action → Antiinflammatory (Fig.52)

- Airway inflammation is present in early phase and mild bronchial asthma. Bronchial remodelling starts developing from the beginning. So inhaled steroid is given for all asthma patients from the beginning to prevent inflammation.

Clinical uses :

- In chronic bronchial asthma. (By inhalation)

Adverse effects:

- Hoarseness of voices, sore throat, oropharyngeal candidiasis are the most common adverse effects.

CROMOLYN SODIUM / SODIUM CROMOGLYCATE

- It is not bronchodilator.
- It prevents bronchoconstriction due to external stimuli.
- It is the mast cell stabilizer.

Mechanism of action: (Fig.52)

- Normally antigen (allergen)-antibody reaction takes place on mast cells → degranulation of mast cells → release of mediators like Histamine, SRS-A (Slow Reacting Substance-A), Kinins, PAF (Platelet Activating Factor), LTs etc., → All are powerful bronchoconstrictors.
- Cromolyn sodium stabilizes the mast cells and prevents degranulation of mast cells → prevents the release of mediators → prevents bronchconstriction.

Dose and administration: By inhalation 1 mg metered dose.

Clinical uses :

1. In bronchial asthma: As long term prophylactic (in acute attack –not useful)
2. In allergic rhinitis: As nasal spray. It is not nasal decongestant. But gives symptomatic relief.
3. In allergic conjunctivitis: As eye drops

Adverse effects: systemic absorption is minimum. bronchospasm, cough occur.

LEUKOTRIENE (LT) ANTAGONISTS: (Zafirlukast, Montelukast)

Zileuton – inhibits leukotriene synthesis

Mechanism of actions: (Fig.52) of LT antagonists

LTs are powerful bronchoconstrictor. LTs are released during the allergic reaction.

LT antagonists do not inhibit the release of brochoconstrictor mediators, but block the LT receptors in the bronchial muscles and prevent bronchoconstriction.

Zafirlukast, Montelukast – Leukotriene Receptor Antagonists – blocks LT Receptors in the bronchial smooth muscles → relieve bronchospasm

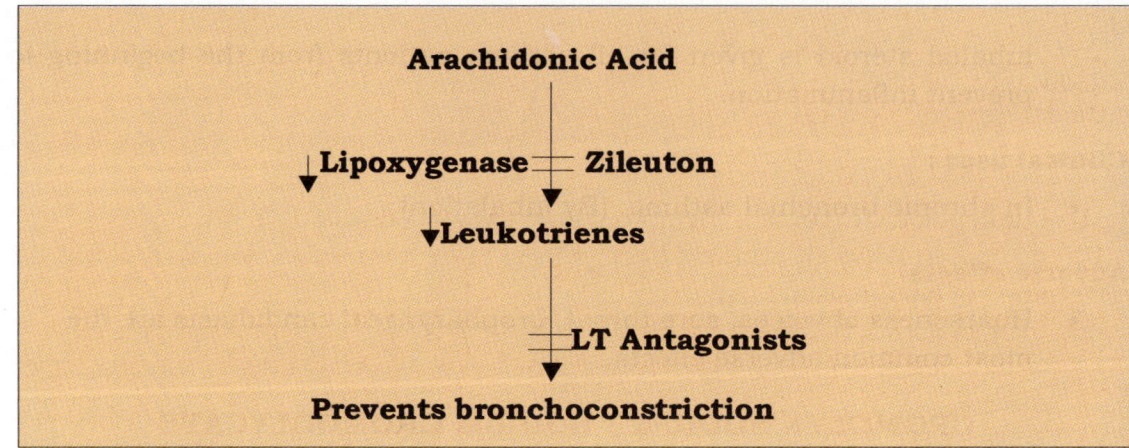

Arachidonic Acid

↓Lipoxygenase ═ Zileuton

↓**Leukotrienes**

═LT Antagonists

Prevents bronchoconstriction

Clinical use:

1. Mainly used as prophylactic as adjuvant with inhaled corticosteroids in poorly responding cases of asthma patients. They also reduce the dose of β_2 agonists.
2. Also useful in allergen induced and NSAIDs induced bronchoconstriction

Dose: Zafirlukast - 10-20 mg/orally /day, Montelukast – 5 – 10 mg/day

Adverse effects: Zileuton is a hepatotoxic (use is restricted)

Zafirlukast is an enzyme inhibitor. It increases the toxicity of warfarin (bleeding), whose dose is to be reduced, GIT upset, Headache.

OMALIZUMAB

It is a monoclonal anti-Ig-E antibody:

Mechanism of Action (Fig.52)

It is a new approach in which monoclonal antibody targeted to IgE. So that the latter cannot bind to its receptors present in the mast cells. It is not a bronchodilator. Omalizumab is a recombinant monoclonal antibody, which
1. Inhibits the binding of IgE to mast cell

2. Inhibits the activation of IgE, which is already bound to mast cells and thus prevents their degranulation

3. Neutralizes the free IgE in circulation by forming IgE – omalizumab complex.

Clinical uses: Omalizumab is indicated in asthamatic patients who are not adequately controlled by inhaled corticosteroids. It is not suitable in acute attacks. Its high cost discourages its used as first line drug.

TREATMENT OF BRONCHIAL ASTHMA

1) Mild episodic asthma – (Symptoms are expressed less than once daily, normal in between attacks) Short acting β_2 agonist inhalation, only at the start of each episode. (step-1)
2) Seasonal asthma : Start regular inhaled steroid / sodium cromoglycate, 2-3 weeks before anticipated seasonal attack and continued 3-4 weeks after the season is over. If any attack occurs meanwhile it is treated with inhalational β_2 Agonists.
3) Mild chronic asthma (Symptoms once daily): Regular inhaled steroid / sodium cromoglycate. If any attack, treat with inhaled β_2 agonist. (Step -2)
4) Moderate asthma with frequent exacerbation. Inhaled long acting β_2 agonist (Step-3) during attack and If not controlled, addition of theophylline (oral) is given.
5) Severe asthma (Continuous attack): hospitalization, Inhaled salmeterol + Inhaled steroid 1000-2000 mg/day. If not controlled, LT antagonist + theophylline (oral) + oral β_2 agonist + inhaled ipratropium bromide are given. (Step-4) If not controlled – instead of inhaled steroid, oral steroid is instituted. (Step – 5)
6) Status asthmaticus : Life threatening condition with upper RTI.

TREATMENT OF STATUS ASTHMATICUS/REFRACTORY ASTHMA:

Any individual can develop status asthmaticus. It is life threatening. Respiratory tract infection and inflammation are the commonest problem.

They are refractory to the conventional bronchodilator.

1. Antiinflammatory drug: Hydrocortisone IV 100 mg (or another equivalent GC)
2. Bronchodilators : Nebulized Salbutamol+Ipratropium bromide
3. Oxygen inhalation
4. Intubation and mechanical ventilation, if needed.
5. Correct dehydration and acidosis : by saline and sodium bicarbonate.

CHRONIC OBSTRUCTIVE PULMONARY DISEASE (COPD)

COPD is a disease state, characterized by the progressive obstruction of air flow in the bronchial tube and unlike in asthma, the obstruction is not satisfactorily reversed. The conventional bronchodilator alone may not be effective. There is a decline in the forced expiratory volume in one second (FEV_1).

CAUSES: Cigarette smoking, chronic bronchitis chronic respiratory infections, environmental pollution and occupational exposure (in persons working in cement or cotton industries). COPD is usually associated with chronic bronchitis and later stages emphysema (Characterized by accumulation of air in the spaces, loss of lung elasticity, closure of smaller airways, which will lead to dyspnoea (dyspnea = both are correct) productive cough, wheezing, recurrent respiratory infection.

- The inflammatory component of COPD is due to increased neutrophil activation, but in asthma, it is due to eosinophil and mast cell activity.
- COPD → activation of macrophages → release of LTs / IL-8 from neutrophils → destroy the tissues of alveolar wall.

Management of COPD:

Most patients have irreversible airway obstruction. The treatment by drugs are only symptomatic without removing the underlying causes.

AIMS of treatment:

1) To minimise airway obstruction as much as possible.
2) To reduce respiratory symptoms and improve the quality of life.
3) To prevent or treat secondary infection, cor pulmonale.

TREATMENT:

1. Stop smoking: Voluntarily or by pharmacological intervention by drug.
2. First line drug treatment is by Salbutamol – 100μg metered dose (inhalation). Now, the anti-muscarinic bronchodilator like Ipratropium is found to be better than β_2 agonist. Since the airway muscle is predominantly under para-sympathetic control (combination is better.) Duolin inhaler 100μg Salbutamol + 20μg Ipratropium (Fixed dose drug combination)
3. In addition to the above, Theophylline is prescribed particularly effective in relieving dyspnea and in the presence of inflammatory mediators – 200mg SR cap.
4. Corticosteroid/ orally / (for one week), inhalational Beclomethasone (preferred): – 100-200 μg metered dose.
5. O_2 administration, if needed.

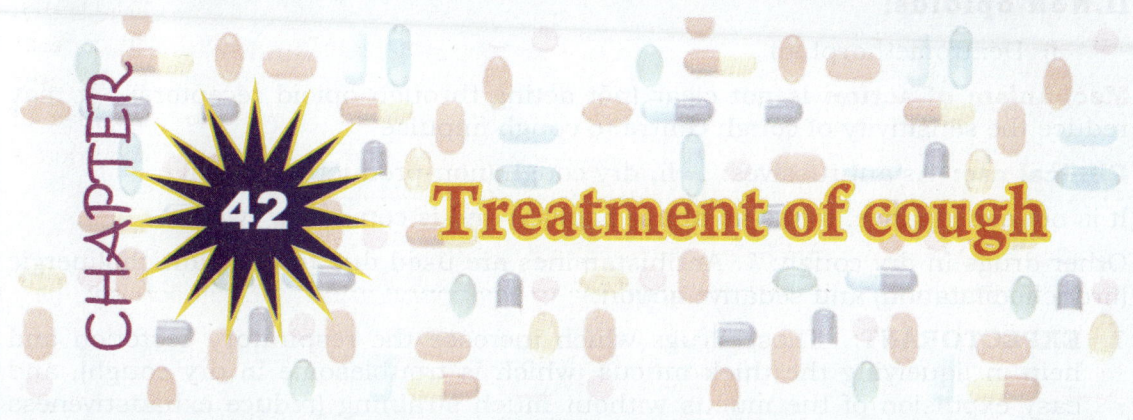

Treatment of cough

CHAPTER 42

Cough is normally protective to expel the unwanted substances (irritants, foreign materials etc.,). But if it is disproportionate → will be troublesome → abdominal pain, disturbance of sleep.

Cough is of two types:

1. Productive: Cough is accompanied by expulsion of mucus, secretion, bacteria, foreign materials, cellular debris etc., It is essential and should not be suppressed.

2. Non-productive (dry cough) cough is troublesome, disturbs the sleep, produces abdominal pain and causes exhaustion. Drugs are needed to suppress it (antitussives).

ANTITUSSIVES are drugs which inhibit the cough centre situated at the brain stem and suppress cough.

Classification of antitussives:

I. Opioid antitussives:

 i) Codeine

 ii) Pholcodeine

Mechanism of action They ↑ (stimulate) opioid receptors in the cough centre → ↓ (inhibit) cough centre → suppress cough

- They produce constipation.
- Abuse liability is more for them.
- They are not used commonly.

 iii) Noscapine

   Mechanism of action : similar to Opioids

- It is a powerful antitussive
- It is also an opioid
- It is commonly used
- Since there is no constipation, no abuse liability

II. Non-opioids:

    i) Dextromethorphan

Mechanism of action is not clear (not acting through opioid receptors). It may reduce the sensitivity of cough centre to cough impulse.

Clinical use: As antitussives: 1. In dry cough (non-productive cough)

It is not constipative, it has no abuse liability, and is commonly used.

Other drugs in dry cough: 1. Antihistamines are used due to their anticholinergic (bronchodilatation) and sedative action.

1. **EXPECTORANT:** Those drugs which increase the respiratory secretion and help in liquefying the thick mucus (which is troublesome in dry cough), and easy expulsion of the mucus without much straining (reduce exhaustiveness and abdominal pain). Dry cough will become productive.
2. **Clinical use :** In cough

Example : Vasaka (guaiphenesin), Ammonium chloride

3. MUCOLYTIC AGENTS:

    i) Bromhexine ii) Acetyl cysteine

Mechanism of action: They depolymerise polysaccharides → net work of tenacious sputum is broken → thin copious bronchial secretion → cough will become less troublesome.

Clinical use: In dry cough (used as cough expectorant in various cough mixtures)

4. PHARYNGEAL DEMULCENTS: Honey, lozenges allay dry cough by preventing the action of irritants on pharyngeal epithelium.

SECTION

VII

CENTRAL NERVOUS SYSTEM

CENTRAL NERVOUS SYSTEM

Learning objectives

- To know about the various neurotransmitters, receptors and drugs modulating them in the Central Nervous System
- To enumerate the general anaesthetics and advantages and disadvantages of them
- Able to remember pre-anaesthetic medications and their aims
- To be aware of antiepileptic drugs, opioid analgesics and their clinical uses
- Able to remember sedative-hypnotics and their uses
- To be aware of antipsychotics drugs, antidepressant drugs and antianxiety drugs
- To know about substance abuse and management

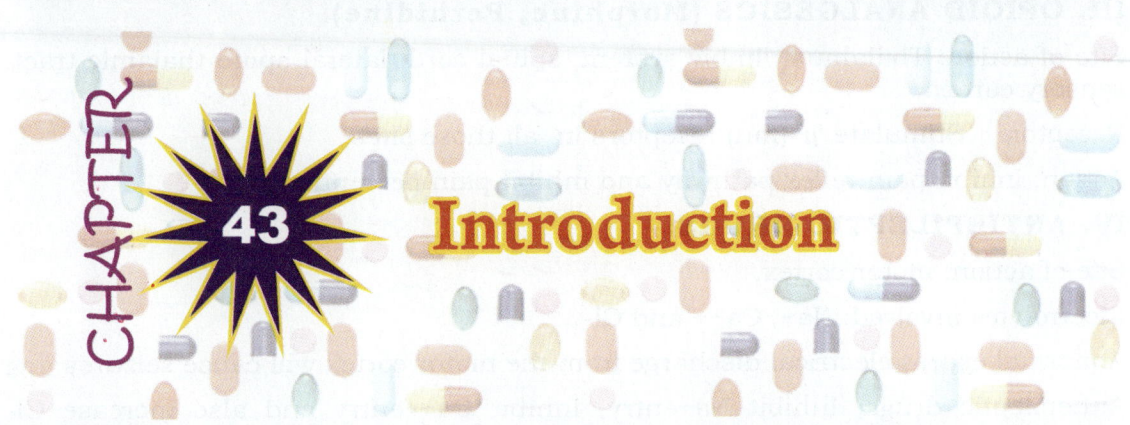

CHAPTER 43 — Introduction

All the drugs are acting through neurotransmitters, respective receptors and electrolytes/ions.

Important neurotransmitters:

1. Dopamine (important receptor DA_2) - Inhibitory
2. 5 HT/SEROTONIN ($5 HT_3$, $5 HT_1$ receptors) – Inhibitory & Excitatory
3. Glutamate NMDA (N-methyl D Aspartate) receptor - Excitatory
4. Noradrenaline (α receptor) - Excitatory
5. Gamma Amino Butyric Acid ($GABA_A$) – Inhibitory
6. ACh (Acetylcholine) – (Muscarinic receptor) excitatory

Mechanism of action of DRUGS ACTING ON CNS; (IN BRIEF)

I. GENERAL ANAESTHETICS:

Site of action: whole CNS.

Stimulate $GABA_A$ receptors in CNS.

GABA is the inhibitory transmitter.

Action: Reversible unconsciousness. Inhibit pain and other reflexes, reduce skeletal muscle tone.

II. SEDATIVE-HYPNOTICS:

Site of action: Reticular Activating System (concerned with sleep-wakefulness).

Receptor: Stimulate BDZ (Benzodiazepine) receptors, in turn stimulate $GABA_A$ receptors, which are situated nearby.

Action: Sedative-hypnotic.

Examples: Diazepam, Zolpidem, Zopiclone.

III. OPIOID ANALGESICS (Morphine, Pethidine).

Site of action: Thalamus, limbic system, spinal cord, lateral spino thalamic tract, sensory cortex.

Receptor: Stimulate 'μ' (mu) receptors in all those sites.

Action: inhibit pain reflex pathway and inhibit pain perception.

IV. ANTIEPILEPTIC DRUGS:

Site of action: motor cortex.

Electrolytes involved: Na+, Ca++ and Cl-.

Abnormal excess electrical discharge from the motor cortex will cause seizures.

Antiepileptic drugs: Inhibit Na+entry, inhibit Ca++entry and also increase Cl-entry.

V. ANTIPARKINSONISM DRUGS (L-DOPA).

Site of action: Extra Pyramidal System (EPS).

Transmitter: Dopamine.

Action: Increase the concentration of Dopamine in the Extra Pyramidal System.

Deficiency of Dopamine in EPS will lead to Parkinsonism.

VI. Alzheimer's disease.

Due to deficiency of ACh (Acetylcholine) at hippocampus.

Tacrine (anticholinesterase) increases the concentration of ACh at that site and useful in Alzheimer's disease.

VII. ANTIEMETICS; ONDANSETRONE AND DOMPERIDONE.

Site of action: Mainly at the relay stations for vomiting impulses (CTZ AND NTS-Chemoreceptor Trigger Zone and Nucleus Tractus Solitorius).

Receptors: Stimulation of DA_2, $5 HT_3$ and $5 HT_1$, M_1, H_1, which are present in the relay station → vomiting.

Antiemetic action: Inhibit one or more receptors, at the relay stations.

VIII. Psychosis is due to the increased concentration of Dopamine and 5 HT in the mesolimbic area of the brain.

Antipsychotic drugs inhibit Dopamine and/or 5 HT.

Receptors: DA_2, $5 HT_1$.

IX. ANTIDEPRESSANTS:

Depression is due to deficiency of N.Adr or 5 HT at limbic system in the brain.

Antidepressants increase the concentration of N.Adr/ 5 HT.

Receptors involved: α receptor, $5 HT_1$

X. Sedatives antianxiety: Act by stimulating GABA receptors.

XI. Migraine: due to extra cerebral vasodilatation. (Sumatriptan, Ergotamine).

Receptor involved: 5 HT.

Symptom (mainly headache) is due excess concentration of 5 HT at the extra cerebral vessels → vasodilatation → Headache.

Sumatriptan and Ergotamine are 5 HT agonists and cause extra cerebral vasoconstriction, useful in migraine.

XII. Dopamine is Prolactin Release Inhibitory Hormone.

Action: Dopamine agonist (Bromocriptine) inhibits prolactin secretion and is useful in breast engorgement.

Actions of Dopamine on CNS (in nutshell)

Dopamine is an important neurotransmitter in CNS. The important Dopamine receptor is DA2.

	Site	Dopamine / Dopamine agonist action	Antidopaminergic / dopamine antagonist
1.	Mesolimbic area	Genesis of psychosis	Antipsychotic action
2.	Hypothalamus	Prolactin release inhibitory harmone. ↓ prolactin. Dopamine agonist (Bromocriptine) is useful in breast engorgement	↑ prolactin secretion → galactorrhoea, infertility
3.	CTZ	Vomiting	Antiemetics
4.	BG/EPS	Antiparkinsonism	Parkinsonism

Fig. 52A Substance abuse on behaviour

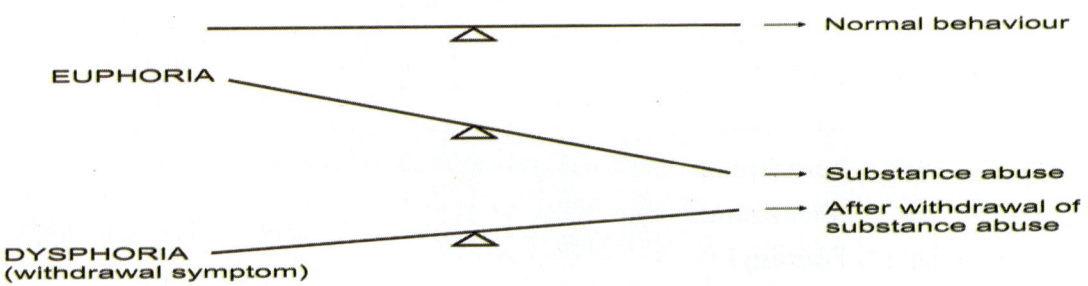

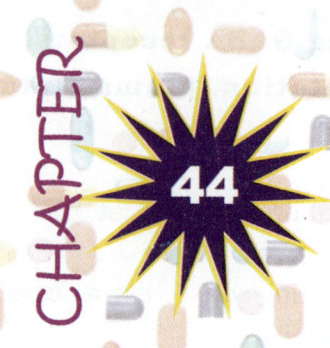

CHAPTER **44**

General anaesthetics and preanaesthetic medication

GENERAL ANAESTHETICS:

General anaesthetics are drugs which produce the following characteristic actions:

1. Loss of consciousness (reversible)
2. Loss of pain and other sensory reflexes
3. Loss of skeletal muscle tone

CLASSIFICATION OF GENERAL ANAESTHETICS:

I.   Inhalational anaesthetics:

  1. Volatile liquids

      i)   Halothane

      ii)   Isoflurane

      iii)   Enflurane

  2. Gas: Nitrous oxide

II.   IV General anaesthetics (inducing agent)

  1. Fast inducers

      i)   Thiopentone sodium
      ii)   Propofol
      iii)   Etomidate

  2. Slow inducers

      i)   Diazepam

      ii)   Lorazepam

      iii)   Midazolam

      iv)   Fentanyl

  3. Dissociative anaesthetic: Ketamine

Ideal general anaesthetics

1. Should produce rapid and pleasant induction.
2. Should produce rapid recovery.
3. Should not irritate respiratory tract.
4. Should not cause nausea and vomiting.
5. Should not be inflammable.
6. Should not be explosive.
7. Should produce sufficient skeletal muscle relaxation for major operation.
8. Should produce sufficient analgesia.
9. Should not react with rubber tubing of soda lime.

No single drug satisfies all the above characters. Now, a balanced anaesthesia is preferred.

For smooth and rapid induction: One IV general anaesthetic is given followed by one inhalational anaesthetic and is maintained in surgical anaesthesia as long as required +analgesic. If needed, one skeletal muscle relaxant for major operation with proper preanaesthetic medications are given.

Now, the surgical anaesthesia stage is divided into light anaesthesia and deep anaesthesia.

Deep anaesthesia is characterized by the absence of corneal reflex, fall in BP, respiratory depression etc., Light anaesthesia is characterized by reflux increase in respiration and BP after making an incision of the skin

Deep anaesthesia is required for major surgery.

Light anaesthesia is required for minor surgery.

HALOTHANE

It is the most commonly used volatile inhalational anaesthetic.

Mechanism of action :

Potentiates GABA (Gamma Amino Butyric Acid), the inhibitory transmitter in the CNS.

Dose: Inhalant solution: For induction- 2-4% and for maintenance-0.5-1%. Administered slowly by inhalation till the surgical anaesthesia stage is reached and then maintained by maintenance dose.

HALOTHANE/ISOFLURANE/ENFLURANE

Advantages:

1. Non inflammable
2. Non explosive
3. Rapid and pleasant induction and recovery
4. Sweet odour and non irritant

5. Potent anaesthetic

6. They produce bronchodilatation and are useful in asthmatic

7. Inhibit intestinal and uterine contraction, which are useful for assisting internal or external version during late pregnancy.

Disadvantages:

1. Not good analgesic / skeletal muscle relaxant

2. COP (Cardiac Out Put) is reduced with deepening of anaesthesia.

3. Depression of respiration.

4. Prolong delivery and increase post partum haemorrhage.

5. Urine formation is reduced due to reduced GFR.

6. Malignant hyperthermia (Dantrolene is given).

7. Psychomotor performance and mental ability remain depressed several hours after regaining consciousness.

Opioid analgesic like Fentanyl and skeletal muscle relaxant are administered along with them.

Clinical uses :   1. In surgical procedure.

Adverse effects: Hepatotoxic, kidney damage, delirium, convulsion, nausea and vomiting after anaesthesia.

NITROUS OXIDE

It is a gaseous general anaesthetic.

Administered by inhalation in the dose of 70%+30% Oxygen (to prevent hypoxia due to Nitrous Oxide).

Advantages:

1. Non inflammable gas.

2. Good analgesic.

3. Rapid and pleasant induction.

4. Little effect on respiration, heart and BP.

5. As a sole agent with 30% Oxygen is used for dental and obstetric analgesia

6. Very cheap and commonly used

Disadvantages:

1. Low potency anaesthetic.

2. Hypoxia (30% Oxygen is given).

3. Poor skeletal muscle relaxant (a skeletal muscle relaxant is needed in case of major surgeries).

Clinical uses : 1. In surgical procedure.

Adverse effects: liver, kidney damage, nausea and vomiting after anaesthesia.

INTRAVENOUS GENERAL ANAESTHETICS (INDUCING AGENTS)

These drugs are mainly used as inducing agents before giving general anaesthetics because of their rapid, pleasant induction and there is no respiratory tract irritation. They produce unconsciousness within 15 to 20 seconds and lasts for 15 to 20 min.

They also reduce the amount of general anaesthetics for maintenance (after induction by inducing agents)

PROPOFOL

- it is a IV general anaesthetic.
- commonly used as inducing agent.
- its injection is painful, but adding 20mg of lignocaine to an ampoule of Propofol overcomes this drawback.
- currently propofol is superseded thiopentone as an IV general anaesthetic, both for induction as well as maintenance.
- Unconsciousness after Propofol occurs in 15-30 sec.and lasts for 5-10 min. Shorter duration of action is due to its rapid metabolism.
- Repeated injection can be given for prolonged anaesthesia unlike for Thiopentone.
- There is no respiratory irritation.
- There is smooth and pleasant induction
- There is no nausea, vomiting after anaesthesia
- It is very much suited for outpatient surgery
- In subanaesthetic dose, it is the drug of choice for sedating intubated patients in intensive care unit.
- It does not have analgesic, skeletal muscle relaxant properties

Other uses: In status epilepticus and as inducing agents, in minor surgical procedures.

Adverse effects:Patient's acceptability is good. Pain during I.V infusion is frequent. (lignocaine is mixed with Propofol).

ETOMIDATE : All are similar to Propofol.

THIOPENTONE SODIUM

- It is an I.V general anaesthetic
- Fast inducer, **Mechanism of action** → potentiates GABA
- It produces unconsciousness within 20 seconds and the consciousness is regained within 10 minutes.

- The shorter duration of action is due to its rapid redistribution into fatty tissues, not due to its rapid metabolism or excretion
- Repeated injection will cause saturation of fatty tissues → Thiopentone will leak out→ increase plasma concentration of Thiopentone → prolonged apnoea
- This drug is not suitable for any surgical procedure takes more than 10 minutes. For prolonged anaesthesia either Propofol or Ketamine is preferred.

Other uses: In status epilepticus, for minor surgical procedures.

KETAMINE

It is called as 'dissociative anaesthetic' characterized by amnesia with light sleep and feeling of dissociation from one's own body and surrounding. It is an hallucinogen, hence drug abuse is common.

Clinical uses :

1. Used for operation of head and neck in patients who have bled, in asthmatics, for angiographies, for cardiac catheterization, in short surgery, burn dressing. C/I in hypertensive individual, because of its vasoconstrictor action.

FENTANYL

- It is an opioid analgesic.
- It is an inducing agent and very much useful in painful surgical procedures including burn dressing.
- It reduces the dose of inhalational general anaesthetics.
- Disadvantage- nausea and vomiting.

PREANAESTHETIC MEDICATIONS

Drugs given prior to the administration of general anaesthetics are called 'Preanaesthetic medication'.

AIMS:

1. For relief of anxiety and apprehension (Diazepam or Midazolam is given). They are good amnesic (loss of recall of perioperative events).

2. Anticholinergics like glycopyrrolate is mainly used as prophylatic to prevent laryngospsasm, vagal bradycardia and hypotension which occur refluxly in certain surgical procedure.
3. For relief of pain: Opioid analgesic like Fentanyl is given.
4. For Hypnotic : Diazepam or Zolpidem is given night before operation to have a comfortable sleep.
5. Antiemetic: Domperidone or Ondansetron is given to prevent post-operative nausea and vomiting due to general anaesthetics.
6. To prevent acid regurgitation during caesarean section and other prolonged operations. (Lansoprazole or H_2 antagonist like famotidine)

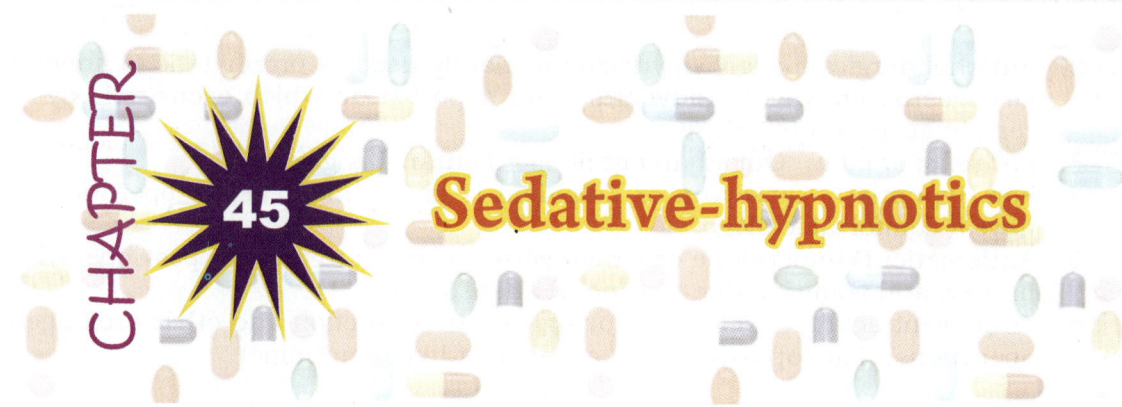

CHAPTER 45 Sedative-hypnotics

- Both are discussed together, because low dose of hypnotic will also act as sedative.
- Sedatives: The drugs which subdue excitement and produce drowsiness without inducing sleep.
- Hypnotics: The drugs which induce sleep (more or less resembling natural sleep, not exactly the natural sleep).
- Sedative action is mainly useful in anxiety.
- Hypnotics are mainly useful in insomnia (loss of sleep).

PHYSIOLOGY OF SLEEP:

Depending upon the movement of eye, the sleep is divided into REM (Rapid Eye Movement) and NREM (Non Rapid Eye Movement). Both types of sleep are important for healthy individuals.

Normally the sleep starts with NREM (light sleep to deep sleep)for about 90 min.and then REM stage starts for 30 min.

Two types of sleep go on alternately throughout the night

NREM : occupy 75% of sleep time, in which the skeletal muscles are relaxed and the maximum growth hormone is secreted. Night walking will be there.

REM SLEEP: dreams and night mares occur, erection of penis etc., Occupy 25% sleep time.Hypnotics suppress this stage more.There is rebound increase in time for REM stage, in which the individuals experience night mare (vivid dream) after withdrawal of hypnotics.

CLASSIFICATION OF SEDATIVES-HYPNOTICS

I. Benzodiazepines:

1. Long acting:
i)   Diazepam (Calmpose, valium)
ii)   Clonazepam
iii)   Nitrazepam, iv) Flurazapam, v) Lorazapam
2.   Short acting:
i)   Alprazolam
ii)   Triazolam,
iii)   Midazolam

Long acting drugs are useful in chronic insomnia, short term insomnia, frequent nocturnal awakenings and night before operation.

Short acting drugs are useful in sleep onset difficulties, unusual timing of sleep.

II. Non Benzodiazepine Derivatives:

1. Zolpidem (zolfresh)
2. Zopiclone

III. Newer Drugs: Ramelteon

IV. Barbiturates: (not used, only toxicological importance)

Earlier Barbiturates (Phenobarbitone) was used as hypnotic. Now, it is completely replaced by Benzodiazepines and Non Benzodiazepines because of the following reasons:

1. Barbiturates are having narrow margin of safety. But Benzodiazepines and Non Benzodiazepines are having wide margin of safety. If anyone takes ten tablets of Barbiturates for suicidal attempts and death is common due to respiratory depression. But even if anyone takes 50 tablets of Benzodiazepines, there won't be any death.
2. Barbiturates inhibit REM stage more. So, they produce rebound increase in REM timings, in which the individuals experience night mares or vivid dreams after withdrawal of the drug. Benzodiazepines will inhibit the REM stage very less and hence less rebound phenomenon.
3. Barbiturates do not have specific antidote. There is only symptomatic treatment in case of poisoning and slow recovery. But Benzodiazepines and Non Benzodiazepines have got specific antidote, Flumazenil, which will reverse the symptoms of overdose Benzodiazepines and Non Benzodiazepines very quickly.
4. Tolerance is common for Barbiturates. But not for Benzodiazepines and Non Benzodiazepines.
5. Barbiturates are enzyme inducers and produce many drug interactions with other drugs. But Benzodiazepines and Non Benzodiazepines are not enzyme inducers.
6. Phenobarbitone poisoning : (Ref. Excretion of drugs)

Pharmacological actions of Diazepam:

I On CNS:

1. Sedative action : Its sedative action is useful in anxiety states. It is produced by half the hypnotic dose of Diazepam.
2. Hypnotic action : Diazepam inhibits REM stage slightly. There will be rebound increase in REM stage time after withdrawal of the hypnotic drug. The individuals experience vivid dreams and night mares.
3. Skeletal muscle relaxation: Spastic muscles are more relaxed, sparing the normal voluntary muscle.

4. Anticonvulsant and antiepileptic actions (convulsion is a violent contraction of skeletal muscles) either tonic (contraction of antagonists muscles simultaneously) or clonic convulsions (contraction and relaxation of skeletal muscles). But epilepsy is convulsions with other symptoms.
5. Analgesia-amnesia (antigrade-loss of memory of recent events) is produced.

BENZODIAZEPINES, DIAZEPAM (CALMPOSE, Valium)

It is mainly sedative-hypnotic.

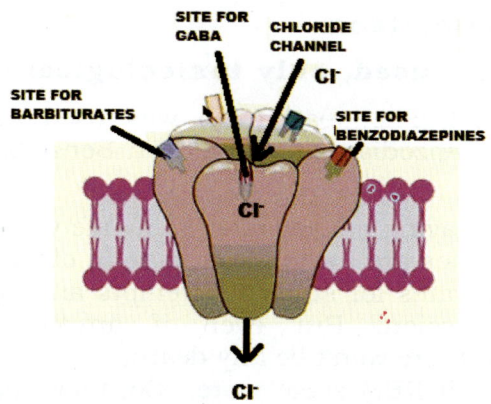

Fig:53 Mechanism of action of Benzodiazepines

Mechanism of action of Benzodiazepines (Fig.53)

Benzodiazepine receptors are present near the $GABA_A$ receptors. GABA is the inhibitory transmitter in CNS.

Benzodiazepines
↓
stimulate the benzodiazepine receptor
↓
enchance GABA binding to $GABA_A$ receptor
↓
modulate (stimulate) the $GABA_A$ receptor which is situated near by
↓
open the chloride channel
↓
increase the flow of chloride ions into the neurons
↓
hyperpolarization of neuronal membrane
↓
decrease synaptic transmission
↓
CNS depressant actions

Anti anxiety (at limbic system)   sedative, hypnotic actions (at RAS)

Sites: Reticular Activating System (hypnotic action), Limbic system (anti anxiety action), Medulla and spinal cord (skeletal muscle relaxant action)

Clinical uses :

I.   As hypnotic : 1.   In insomnia (chronic, short term, and transient). Insomnia refers as in sufficient sleep or poor quality sleep. There is problem of falling asleep (initial insomnia), staying asleep, night awakenings (maintenance insomnia), waking up too early (late insomnia) Long acting drugs are preferred. All the drugs are given at bed time.

i). Chronic insomnia: Lasts longer than 3 weeks due to underlying diseases (malignancy) and psychiatric disorders (long acting drugs are preferred).

ii) Short term insomnia: Lasts for 1 to 3 weeks, due to loss of close relatives (bereavement), loss of job (long acting drugs are preferred)

iii) Transient insomnia: Lasts less than 7 days. It occurs in jet lag, night shift workers, over night train journey (short acting drugs are preferred).

iv) To induce sleep in night before operation to have a comfortable sleep (long acting drugs)

Dose: Diazepam (calmpose, valium) 10 mg/oral

II.   As sedative: To reduce anxiety before surgery (administration of general anaesthetic) as preanaesthetic medication

III.   As anticonvulsant : In drug induced convulsion, in electric shock (given to psychiatric patient) induced convulsion and in febrile convulsion in children (Diazepam suppository)

IV.   As antiepileptic: in status epilepticus (IV Diazepam)

V.   As centrally acting skeletal muscle relaxants: In skeletal muscle spastic disorders like hemiplegia, sprain, dislocation and over stretching of skeletal muscles etc.,

VI.   IV Diazepam produces calmness-amnesia-analgesic actions, are useful in obstetrics.

VII.   In alcohol withdrawal symptoms.

Adverse effects:

Relatively safe drug, hang over and impairment of psychomotor skill in the next day morning are experienced.

Dry mouth, urinary incontinence, slight rebound of REM stage, and hence the individuals will experience vivid dreams (some misuse Alprazolam for this purpose), tolerance, in pregnancy (contraindicated), since it depresses respiration in the neonates.

Antidote: In case of overdose of Benzodiazepines and Non Benzodiazepines: Flumazenil is given by IV route (**other uses** of Flumazenil is to reverse unwanted effects of Benzodiazepines and Non Benzodiazepines)

NON BENZODIAZEPINES: ZOLPIDEM (zolfresh) AND ZOPICLONE

They are Sedative-hypnotic

Mechanism of action

They act through BZD receptors and the mechanism of action is similar to that of Benzodiazepines.

Advantages over Benzodiazepines:

1. They do not alter REM sleep. Hence do not affect the sleep architecture. No rebound phenomenon on withdrawal is seen. They do not cause hangover.
2. They rarely develop tolerance and dependence.
3. Antidote, Flumazenil is available in case of over dose.

But no anticonvulsant/antiepileptic, skeletal muscle relaxant actions for them.

Clinical uses : (very commonly used)

1. In short term insomnia.
2. In sleep onset insomnia
3. To induce comfortable sleep in night before operation.

   Dose : Zolpidem (Zolfresh) – 10 mg/at bed time, Zopiclone – 7.5 mg/at bed time.

Adverse effects: Headache

Hypnotic Dose:

> Diazepam – 10 mg
> Nitrazepam – 5-10 mg
> Lorazepam – 1-2 mg
> Midazolam – 5-10 mg
> Zolpidem – 5-10 mg
> Zopiclone – 5-10 mg

NEWER HYPNOTIC: RAMELTEON (Melatonin analogue)

Melatonin is a hormone secreted from pineal gland during hours of darkness and declines during day time. Ramelteon induces sleep to maintain the circadian rhythm of normal sleep-awake cycle.

Clinical uses :

1. To alleviate the symptoms of jet lag (sleep disturbance will occur, while crossing intercontinental zone by flight). This drug synchronizes to circadian rhythm and induces comfortable sleep in them.
2. In night shift workers (given 2 hrs. before bed time)

Adverse effects: fatigue, dizziness.

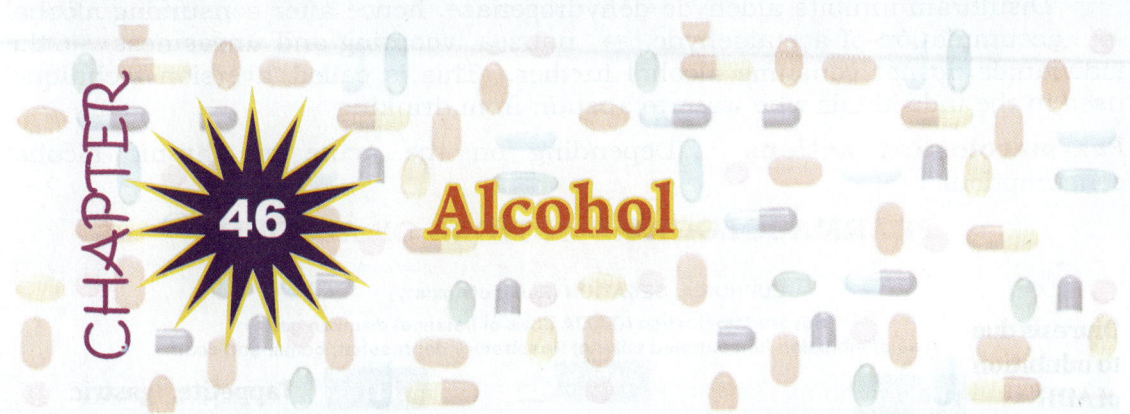

CHAPTER 46 **Alcohol**

It is very important to know by medical graduates to bring public 'awarness' of 'drinking alcohol is injurious to health'

All the liquors available mainly contain ethyl alcohol (ethanol). Methylated spirit , a country liquors contain methyl alcohol, which is highly potent and toxic.

Ethyl alcohol is normally referred as 'alcohol'.

The strength of liquor is expressed as percentage of ethyl alcohol content.

Rum – 50-55% of ethyl alcohol

Brandy, whisky contain- 45-50% of ethyl alcohol

Beer- 5-10 % of ethyl alcohol.

Mechanism of action of Alcohols

Alcohols enhance the action of GABA at $GABA_A$ receptors, which leads to CNS depressant actions.

Also Alcohols inhibit the ability of glutamate to activate NMDA receptors, which leads to CNS depressant actions.

Metabolism of Alcohols:

Ethanol → By alcohol dehydrogenase enzyme → Acetaldehyde → By aldehyde dehydrogenase enzyme → Acetic acid

Clinical significances of metabolism of alcohol: (Mechanism of action of Disulfiram)

Mechanism of action of DISULFIRAM

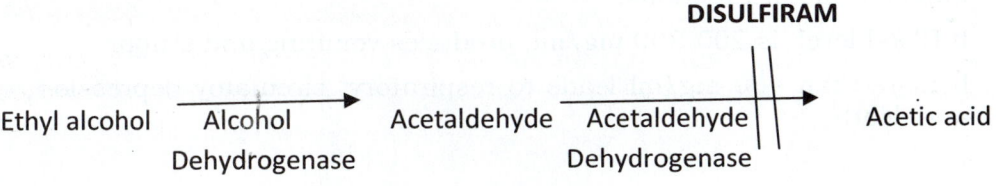

DISULFIRAM

Ethyl alcohol → Alcohol Dehydrogenase → Acetaldehyde → Acetaldehyde Dehydrogenase ⫽→ Acetic acid

Disulfiram inhibits aldehyde dehydrogenase, hence after consuming alcohol → accumulation of acetaldehyde → nausea, vomiting and uneasiness → the individuals do not consume alcohol further. This is called 'aversion technique' used in the individuals who want to abstain from drinking

Pharmacological actions : (Depending on the acute or chronic alcohol consumption)

PHARMACOLOGICAL ACTIONS OF ALCOHOL

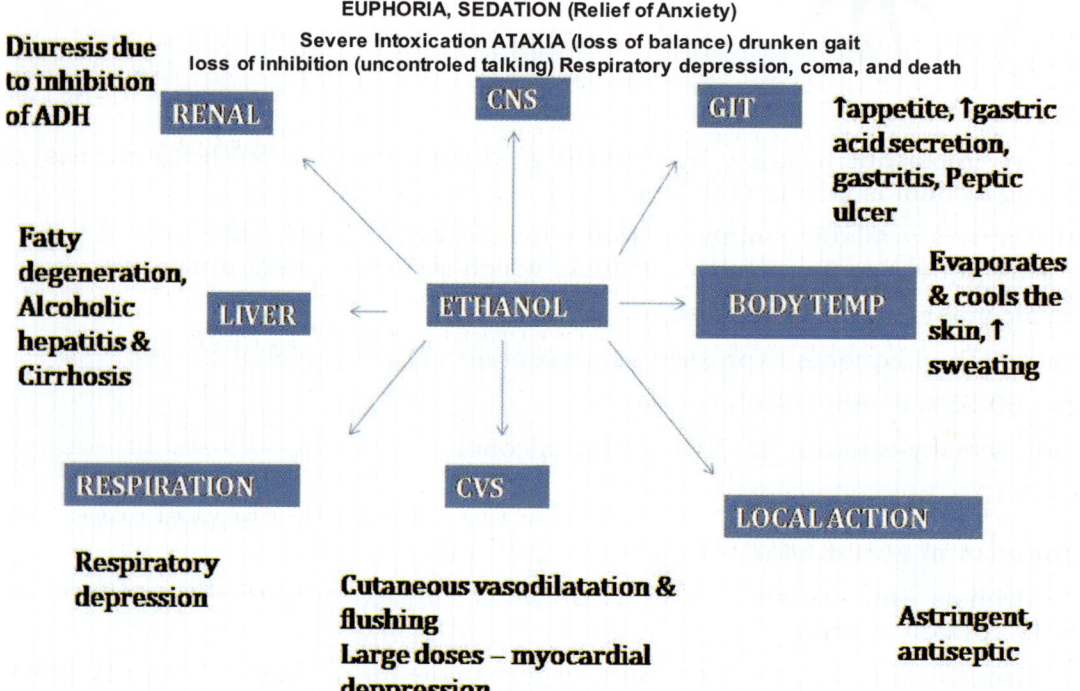

EUPHORIA, SEDATION (Relief of Anxiety)
Severe Intoxication ATAXIA (loss of balance) drunken gait
loss of inhibition (uncontroled talking) Respiratory depression, coma, and death

Diuresis due to inhibition of ADH — **RENAL**

CNS

GIT — ↑appetite, ↑gastric acid secretion, gastritis, Peptic ulcer

Fatty degeneration, Alcoholic hepatitis & Cirrhosis — **LIVER** ← **ETHANOL** → **BODY TEMP** — Evaporates & cools the skin, ↑ sweating

RESPIRATION

CVS

LOCAL ACTION

Respiratory depression

Cutaneous vasodilatation & flushing
Large doses – myocardial deppression

Astringent, antiseptic

Acute Alcohol consumption

1. On CNS: Euphoria → feeling of well being (for which individuals are taking alcohol) Sedation and hence relief of anxiety, loss of inhibition (uncontrolled talking), impaired judgement and driving skill (the blood level is between 50 and 100 mg/dl)

   Gross drunkenness: If blood level is 120-160 mg/dl, then characterized by ATAXIA (loss of balance)- 'drunken gait', mental clouding and grossly impaired motor functions.

   If Blood level is 200-300 mg/ml, produces vomiting and stupor

   If more than 400 mg/ml leads to respiratory, circulatoy depression, coma and death.

2. On smooth muscles and other effects: Cutaneous vasodilatation (feeling of warmth), watery diuresis, aphrodisiac action (provokes sexual desire but takes away performance}

Management of Acute Alcohol Poisoning:

- Only symptomatic.
- Prevent the aspiration of vomitus.
- Maintenance of vital signs.
- Maintenance of electrolyte balance- IV electrolytes.
- Treatment of hypoglycaemia- IV Glucose.
- For vitamin deficiency –IV/IM Thiamine.

Chronic alcohol consumption:

1. On CNS: Tolerance and physical dependence → withdrawal symptoms appear, if they stop taking alcohol. The main withdrawal symptoms are nausea, tremor, hallucination, delirium tremons (confusion, agitation, aggressiveness, hallucination, dysphoria)
2. Neurotoxicity : ATAXIA, dementia and peripheral neuropathy (Thiamine deficiency) in chronic alcoholics, there is impairment of visual acuity with blurring of vision.
3. LIVER AND GIT: HEPATITIS, CIRRHOSIS OF LIVER, BLEEDING OESOPHAGEAL VARICES, CHRONIC PANCREATITIS, INHIBITS ABSORPTION PROCESS- leads to NUTRITIONAL DEFECIENCY, PEPTIC ULCER, ASCITIES AND OEDEMA.
4. CVS: Dilated cardiomyopathy, atrial and ventricular arrhythmias
5. Blood: Alcohol causes Megaloblastic anaemia
6. Endocrines: Testicular atrophy, gynaecomastia, impotence etc., are produced by alcohol.
7. Carcinogenic effect.
8. Precipitate gout.

Management of Chronic Alcohol Toxicity:

For physical dependence and withdrawal symptoms → Diazepam/clonidine.

Management of alcohol dependence:

1. Aversion therapy – Disulfiram (ref: mechanism of action of Disulfiram)
2. Use drugs to reduce 'craving' with similar pharmacological actions and less abuse liability will be substituted → Diazepam is given.
3. To prevent accompanying side effects.
   For depression- anti depressant → Fluoxetine (Selective Serotonin Reuptake Inhibitor) is given.
   For vomiting- antiemetic → Ondansetron is given.

Clinical uses of ETHYL ALCOHOL:

1. As skin antiseptic (Before giving IM/IV injection).
2. As astringent → precipitate superficial protein and hardens the skin → useful to prevent bed sore.

METHYL ALCOHOL (METHANOL)

The illicit liquors mainly contain methyl alcohol

Good euphoric effect, quick onset, very potent and highly toxic.

Metabolism of Methyl alcohol and Treatment of methanol poisoning.

1. Ethyl alcohol competes with Methyl alcohol for the enzyme Alcohol dehydrogenase, prevents the conversion of Methyl alcohol to Formaldehyde (retinal damage) and then Formic acid. Instead of that ethyl alcohol is converted into less toxic Acetaldehyde.
2. Fomepizole- a competitive inhibitor of Alcohol dehydrogenase, prevents the conversion of Methyl alcohol to toxic formaldehyde.

Mechanism of action of FOMEPIZOLE

FOMEPIZOLE

Methyl alcohol $\xrightarrow[\text{Dehydrogenase}]{\text{Alcohol}}$ ⫽→ Formaldehyde ⟶ Formic acid ⟶ **Blindness Death**

3. Dialysis- To eliminate Methanol and its metabolite.
4. Protect eye from light.

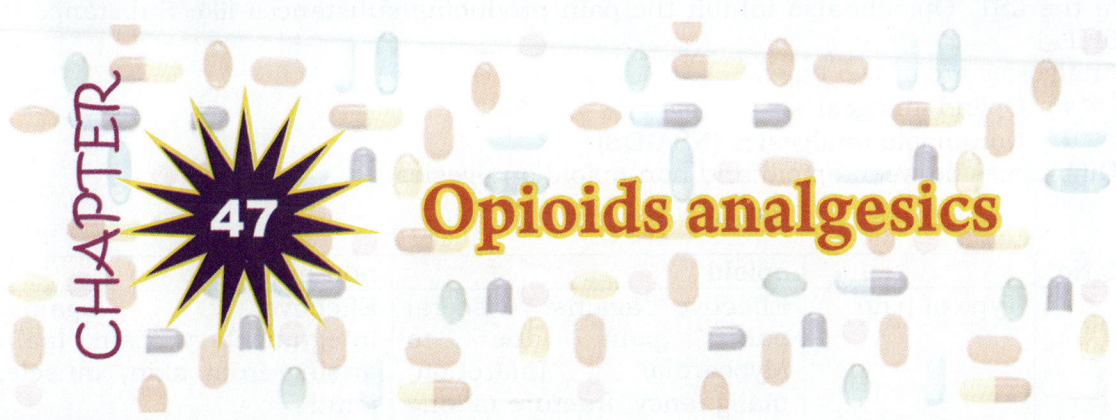

CHAPTER 47 Opioids analgesics

They are opium alkaloids like drugs with analgesic action acting on opioid receptors (mu, kappa, delta).

Opioid alkaloids are obtained from *Papaver somniferum* (poppy seeds)

Opioid alkaloids are

- Morphine
- Codeine
- Thebaine
- Noscapine
- Papaverine

The important opioid analgesic is MORPHINE

Analgesic – the drugs which relieve pain without affecting the consciousness.

Pain transmission:

There are some natural analgesic peptides synthesized and released in the CNS. They are released in response to visceral pain (pain due to Myocardial Infarction, Malignancy, and Fracture of long bone, biliary and renal colic pain). The endogenous opioid peptides are endorphins, enkephalins, dinorphins. They act as opioid analgesic by stimulating opioid receptors – mu, kappa.

Pain impulses are carried from the periphery to the sensory cortex via spinal cord through Lateral Spinothalamic tract (LST) and Thalamus, if the pain is arising from the skin, muscle and joint. But in case of pain arising from the viscera is carried through LST and one part of the impulse from LST goes through Limbic system, where the pain is felt more due to psychological reactions (fear, anxiety and apprehension) to pain. The visceral pain is due to two components i.e., nociceptive component (actual pain) and affective component due to psychological reaction to pain. So, in case of visceral pain the individual experience pain much more than the actual pain. There is also descending nociceptive component, which ends in spinal cord and releases the pain producing substances like Substance P, 5HT etc., Opioid receptors (μ, kappa) are present all over CNS. Stimulation of those receptors will produce analgesic action by inhibiting both the nociceptive component and affective component. Opioids are also increase the pain threshold in the LST. Opioids also inhibit the pain producing substances like Substance P, 5HT.

Analgesics are of two types
- Opioid analgesics
- Non-opioid analgesics (NSAIDS)

Differences between opioid and non-opioid analgesics

S.No.		opioid	non-opioid
	Type of pain	Effective against visceral pain (pain due to Myocardial Infarction, malignancy, fracture of long bones)	Effective against integumentary pain (pain arising from skin, muscle, joints)
	Action on CNS	CNS depressant (Sedative-Hypnotic)	No CNS depressant action (No sedative or Hypnotic)
	On psychological effect	Cause physical dependence tolerance	No tolerance, do not cause physical dependence
	Site of action	Mainly central - ↑pain threshold in LST - ↑μ receptors in thalamus, Limbic system, sensory cortex	Peripheral: They inhibit PGs (pain producing substances) synthesis. They also antipyretic, anti-inflammatory

Classification of opioid analgesics

1. Natural opium alkaloids

- Morphine

- Codeine

2. Semisynthetic Opioids

- Dextropropoxyphene

- Heroin (Diamino morphine) – highly abuse liability, not used clinically

3. Synthetic opioid analgesics

- Pethidine

- Methadone

- Fentanyl

- Tramadol

4. Partial agonist

- Pentazocine

5. Opioids like drugs with no analgesic action

- Loperamide

- Diphenoxylate
- Noscapine
- Pholcodeine

MORPHINE

It is a natural opium alkaloid from papaver sommiferum (poppy seed)
It is one of the most important and potent opioid analgesic.

Orally not effective due to high first pass metabolism (mainly given by S.C. injection)

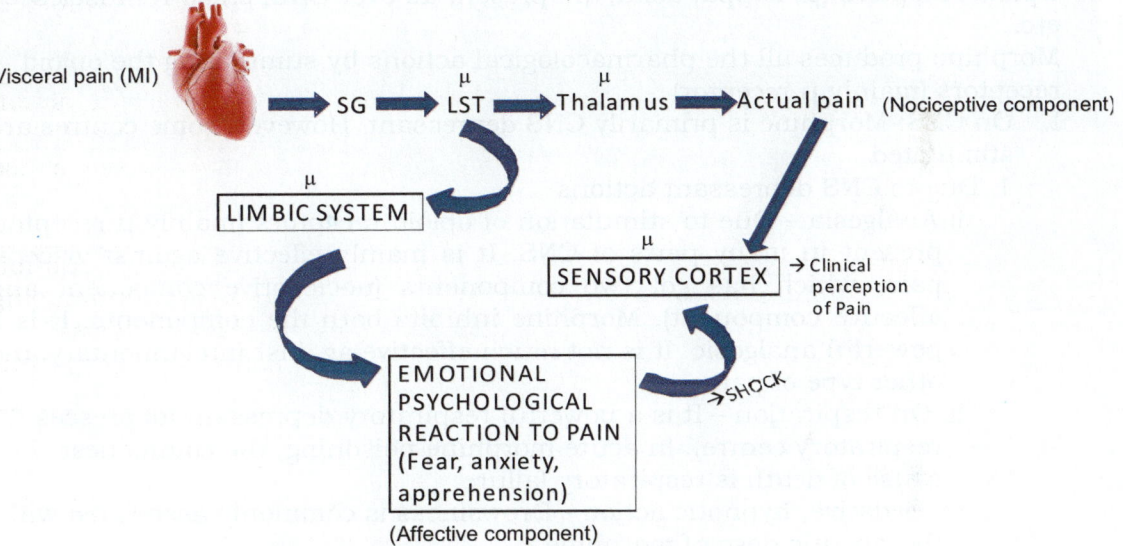

LST – Lateral Spinothalamic tract, SG – Substantia Gelatinosa

Clinical Perception of pain = Nociceptive component + Affective Component

Fig.54 Mechanism of action of Opioid analgesics

Mechanism of action of Opioids (Morphine) (Fig.54)

Sites: Sensory cortex, thalamus, limbic system and LST (Lateral Spino Thalamic Tract)

Receptors: Stimulate 'μ' (mu) receptors present in all the above sites.

1. Inhibits LST, which carry the pain impulse from spinal cord to the cortex (by increasing pain threshold).
2. Very effective against visceral pain (MI, malignancy pain and fracture of long bone etc)
3. Pain from the viscera is felt as two components. One is nociceptive component (actual pain) through Thalamus and another one is psychological reaction to pain (affective component) due to anxiety, fear

and apprehension, through limbic system. Morphine inhibits both the components by stimulating 'μ' receptors.

4   It should not be used against mild pain like headache, because of the danger of dependence.

5   Hypnotic action as synergestic action for analgesic.

6.   Euphoric action (feeling of well being): The individuals feel that pain is no longer unpleasant.

ORALLY NOT EFFECTIVE-GIVEN BY SC INJECTION

Pharmacological actions of Morphine

Opioid receptors (μ, kappa, delta) are present all over CNS, smooth muscles etc.,

Morphine produces all the pharmacological actions by stimulating the opioid receptors (mainly μ receptor)

I.   On CNS: Morphine is primarily CNS depressant. However, some centres are stimulated

   1. Due to CNS depressant actions

      i. Analgesia – Due to stimulation of opioid receptors (mainly μ receptor) present in many parts of CNS. It is mainly effective against visceral pain, which has got two components (nociceptive component and affective component). Morphine inhibits both the components. It is a powerful analgesic. It is not much effective against integumentary and other type of pains.

      ii. On respiration – It is a powerful respiratory depressant (depresses respiratory centre). In acute morphine poisoning, the commonest cause of death is respiratory failure.

      iii. Sedative, hypnotic action - Drowsiness is commonly associated with therapeutic dose of morphine.

      iv. Cough suppressant – morphine inhibits cough centre. But cannot be used because of danger of dependence.

      v. Vasomotor centre – morphine depresses slightly the vasomotor centre – will lead to fall in BP

      vi. Euphoria (feeling of well being) – is due to its action on limbic system. It helps for analgesic action.

   2. Due to CNS stimulant actions:

      i. On CTZ – due to stimulation on CTZ - it produces vomiting, which is one of the most common adverse effects of morphine.

      ii. On eye – pin point pupil – Morphine produces miosis by stimulating the III nerve nucleus. There is no miosis by direct appilication of morphine on eye. The pin point pupil is a diagnostic with respiratory depression in morphine poisoning.

      iii. On vagus – stimulation of vagus centre by morphine causes bradycardia.

II. On smooth muscle

   1. On GIT (μ receptors)

      •   Morphine reduces the gastric motility

- It increases the tone of antrum
- It delays gastric emptying
- It delays the absorption of many drugs
- It reduces the motility of intestine
- It constricts sphincters all over the intestine
- It increases the tone of intestinal muscle
- It reduces the intestinal secretion
- More absorption of water from the intestine
- The intestinal contents become more solid
- It inhibits the sensory defecation reflex, decreases the awareness for the necessity to defecate
- All the above actions lead to spastic constipation

2. On urinary bladder and ureter
   - Morphine constricts external sphincter of urinary bladder
   - Morphine increases tone of ureter
   - It increases the release of ADH and causes urinary retention

3. Biliary tract
   - Morphine constricts the sphincter of oddi
   - Increases intrabiliary pressure. Morphine aggravates biliary colic pain

4. On bronchus
   - Morphine causes bronchoconstriction due to the release of Histamine.

II. On CVS
   - Morphine produces fall in BP (due to histamine release and inhibition of vasomotor centre)

V. On endocrine
   - Morphine inhibits the release of gonadotrophin release hormone and Corticotropin Release Hormone from hypothalamus

Clinical uses of Morphine

1. Mainly as analgesic in visceral pains. It is not much effective in integumentary and other types of pain. In malignancy pain, it is given ORALLY in high dose, since daily injection is troublesome in them.

2. In left ventricular failure
   i. It is effective in relieving dyspnea.
   ii. It relieves anxiety due to dyspnea
   iii. The exact mechanism of action is not clear. However, due to reduction in the workload on heart (reduce preload and afterload) increase the efficiency of ventricles → relieve pulmonary oedema and dyspnea.

   Dose: 5-10 mg/SC, high oral dose is also possible.

Adverse effects:

Vomiting, constipation, urinary retention, bronchoconstriction, miosis, respiratory depression, fall in BP, tolerance and dependence (on prolonged usage).

Contraindications:

1. Head injury:

It is contraindicated to relieve pain due to head injury because Morphine increases intracranial pressure (increased intracranial pressure will be in head injuries). The second reason is that the diagnosis of site of head injury by the eye sign is affected by Morphine.

2. Biliary and ureteric colic pain:

Morphine alone is contraindicated. However, it is given along with atropine.

3. Pancreatitis:

Morphine holds back pancreatic juices and increases serum amylase concentration. Hence it should be avoided in pancreatitis.

4. Bronchial asthma

Morphine aggravates bronchial asthma due to its brochoconstriction action.

5. Pregnancy

Morphine is contraindicated in pregnancy, since it depresses the foetal respiration. (Pethidine depresses very little foetal respiration and hence is preferred as obstetric analgesic to Morphine)

6. In enlarged Prostate

Prolonged administration of Morphine, lead to hypertrophy of prostate.
Acute poisoning: it may be accidental, suicidal or in drug addicts who consume overdose of morphine (more than 50 mg/IM).
Symptoms: Pin Point Pupil, hypotension, respiratory depression, coma → pulmonary oedema →respiratory failure → death.

Treatment of acute Opioids poisoning

Rx
1. Supportive measures
2. Gastric lavage with Potassium permanganate is given to remove unabsorbed Opioids from GIT, if the patient consumed Opioids orally.
3. Specific antidote – Naloxone 0.4-0.8 mg/IV

PETHIDINE

➤ Synthetic opioid analgesic
➤ Less respiratory depression in foetus, hence it is preferred as obstetric analgesia
➤ No cough suppression
➤ Orally effective

Mechanism of Action and clinical uses:

Same as that of Morphine and useful in conditions where Morphine is contraindicated (as obstetric analgesia, where morphine is C/I in pregnancy)

Adverse effects - Resperatory depression

It causes mydriasis but morphine causes miosis

Dose: 50-100 mg/oral, 50 mg/IM

TRAMADOL

ORALLY EFFECTIVE.

Mechanism of action: Similar to that of Morphine and it also stimulates 5 HT release and thus activates spinal inhibition of pain.

Clinical uses :

1. AS ANALGESIC: In visceral pain as alternate to Morphine and Pethidine, because of least physical dependence. It is also suitable in post operative pain and in moderate short lasting pain due to diagnostic procedure, injury and in chronic pain like in malignancy.

Dose: 50-100 mg/oral/IM/IV infusion

Adverse effects: It is well tolerated, nausea, sleepiness, dry mouth, lower seizure threshold and hence it is contraindicated in epilepsy.

FENTANYL (Ref: IV general anaesthetics)

METHADONE

ORALLY EFFECTIVE.

Mechanism of action : Similar to that of morphine.

Less potent, LESS ABUSE LIABILITY (HENCE, IT IS USED IN OPIOID WITHDRAWAL SYMPTOMS)

NALOXONE AND NALTREXONE

- They are specific antidote for opioid poisoning
- They block opioid receptors.
- In opioid poisoning, the death is mainly due to respiratory depression.
- They first reverse the respiratory depression due to opioids poisoning.
- They are not effective to reverse respiratory depression due to any other CNS depressants.
- They reverse all the actions of opioids including analgesic action.
- It will aggravate the opioid withdrawal symptoms, if it is given to opioid dependence (opioid addicts)
- These drugs are given by IV route in opioid poisoning

Clinical uses : ONLY IN OPIOIDS POISONING

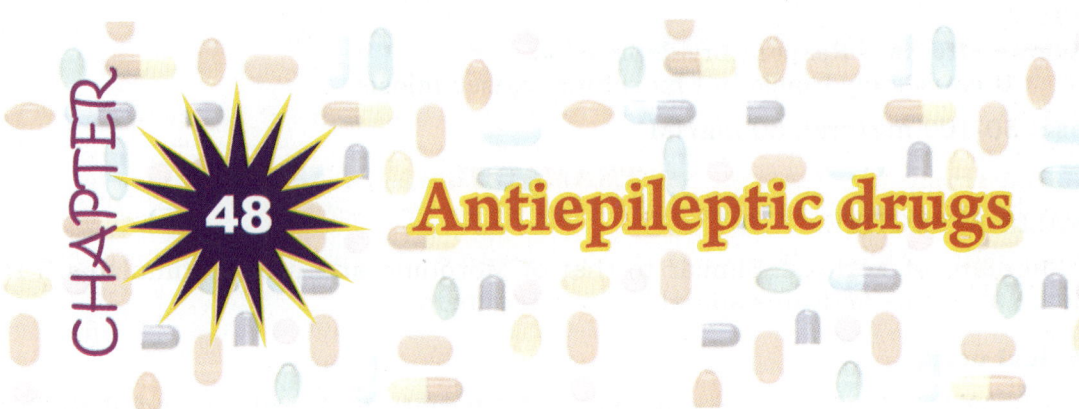

CHAPTER **48** **Antiepileptic drugs**

Types of EPILEPSY

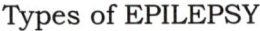

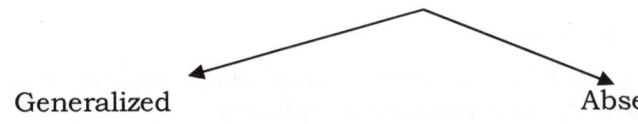

Generalized

(1) Tonic – clonic seizure
    (grandmal epilepsy)
(2) Clonic seizure (petitmal epilepsy)

Absence seizures

1. Psychomotor epilepsy
2. Temporal lobe epilepsy

EPILEPSY is characterized by convulsion and other symptoms depending upon the abnormal, excessive electrical discharge to the surrounding areas of cortex.

- Epilepsy is different from convulsion.
- Convulsion: Violent involuntary contraction of skeletal muscles.
- Tonic convulsion: Both antagonistic muscles are contracted simultaneously.
- Clonic convulsion: Contraction and relaxation of skeletal muscles.

Anti epileptic drugs, which are used to prevent / control epilepsies.

CAUSES of epilepsy:

1   Abnormal foci in the motor cortex are formed due to brain tumour, brain surgery and brain trauma. The excessive electrical discharge from abnormal foci spreads to the surrounding areas of cortex and hence the symptoms other than the seizure.

2 It may be due to genetic factors.

3 Metabolic disorders may also cause epilepsies.

4. Sudden withdrawal of antiepileptic drugs, will lead to status epilepticus.

The important and common form of epilepsy is 'grand mal epilepsy'. (Tonic-clonic seizure) The sequences of grand mal epilepsy are as follows:

First it may precede with an aura or may not. Then the patient undergoes a violent tonic convulsion. The patient falls down. The person becomes unconcious for few minutes and followed by violent clonic convulsion. During clonic convulsion, he may bite his tongue or hurt himself (to prevent biting of tongue, a hard object should be placed in between the teeth, and the tongue is pulled out to prevent respiratory obstruction). He will remain in the ground for few minutes. Then he will regain conscious and get up. He will become normal.

Drugs either inhibit the abnormal foci or spread the electrical discharge by any one of the following mechanisms:

Mechanism of action of antiepileptic drugs

1. Inhibit conductance: Antiepileptic drugs block Na⁺ channel → inhibit the Na⁺ entry into the neurons → prolong the refractory period of the neurons → inhibit the generation and propagation of abnormal electrical impulses (discharge) through neurons. They also produce membrane stabilizing action on neurone → protect the normal neurons → inhibit the conductance of impulses in the neurons, just like the action on heart by Na⁺ channel blockers.

2. Stimulation of NMDA receptors → depolarization of neurons → initiate seizure.

   NMDA receptor blockers → inhibit depolarization → suppress seizure (valproate, lamotrigine)

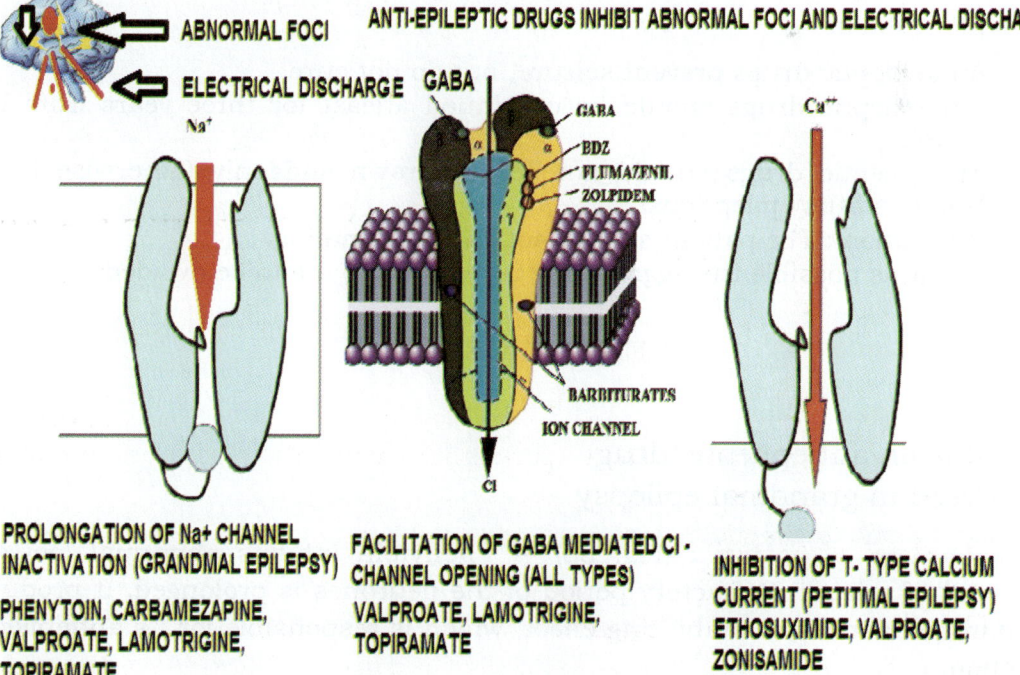

Fig.55 Mechanism of action of Antiepileptic drugs

3   Enhancement of GABA ergic, an inhibitory neurotransmission by opening Cl-channel. (Valproic acid, Vigabatrin).

4   Ca++ entry stimulates neurons. Antiepileptic drugs act by inhibiting Ca++ channel and preventing the entry of Ca++ (Valproic acid, Lamotrigine, Gabapentine) inhibit neurons.

CLASSIFICATION OF ANTIEPILEPTIC DRUGS ACCORDING TO THEIR CLINICAL USES :

I   Drugs effective only in grand mal epilepsy

　1 Phenytoin

　2 Carbamazepine(not used now)

II   Drugs are effective only in petit mal epilepsy: Ethosuximide (not used now)

III   Drugs are effective both in grand mal and petit mal (broad spectrum anti epileptics)-commonly used

　1 Valproic acid

　2   Newer anti epileptics

　　i) Lamotrigine

　　ii) Gabapentine

　　iii) Vigabatrin

　　iv) Pregabalin

- Antiepileptic drugs prevent seizure, but do not cure.
- Antiepileptic drugs should be continued atleast for three years from last attack.
- Antiepileptic drugs should not be withdrawn suddenly (otherwise it will lead to status epilepticus).
- Precaution : The patient should not go for swimming.
- As far as possible the aggravating factors (aura) are to be avoided.

PHENYTOIN SODIUM

- It is an antiepileptic drug
- Used in grandmal epilepsy

Mechanism of action : (Fig. 55) → Phenytoin inhibits abnormal foci and spread of seizure. Refractory period of the neurones is prolonged. It produces neuronal membrane stabilizing effect, which is responsible for its antiepileptic action.

Clinical uses :

1. In grandmal epilepsy ⎤ first line antiepileptic drug,
                              ⎟ but less commonly used now
2. In psychomotor epilepsy ⎟ because of side effects
3. In cardiac arrhythmias ⎦
4. In trigeminal neuralgia (second choice to carbamazepine)

It aggravates petitmal epilepsy.

Adverse effects: are numerous

1. Enzyme induction → reduce the efficacy of many drugs (reduce efficacy of oral contraceptive → failure of contraception), osteomalacia, megaloblastic anaemia (due to increased metabolism of endogenous Vit. D and Folic acid)
2. CNS : cerebellar and vestibular manifestations. ATAXIA, vertigo, nystagmus, diplopia, mental confusion, hallucination etc.,
3. Gum hyperplasia, hirsutism, hyperglycemia
4. In pregnancy→ fetal hydantoin syndrome (cleft palate, hare lip, microcephaly)

Carbamazepine

Carbamazepine is not preferred in epilepsy. Better drugs are available.

Mechanism of action : (Fig.55)

Other Clinical uses:

1. In trigeminal neuralgia → first line drug
2. In manic depressive illness and acute mania (as alternate to Lithium)

Adverse effects: Similar to Phenytoin except gum hyperplasia

VALPROIC ACID

Broad spectrum antiepileptic.

Mechanism of action (Fig.55)

1 It produces prolongation of Na+ inactivated channel by incresing the refractory period of the neurons

2 It causes enhancement of GABAergic activity.

3 It blocks Ca++ channel.

4 It decreases the excitatory transmitter, Glutamate.

Clinical uses :

1 In grand mal epilepsy.

2 In petit mal epilepsy.

3   In infantile spasm.

4   Non anti epileptic use:

   i.   Prophylaxis in migraine.

   ii.   Manic-depressive bipolar disorder (it suppresses mainic phase).

   iii. In trigeminal neuralgia (alternate to Carbamazepine).

Dose : 500 mg – 1 g. (The dose is slowly increased from 500 mg till optimal therapeutic effect is achieved.)

Adverse effects: C/I in pregnancy, long term use → ATAXIA, HYPOALBUMINEMIA, HEPATOTOXIC (REGULAR LIVER FUNCTION TEST IS TO BE DONE), pancreatitis in some

Regular plasma valproic acid to be monitored to keep plasma concentration in steady state level. (80-100 mg/ml.) (Therapeutic drug monitoring is needed)

NEWER ANTI EPILEPTICS

1   Vigabatrin

2   Lamotrigine

3   Gabapentine

4   Pregabalin

Mechanism of action (Fig.55)

1   They activate GABA receptors (Vigabatrine)

2   They inhibit NMDA (N-methyl D Aspartate) receptors (Lamotrigine)

3 They block voltage gated Ca++ channel (Lamotrigine, Gabapentine, Pregabalin)

    The newer anti epileptics drugs are NOT CONTRAINDICATED IN PREGNANCY

Clinical uses :

1   Broad spectrum anti epileptics. (used both in grand mal and petitmal epilepsies)

2 In trigeminal neuralgia (in pregnancy, where Carbamazepine is contraindicated) Pregabalin, Gabapentine are used.

3. In mania

DRUGS USED IN STATUS EPILEPTICUS:

-   It may be due to sudden withdrawal of antiepileptic drug.

1. Lorazepam (IV)

2. Diazepam – 10mg (IV) → standard therapy, repeated after 10 min, if required

3. Fosphenytoin (IV) → 100-150 mg/min/IV infusion

4. Phenobarbitone sodium (IV) 50-100 mg

5. IV general anaesthetics: Propofol, Thiopentone sodium (IV)

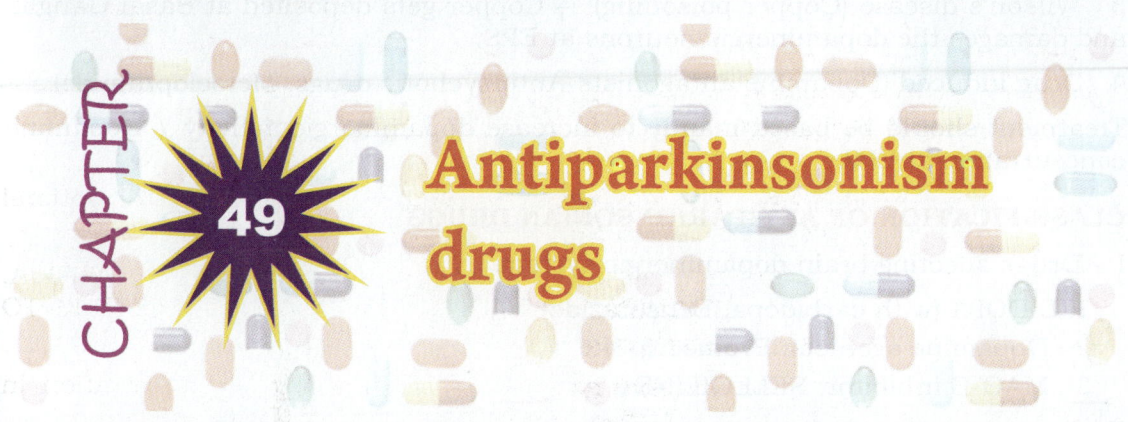

CHAPTER **49**

Antiparkinsonism drugs

Parkinsonism (Paralysis agitans) is a neurodegenerative disorder (disease) of Extra Pyramidal System (Basal ganglia) characterized by bradykinesia (slowness of skeletal muscles movement), rigidity and tremor.

Parkinsonism is due to deficiency of Dopamine or over activity of cholinergic system in the Extra Pyramidal System. Normally over 90% of cases are due to deficiency of Dopamine.

The treatment of Parkinsonism is either by increasing Dopamine concentration or by reducing cholinergic activity or by both in extra pyramidal system.

But Dopamine doesn't cross BBB (Blood Brain Barrier). So, the precursor of Dopamine, L-Dopa, which cross BBB is given

EPS (Extra Pyramidal System) controls finer movement of skeletal muscles.

Symptoms of Parkinsonism:

1   Bradykinesia.
2   Muscular rigidity.
3   Tremor (pill rolling movement).
4   Abnormal gait (No swing movement of hands while walking).
5   Mask like face (expressionless).
6   Oculogyric crisis (eyes are fixed for long time-mechanism is not known)
7   Sialorroea (excessive salivation → due to over activity of cholinergic system)
8   Dementia (unknown reason)
9   If it is not treated in time leads to i)rigid ii) unable to move iii) unable to breath iv) chest infection v) embolism and death.

Possible causes:

1   Mainly loss or damage to dopaminergic neurons at EPS

2 It may be due to toxin, MPTP (N-Methyl 4 Phenyl Tetra hydro Pyridine), causes degeneration of dopaminergic neurons at EPS

3   Wilson's disease (Copper poisoning) → Copper gets deposited at Basal Ganglia and damages the dopaminergic neurons at EPS.

4   Drug induced (Dopamine antagonists-Antipsychotic drugs, Metoclopramide)

Treatment should be based mainly to increase dopaminergic activity / Dopamine concentration at EPS

CLASSIFICATION OF ANTIPARKINSONIAN DRUGS

I   Drugs affecting brain dopaminergic system

1. L-DOPA (with carbidopa, Benserazide)
2   Dopamine agonists: Bromocriptine
3   MAO-B inhibitor: SELEGILINE

II   Drugs affecting cholinergic system

1   Central anticholinergics: i) Trihexyphenidyl (Benzhexol), Benztropine
2   Antihistamines (due to their anticholinergic property): Promethazine

L-DOPA

It is precursor of Dopamine. It is the first choice drug

Mechanism of action (Fig.56)

Dopamine doesn't cross BBB.

L-dopa crosses the BBB and converted into Dopamine by dopa decarboxylase enzyme in the EPS.

But 90% of L-dopa is converted to Dopamine by that enzyme in the periphery. So bioavailabilty is less when L-Dopa is given alone. It is combined with PERIPHERAL Dopa Decarboxylase Inhibitor. Now more than 90% of L-Dopa is available for action at EPS, since peripheral conversion is inhibited by peripheral dopa decarboxylase inhibitors (Carbidopa and Benserazide), which do not cross BBB. Now more L-Dopa crosses BBB and converted into Dopamine by dopa decarboxylase present at EPS. (Fig.56)

Pharmacological actions of L-Dopa with carbidopa: (since L-Dopa is not used alone)

I   On B.G (Basal Ganglia):

Increases DA concentration at B.G → relieve all the symptoms of Parkinsonism like bradykinesia, rigidity resolve first, then tremor and other symptoms gradually disappear.

The secondary symptoms like gait, handwriting, posture, speech and facial expression become normalized.

Life long treatment is needed.

Surgery is preferred for permanent cure in severe cases.

II On mesolimbic system: Frank psychosis (due to increased concentration of dopemine in mesolimbic system).

III On CTZ: Vomiting (Domperidone-anti emetic is given) (ref:anti emetic)

IV Prolactin Release Inhibitory hormone is Dopamine: inhibits Prolactin secretion and milk secretion.

Adverse effects: Facial tick, grimacing, mental confusion, frank psychosis (increase the concentration of Dopamine in mesolimbic area), vomiting etc.,

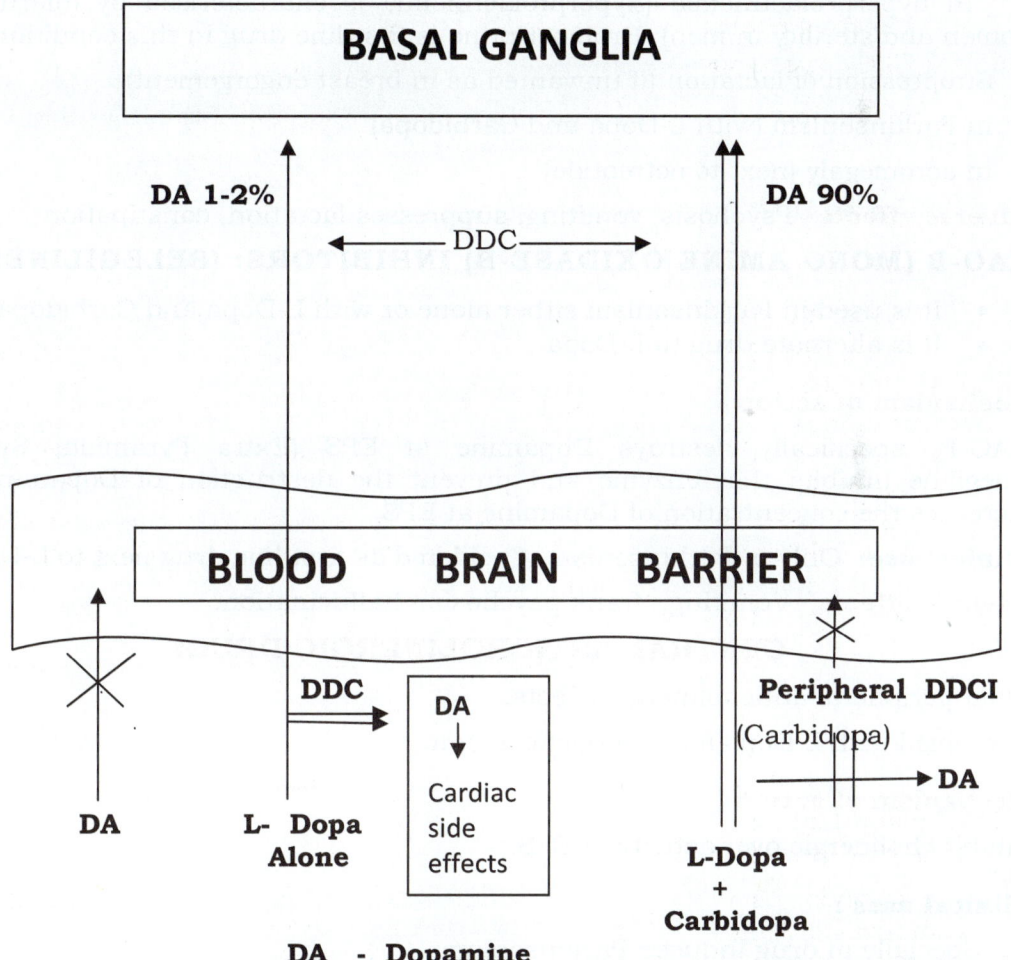

DA - Dopamine
DDC- Dopa Decarboxylase
DDCI – Dopa decarboxylase Inhibitor

Fig.56 Mechanism of action

DOPAMINE AGONIST (BROMOCRIPTINE)

Pharmacological actions :

1   It is a strong antigalactorrhoea (for which it is commonly used)
2   It inhibits Growth hormone in acromegaly.
3   It is a antiparkinsonism drug.
4   It stimulates CTZ and produces vomiting.
5   It stimulates DA_2 receptors in the mesolimbic area causes frank psychosis
6   It inhibits gastric motility and causes constipation.

Clinical uses :

1   In hyperprolactinemia (hyperprolactinemia is characterised by infertility in women and sterility in men). Bromocriptine is first line drug in this condition.

2   Suppression of lactation (if unwanted as in breast engorgement)

3· In Parkinsonism (with L-Dopa and Carbidopa)

4   In acromegaly (next to octreotide)

Adverse effects: Psychosis, vomiting, suppresses lactation, constipation

MAO-B (MONO AMINE OXIDASE-B) INHIBITORS: (SELEGILINE)

- It is used in Parkinsonism either alone or with L-Dopa and Carbidopa.
- It is alternate drug to L-Dopa.

Mechanism of action

MAO-B, specifically destroys Dopamine at EPS (Extra Pyramidal System) Selegiline inhibits that enzyme and prevent the destruction of Dopamine and increases the concentration of Dopamine at EPS.

Clinical use: Only in Parkinsonism. Cosidered as first line drug next to L-Dopa.

Adverse effects: Vomiting, frank psychosis, hallucination.

CENTRAL ANTICHOLINERGIC DRUGS

Least peripheral anticholinergic effects.

Combined with L-Dopa for synergistic action.

Mechanism of action

Inhibit cholinergic over activity at EPS.

Clinical uses :

1   Specially in drug induced Parkinsonism
2   In Parkinsonism along with L-Dopa and Carbidopa

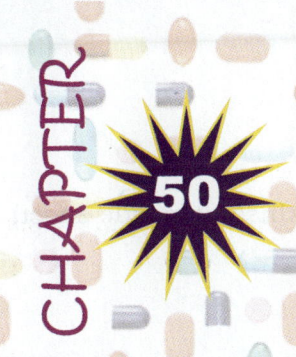

CHAPTER 50

Psychopharmacology-Antipsychotic drugs, antidepressants, antimaniac, antianxiety drugs, substance abuse, cerebroactive drugs and cognitive enhancers

ANTIPSYCHOTIC DRUGS

The Antipsychotic drugs are used in psychosis (Schizophrenia, a common disorder) and other agitated states.

The common features of Schizophrenia include two types of symptoms.

Positive symptoms are characterized by delusions (false belief), hallucinations, visual or auditory (abnormal sensation of vision or sound) or at times aggressive behaviour.

Negative symptoms are characterized by poor socialisation, emotional blunting, lack of motivation, lack of attention and loss of memory. So, disturbances of reasoning or thought process, withdrawal from the surroundings.

- NEUROTRANSMITTERS THEORY OF schizophrenia (split mind) and causes:
- Increased DOPAMINERGIC OR SEROTONINERGIC activity at MESOLIMBIC AREA OF BRAIN
- Organic psychosis is due to some organic diseases like cerebral infection by rabies, brain injury, heavy metal poisoning (anti psychotic drugs are not much useful).
- Functional psychosis: (Schizophrenia- split mind) is a psychiatric disorder characterized by distortion of thought, behaviour (usually aggressiveness) and capacity to recognize realty and distortion of perception (hallucination-visual or auditoty} and delusion (false belief)- (POSITIVE SYMPTOMS)
- Unable to meet ordinary demands due to cognitive deficit, lack of attention, loss of memory, loss of education, loss of interest in neighbours (NEGATIVE SYMPTOMS).
- Antipsychotic drugs are effective only in functional psychosis.
- They are not much effective in organic psychosis.

CLASSIFICATION OF ANTIPSYCHOTIC DRUGS:

 I. Classical/Typical antipsychotic drugs (Since they produce typical parkinsonism side effect)

1) Phenothiazine derivatives
   - Chlorpromazine
   - Trifluperazine
   - Fluphenazine
2) Haloperidol
3) Pimozide

II. Atypical/Novel antipsychotic drugs (No parkinsonism side effect)
   1) Clozapine
   2) Olanzapine
   3) Quetiapine
   4) Risperidone

CHLORPROMAZINE (LARGATIL)

- It is commonly used drug in schizophrenia, since it is cheap. But now a days, it is largely replaced by less toxic atypical antipsychotic drugs.
- The trade name is 'Largactil', since it has got wide range (large number) of pharmacological actions.

Mechanism of action:

As already discussed, the schizophrenia is due to excess dopaminergic activity at mesolimbic area. All typical antipsychotic drugs inhibit DA_2 receptor at mesolimbic area and reverse all the aymptoms of schizophrenia.

- It also inhibits DA_2 receptors at basal ganglia (extra pyramidal systems) and cause parkinsonism symptoms.
- Dopamine is considered as PRIH (Prolactin release inhibitory hormone) from hypothalamus. Since these drugs are antidopaminergic, will produce galactorrhoea (spontaneous milk flow).
- Dopamine stimulates DA_2 receptors at CTZ produce vomiting. Since chlorpromazine is antidopaminergic acts as antiemetic (But not used, since better drugs are available).

Pharmacological actions of chlorpromazine:

I. On CNS:
    1) In schizophrenia : It reverses all the symptoms of schizophrenia slowly. In normal individuals, it produces indifference to surroundings, emotional quitening, reduction in initiative and feeling sleepy.

2) Parkinsonism like symptoms (inhibits DA_2 receptors at Basil ganglia)
3) It is antiemetic (inhibits DA_2 receptors at CTZ)
4) It produces tolerance and dependence

II. On ANS
1) Its α – adrenergic blocking action leads to vasodilatation and fall in B.P.
2) It has got anticholinergic properties : Dryness of mouth, urinary retention, constipation etc.,
3) It has got antihistamine action, local anaesthetic action – not useful clinically.
4) On endocrine
   i. It inhibits the release of PRIH and causes galactorrhoea, gyneacomastia
   ii. It inhibits gonadotropin causes infertility
   iii. It inhibits ADH and increases urine volume.

Trifluoperazine

Fluphenazine, haloperidol are best used in case of acute, severe schizophrenia to control the symptoms immediately. They are given by parenteral administration.

Dose: Chlorpromazine – 100-800mg/oral.

Clinical uses of chlorpromazine:

1) In Schizophrenia: It is not curative. It has to be continued lifelong. It controls the positive symptoms better than negative symptoms. 90% of patients will lead to normal life. It is only for symptomatic treatment. The actual cause is not removed.
2) In intractable hiccups: The mechanism is not known (respond to parenteral therapy).

Adverse effects:

Drowsiness, mental confusion, extra pyramidal disturbances.

Parkinsonism symptoms:

Rigidity, tremor, bradykinesia (partly controlled by centrally acting anticholinergic antiparkinsonism drugs).

Endocrine side effects:

- Galactorrhoea, gynaecomastia, infertility.
- Weight gain.
- α – adrenergic blocking effects : Postural hypotension, impotency.

- Anticholinergic side effects: Dry mouth, blurring of vision, urinary retention and constipation etc.,

ATYPICAL ANTIPSYCHOTIC DRUGS

They are called as atypical antipsychotic drugs because they do not produce typical PARKINSON SYMPTOMS (UNLIKE ATYPICAL ANTIPSYCHOTIC DRUGS). THE MECHANISM OF ACTION IS DIFFERENT FROM TYPICAL ANTIPSYCHOTIC DRUGS.

Examples : OLANZAPINE, RISPERIDONE, QUETIAPINE

Mechanism of action

- They mainly inhibit $5 HT_2$ receptors.
- They produce minimum/no inhibition of DA_2 receptors.
- They do not produce EP side effects/Parkinsonism.
- There are not antiemetic
- They do not produce galactorrhoea action.

Clinical uses :

1 In schizophrenia: They suppress both +ve and –ve symptoms. Paranoid schizophrenia: A form characterized by delusion, often with auditory hallucination with relative preservation of affect and cognitive functions. This condition is treatable by long term use of antipsychotic drugs.

2 In mania.
3 In drug induced hallucination - LSD (Lysergic acid Diethylamide) induced.
4. In trigeminal neuralgia (Where Carbamazepine is contraindicated in pregnancy)
Dose : Olanzapine – 5-10 mg/daily and slowly increased upto 20 mg/daily
Clozepine – initially 12.5 mg/daily slowly increased upto 100 mg/daily.
Risperidone – 1mg twice daily and slowly increased upto 3 mg twice daily.

Adverse effects:

Olanzepine : weight gain, worsening of diabetes, increased incidence of stroke
Clozepine : Sedation, tachycardia, weight gain
Risperidone : increased risk of stroke in elderly.

ANTIDEPRESSANT DRUGS (MOOD ELEVATORS)

- Unipolar depression is a disorder of MOOD (not disorder of THOUGHT PROCESS AS IN SCHIZOPHRENIA).
- Common one is reactive depression, characterized by disproportionate feeling of grief, anxiety and sadness as a consequence of physical illness (like cancer), unemployment, bereavement of loved one (death of close relatives) or due to some social problems.

Endogenous depression:

- Bipolar depression (Manic Depressive Illness-MDI) is characterized by alternate of depression and mania.
- Drugs used in unipolar depression (Antidepressants are useful)
- Neurotransmitters theory of depression:
- Reduced NORADRENERGIC and 5 HT activity IN MESOLIMBIC AREA, leads to MENTAL DEPRESSION.
- Antidepressants increase Noradrenaline or 5 HT concentrations / activity in Mesolimbic area of the brain.

ANTIDEPRESSANT DRUGS:

I. Classical/typical antidepressants:

1. Tri Cyclic Antidepressant (TCA): Imipramine like drugs

II. Atypical antidepressants:

1. SSRI (Selective Serotonin Reuptake Inhibitors): FLUOXETINE, Duloxetine

2. Newer antidepressants:

i) Trazadone

ii) Nafazodone

iii) Mirtazapine

iv) Bupropion

TYPICAL ANTIDEPRESSANTS; IMIPRAMINE

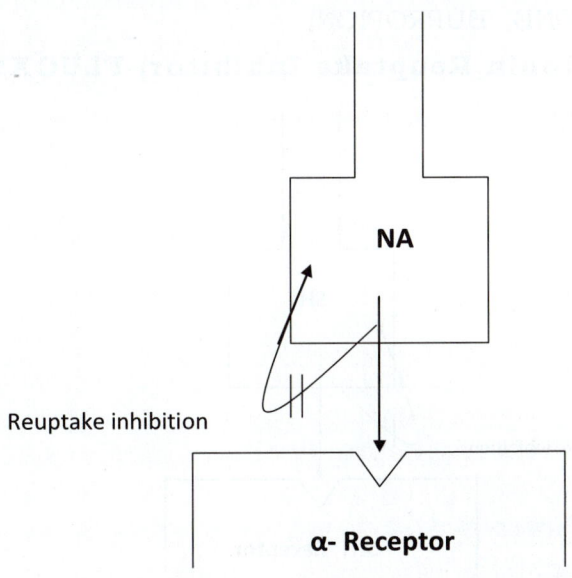

Fig.57 Noradrenaline reuptake inhibition

MEHANISM OF ACTION OF TCA (Fig.57)

Inhibits reuptake of Noradrenaline from the nerve ending.

Increase the concentration of Noradrenaline in the mesolimbic area of the brain and periphery.

Other effects:

1. Anticholinergic: Dry mouth, blurring of vision, photophobia, urinary retention etc.,

2. α blocking action: postural hypotension, impotence etc.,

Slow onset of action

Clinical uses :

1. In endogenous depression

2. In Attention Deficit Hyperkinetic Disorder in children (ADHD)

3. In phobic states

4. Obsessive-compulsive disorder

5. Enuresis and bed wetting in children

6. In neuropathic pain

Adverse effects: 1. Anticholinergic 2. α_1 blocking actions

ATYPICAL ANTIDEPRESSANTS

They are called 'atypical', since they do not produce the adverse effects of typical antidepressant and the mechanism of action is different from that of typical antidepressants.

DRUGS: (SSRIs, TRAZODONE, BUPROPION)

SSRI (Selective Serotonin Reuptake Inhibitor)-FLUOXETINE:

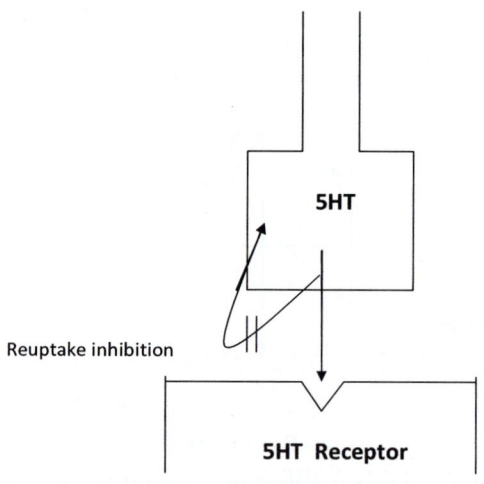

Fig.58 5HT reuptake inhibition

MEHANISM OF ACTION OF SSRI (Fig.58)

Selectively inhibits the reuptake of 5 HT (5 Hydroxy Tryptamine) only from the nerve ending in the mesolimbic area of the brain. Hence, antidepressant action.

Do not inhibit the reuptake of Noradrenaline

It is not anticholinergic and there is no α_1 blocking adverse effects

Clinical uses : 1. In endogenous depression (first choice drug, quick onset of action unlike the typical antidepressants, which are slow in onset)

2. In Obssessive-Compulsive Disorder (OCD)

3. In blumia nervosa (habit of excess eating)

4. In kleptomania (uncontrollable habit of stealing)

5. In phobic states (school phobia, phobia due to public appearance for the first time, afraid of being lonely)

Dose : 10-20 mg/daily

Adverse effects: Nausea, loose stool

NEWER ANTIDEPRESSANTS:TRAZADONE, BUPROPION

Mechanism of action

- Selectively inhibit the reuptake of 5 HT and increase the concentration of 5 HT in the mesolimbic area of brain → antidepressants.
- No anticholinergic/No α blocking adverse effects.
- Quick onset of action.

Clinical uses : In endogenous depression only

ANTI MANIAC DRUGS

Mania is a mental disorder characterized by agitation, hyperexcitability, hyperactivity (mental stimulant).

The causes for mania

1. Increased concentration of DA, 5HT and Noradrenaline in the mesolimbic area of the brain.
2. Increased neuronal activity.

DRUGS:

1. Lithium carbonate (toxic drug and kept as reserve)
2. Antiepileptic drugs – Carbamazepine, valproic acid, newer antiepileptic drugs.
3. Atypical antipsychotic drugs Olanzepine, Risperidone.

Mechanism of action of antimanic drugs:

1. Lithium carbonate
    -   It reduces Dopamine/Noradrenaline concentration at mesolimbic area
    -   It also potentiates GABAergic neuron.
2. Antiepileptic drugs
    -   They inhibit Na^+ entry into neurons → prolong the refractory period in the neurons → inhibit the hyperexcitability and hyperactivity.
    -   They potentiate GABA ergic activity in the neurons
3. Atypical Antipsychotic drugs
    -   They inhibit 5 HT receptors in the mesolimbic area and suppress mania.

LITHIUM CARBONATE (MOOD STABILIZER):

Mechanism of action

The exact mechanism is not known

-   It inhibits IP_3 concentration and reduces the sensitivity of some neurones to the actions of various neurotransmitters.
-   It modifies GABA activity.
-   It inhibits the synthesis of Dopamine and Noradrenaline in the limbic area of brain

Clinical uses :

1. In MDI (toxic drug, so less toxic drugs are preferred- see below)

2. Increases Leukocyte count and hence it is useful in anticancer drugs induced leukopenia

Adverse effects: Fine tremor, hypothyroidism, nephrogenic diabetes insipidus , oedema
Other drugs used in mania.
Carbamazepine, valproic acid, atypical antipsychotic drugs etc.,

ANTIANXIETY DRUGS

-   Anxiety is a feeling of apprehension, uncertainity and fear without apparent stimulus, associated with physiological sympathetic over activity (tachycardia, sweating, tension, tremor and palpitation)
-   Some degree of anxiety is a part of normal life. Treatment is needed when it is disproportionate to the situation.
-   Anxiety is seen in worrying situation and apprehension is associated with examination fear, job interview or public address.

DRUGS:

I. Benzodiazepines: Diazepam, Lorazepam, Oxazepam, Alprazolam etc., (SEDATIVE action is useful in anxiety)

2. β adrenergic blocking agents: (reduce sympathetic over activity in anxiety) Propranolol, Atenolol

3. Atypical anxiolytic: BUSPIRON

- **Mechanism of action** It suppresses 5 HT neurotransmission. Delay in onset. It is not suitable in acute anxiety
- It does not produce SEDATION, REBOUND ANXIETY AND INSOMNIA

Adverse effects: Miosis

SUBSTANCE ABUSE (Fig.52A - Page 215)

Better to call substance abuse, instead of drug abuse. As per the definition of drug is that a drug should be beneficial to the individuals. But here, these substances are producing harmful effects to the individuals. So, better to call as 'substance abuse'

Abuse means, that any misuse of CNS STIMULANTS OR CNS DEPRESSANTS is called as 'abuse'

- Substance dependence is more or less similar to substance abuse.
- Dependence is of two types: 1. psychological dependence and 2. physical dependence
- Psychological dependence: Any individual depending on a substance (not on medical ground) psychologically, examples: coffee, tea, cigarette etc. There won't be any harm to that individual, if they stop taking those substances. Severe psychological dependence → LSD (Lysergic acid diethylamide), Marihuana (Bhang), alcohol. Moderate use of those substances may cause mild physical dependence.

Physical dependence: Any individual is depending on a substance compulsorily (there will be intolerable withdrawal symptoms appear if he stops / withdraws the drugs). There will be substance seeking (craving) behaviour in that individual.

Physical dependence can be called, if the following symptoms appear:

1. Development of tolerance.
2. Distressful withdrawal syndromes after cessation of the substance.
3. Persistent desire to use the drug (craving).
4. Substance use in larger amount than intended.
5. Withdrawal from social, occupational or recreational activities.

Withdrawal symptoms: The symptoms that occur opposite to the previous actions of substance after withdrawal, for example: The individual experience euphoria (feeling of well being, for which the substances are abused) first, and after withdrawal the individual experiences dysphoria (feeling of unwell being) and intolerable tachycardia, tension, nervousness, irritability etc., To prevent the withdrawal symptoms, one has to take the drug continuously. The withdrawal symptoms are due to rebound phenomenon

Example of substances which produce physical dependence:

- Opium alkaloids like Morphine, Pethidine, Heroin etc., and alcohol heavy use

- Severe withdrawal symptoms appear after cessation of the substance.
- In Opioid withdrawal symptoms: Methadone is substituted and then Methadone is withdrawn, since it produces mild withdrawal symptoms.
- In Alcohol withdrawal symptoms: Clonidine, Diazepam are given.
- Site of action of substance abuse: In limbic area, which controls behaviour, emotion etc.
- Receptors involved: 'μ' receptors for opioids, DA, NMDA, GABA receptors for other substances.
- EUPHORIA is the main action produced by all the substances.
- The common withdrawal symptom for all substances abuse is DYSPHORIA.

COGNITION ENHANCERS OR CEREBROACTIVE DRUGS

These drugs are used in dementia and other cerebral disorders.

Dementia: Refers to acquired impairment of cognitive functions (intellect, memory and personality)

Memory: Capacity to solve the problems of day to day life, performance of learned motor skills are primarily affected.

Alzhiemer's disease: A progressive neurodegerative disorder, which normally affects old people and is the most common cause of dementia. There is marked cholinergic deficiency in the cortex and subcortical areas. Atrophy of cortical and subcortical areas is seen.

Receptors involved: Cholinergic, NMDA, GABA

Other causes: cerebral thrombosis and infarct.

DRUGS:

1. Cholinergic activators: Tacrine, Rivastigmine (Anticholinesterases)
2. Glutamate (NMDA receptors) antagonist: Memantine
3. Cerebroactive drugs: Piracetam, Ginkgo biloba

Clinical uses :

1. Senile dementia of Alzheimer type and multi infarct dementia.
2. A memory disturbance in elderly.
3. Mental retardation in children, learning defects, attention deficit disorder.

Possible Mechanism of action of cognition enhancers:

1. Increase cerebral blood flow.
2. Improve neuronal metabolism.
3. Enhancement of neurotransmission.
4. Improvement of cerebral function (memory).

MEMANTINE (new drug)

It is a cerebroactive drug.

Mechanism of action It is a NMDA receptors antagonist.

Clinical uses : as above.

Ginkgo biloba: A Chinese plant extract is a PAF (Platelet Activating Factor) antagonist. It is useful in cerebral thrombosis and infarct. It prevents cerebral impairment of MID (Multiple Infarct Dementia)

SECTION VIII

BLOOD AND BLOOD FORMING ORGANS

BLOOD

Learning objectives

- To know the types of anaemias due to the deficiency of Iron, Vitamin B_{12}, Folic acid and management of them
- To enumerate the drugs used in thrombo-embolic disorders (coagulants, anticoagulants, antiplatelets, fibrinolytics) and their uses

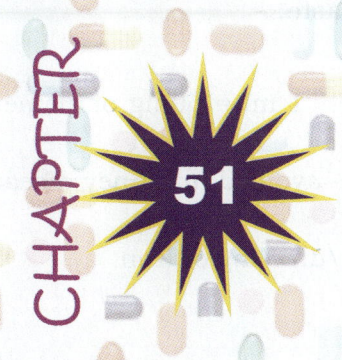

CHAPTER
51

Haematinics- Iron, Vit. B12, Folic acid and Erythropoietin

HAEMATINICS

Haematinics are the drugs which improve the quality/quantity of blood.

1. Iron
2. Vit B_{12} and Folic acid
3. Erythropoietin

IRON

- Iron is necessary for the formation of haemoglobin, which carries Oxygen through blood to all over the body
- Requirement of Iron is increased in women during pregnancy and lactation
- The main use of the Iron salts is in Iron deficiency anaemia/microcytic hypochromic anaemia
- Total body Iron is 3.5-4g (75% circulates in the blood as Hb).
- Each molecule of Hb has 33% of elemental Iron
- Loss of 100 ml of blood=loss of 50mg of elemental Iron
- Daily requirement of Iron in male is 1mg
- But pregnancy, lactating women need higher Iron 3-5mg/daily
- Sources of Iron: liver, egg yolk, chicken, fish are good sources of Iron
- pulses, dry fruits, wheat grain, banana are moderate sources of Iron

IRON PREPARATION

ORAL IRON :

1. Ferrous sulphate (commonly used preparation, it is cheap)=32% elemental Iron
2. Ferrous gluconate= 12% elemental Iron
3. Ferrous fumerate=33% elemental Iron
4. Ferrous succinate =35% elemental Iron (better absorbed, less bowel upset, but expensive)

Clinical uses : 1. In Iron deficiency anaemia

Ferrous sulphate (200mg) for 1-2 weeks, increases Hb by 1g% in 6 months

Adverse effects: due to elemental Iron: Epigastric pain, heart burn, NAUSEA , VOMITING, staining the teeth, constipation, metallic taste.

PARENTERAL IRON:

1. Iron-Dextran(IM/IV)- can be given in renal failure. 1 ml = 60mg of elemental Iron

2. Iron-Sorbitol-Citric acid (only IM) 'Z' track injection- avoided in kidney diseases. 1 ml = 60mg of elemental Iron

Dose calculation=4.4 x Body weight(kg) x Hb deficit (g/dl) = mg of Iron

Indications for parenteral Iron:

1. If oral Iron is not tolerated due to bowel upset

2. Failure to absorb oral Iron

3. Non compliance to oral Iron

4. In the presence of severe Iron deficiency with chronic bleeding

5. Along with Erythropoietin (oral Iron is not sufficient)

Adverse effects: pain at the site of injection, fever, headache, flushing, palpitation

Clinical uses: 1. In Iron deficiency anaemia (microcytic hyprochromic) due to deficient of Hb synthesis as prophylactic and treatment, nutritional deficiency in chronic bleeding from GIT (peptic ulcer, hook worm infestation), pregnancy etc.,

2. In megaloblastic anaemia (along with Vit. B_{12} and Folic acid)

Acute Iron poisoning:

Symptoms: Haematemesis, diarrhoea, abdominal pain, cyanosis, dehydration, acidosis, shock, cardiovascular collapse.

Treatment:

I. To prevent further absorption from GIT

   - gastric lavage with sodium bicarbonate to render Iron insoluble and induce vomiting

   - egg yolk forms insoluble complex with Iron, which is not absorbed

II. To bind and remove already absorbed Iron

   • Desferrioxamine (Iron chelating agent-IV) and also given by orally to prevent further absorption of Iron present in GIT (ref: chelating agents)

MATURATION FACTORS (Vit.B_{12} AND FOLIC ACID)

The deficiency of maturation factors   → megaloblastic anaemia or macrocytic anaemia, due to accumulation of large red cell precursors (megaloblast) in bone marrow and their large and short lived progeny in peripheral blood

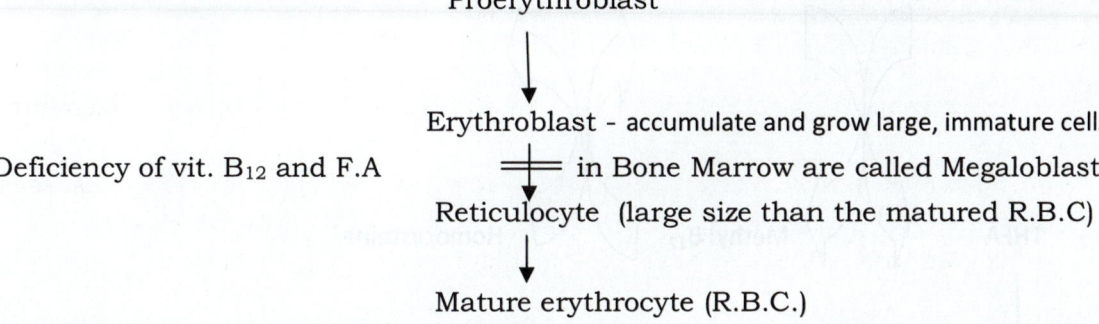

Proerythroblast

↓

Erythroblast - accumulate and grow large, immature cells

Deficiency of vit. B$_{12}$ and F.A ══ in Bone Marrow are called Megaloblast

Reticulocyte (large size than the matured R.B.C)

↓

Mature erythrocyte (R.B.C.)

Basic defect is in DNA synthesis. Deficiency of vit. B$_{12}$ and F.A → inhibit DNA synthesis → ↓ (inhibit) haemopoietic system → ↓ (inhibit) maturation of erythroblast to reticulocyte and also other rapidly proliferating tissues are also affected (GIT)

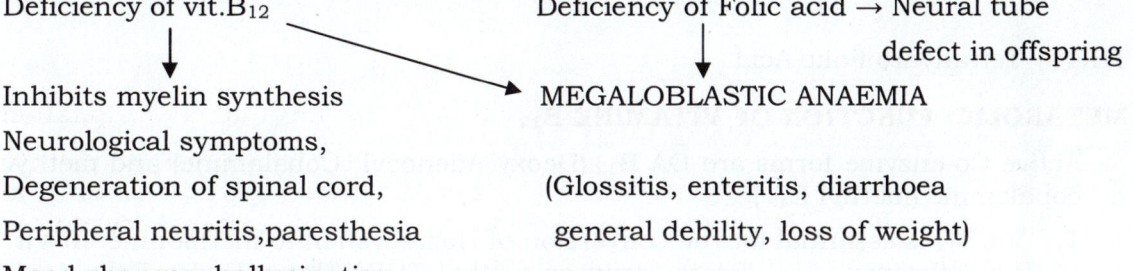

Deficiency of vit.B$_{12}$

↓

Inhibits myelin synthesis

Neurological symptoms,

Degeneration of spinal cord,

Peripheral neuritis,paresthesia

Mood changes, hallucination

Deficiency of Folic acid → Neural tube
defect in offspring

↓

MEGALOBLASTIC ANAEMIA

(Glossitis, enteritis, diarrhoea
general debility, loss of weight)

VITAMIN-B$_{12}$

Preparatiions: Cynocobalamine and Hydroxycobalamine

It is Water soluble vitamin.

It is absorbed from GIT with the help of intrinsic factor synthesized in parietal cells of stomach. In pernicious anaemia, the parietal cells are destroyed due to immune disorders and Vit. B$_{12}$ is not absorbed from GIT.

Daily requirement: 1-3 micro gm. Stored in the liver (4-5 yrs)

Sources:

1. Synthesized in nature only by microorganisms
2. Plants and animals acquire it from them
3. Liver, kidney, sea fish, egg yolk, meat are other sources of vit.B$_{12}$.
4. Only vegetable source is legumes (pulses)-megaloblastic anaemia is common among vegetarians
5. Commercial sources: Streptomycin griseus as a by-product of Streptomycin synthesis

Metabolic functions of Vit. B$_{12}$

Independent function as well as interlinked with Folic Acid

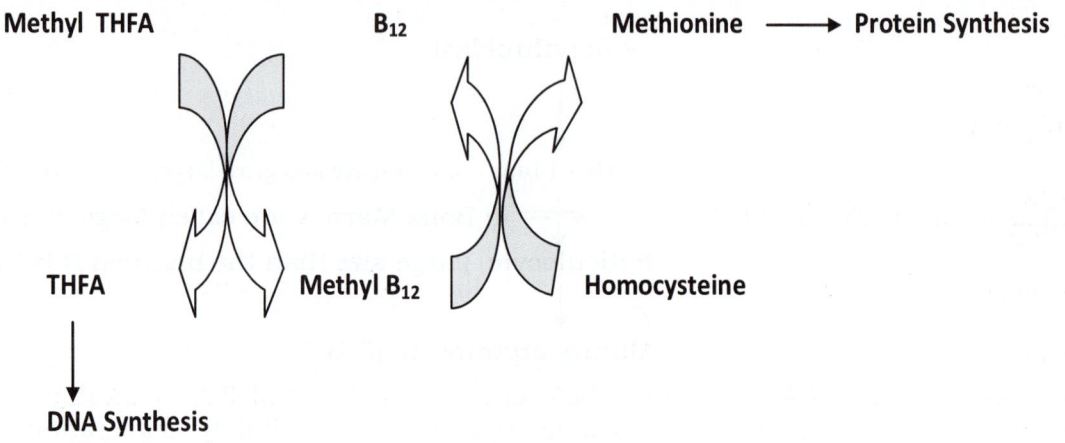

Fig. 59 Synthesis of DNA by Vitamin B$_{12}$

THFA – Tetrahydro Folic Acid

METABOLIC FUNCTION OF VITAMINE B$_{12}$

Active Co-enzyme forms are DA B$_{12}$ (Deoxy Adenosyl Cobalamine) and methyl cobalamine (methyl B$_{12}$)

1. Vit.B$_{12}$ is essential for the conversion of Homocystien to methionine. In Vit. B$_{12}$ deficiency → 'folate ' trap as methyl THFA (Tetra Hydro Folic Acid) → one carbon transfer reaction suffers → ↓ (inhibits) purin-pyrimidine synthesis → ↓ (inhibits) DNA synthesis in BM (Bone Marrow) → ↓(inhibits) maturation of erythroblast to reticulocyte → megaloblastic anaemia

2. Malonic acid $\xrightarrow{\text{DAB}_{12}}$ succinic acid. It links metabolism that is essential for the synthesis of myelin sheath.

3. Methionine $\xrightarrow{\text{DAB}_{12}}$ S-adenosyl methionine needed for the synthesis (folate is not involved) of phospholipids and myelin sheath

Clinical uses : 1. In Vit. B$_{12}$ deficiency (megaloblastic anaemia) (oral) due to gastritis, gastric carcinoma, pregnancy, nutritional deficiency, malabsorption syndrome. The response is dramatic. It is given along with folic acid. It improves apetite and the patient feels better. The neurological symptoms improve slowly

In pernicious anaemia (lack of intrinsic factor, which helps for the absorption of Vit.B$_{12}$ from GIT), it is given by intramuscular injection.

Dose : Cobalamine 500 – 1000 µg/oral 500 µg/IM

Adverse effects: rare

Megaloblastic anaemia

Normal	In Megaloblastic
Vit B_{12}/FA	Deficiency of vit. B_{12} and FA
↓	↓
Synthesis of purine/ pyrimidine bases	reduced formation of Purine / pyrimidine bases
↓	↓
Synthesis of DNA	inhibition of DNA synthesis
↓	↓
Haemopoiesis	inhibits maturation of erythroblast and RBC
	↓
	Megaloblastic anaemia

Metabolic functions of Vit B_{12} / Folic Acid

Deficiency of Vit B_{12}	Deficiency of Folic acid
↓	↓
Inhibits conversion of Homocystien to Methionine	Reduced formation of DHFA
	↓
	Reduced formation of THFA
↓	↓
'folate' trap as methyl THFA (Tetra Hydro Folic Acid)	THFA is essential for the formation of Thymidylate, which is essential for the synthesis of DNA
↓	↓
one carbon transfer reaction suffers	Inhibits the formation of Thymidylate
↓	↓
(inhibits) purin-pyrimidine synthesis	Inhibit DNA synthesis in BM
↓	↓
megaloblastic anaemia	(inhibits) maturation of erythroblast to reticulocyte
↓	↓
(inhibits) DNA synthesis in BM (Bone Marrow)	Accumulation of immature and large sized megaloblast in Bone Marrow
↓	↓
(inhibits) maturation of erythroblast to reticulocyte	megaloblastic anaemia
↓	
Accumulation of immature and large sized megaloblast in Bone Marrow	
↓	
megaloblastic anaemia	

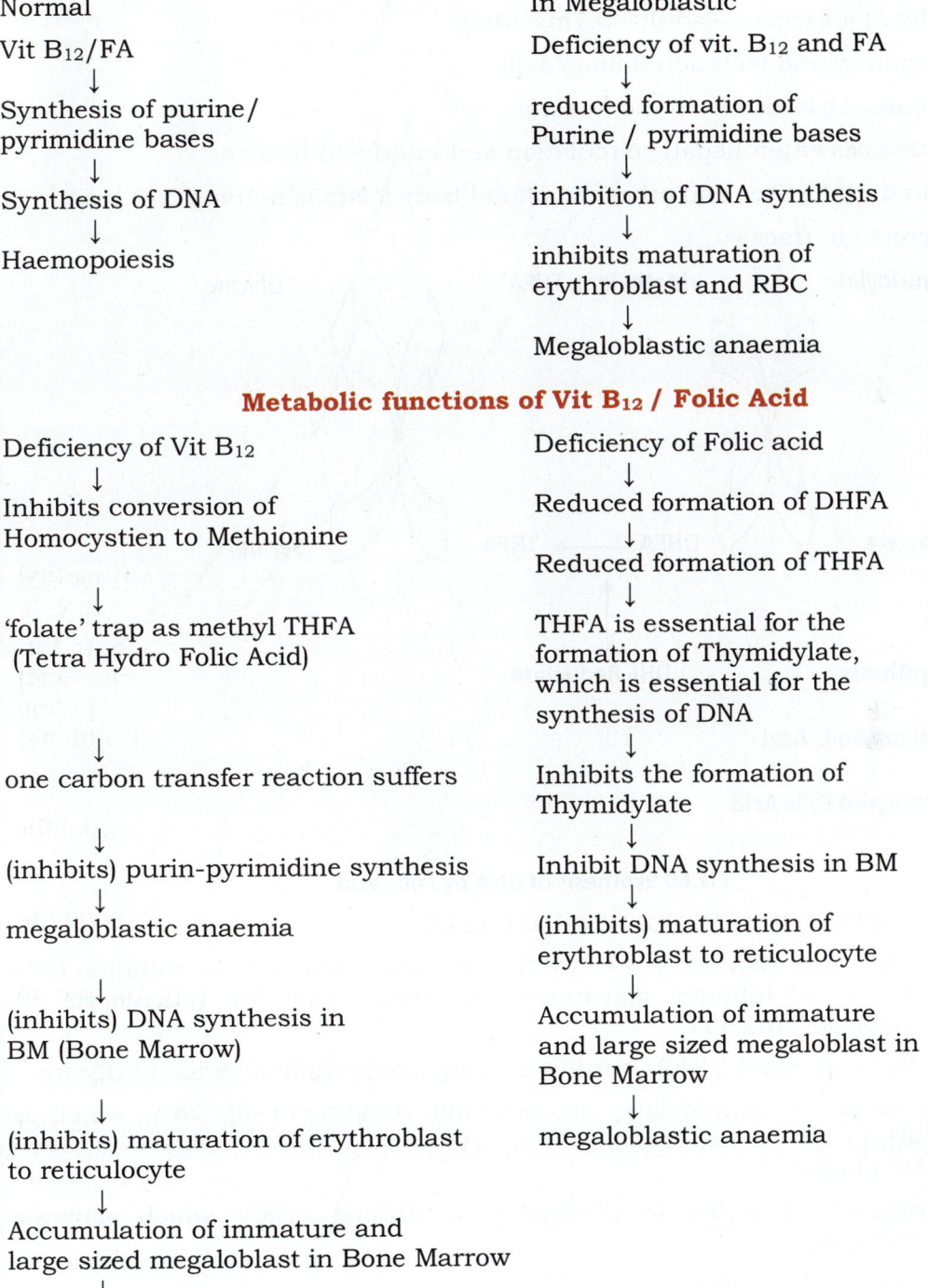

FOLIC ACID (F.A.)

- Dietary sources: Liver, green leafy vegetable (Folia),egg, meat, milk etc.
- Daily requirement – adult- 0.1mg /daily
- Pregnancy and lactation:0.8mg/daily
- Storage: absorbed from the intestine
- Undergoes enterohepatic circulation and interfered by acid
- Stored in the liver and other cells (total body folate is 6-10mg (2-3 yrs)
- Excreted in traces

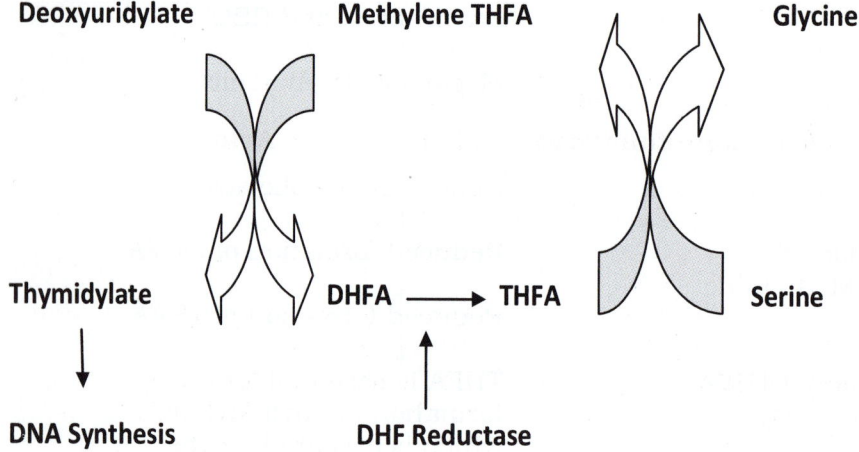

DHFA – Dihydro Folic Acid

THFA – Tetrahydro Folic Acid

Fig.60 Synthesis of DNA by Folic acid

METABOLIC FUNCTION OF FOLIC ACID (Fig.60)

1. In Folic acid deficiency → No thymidylate formation → inhibits DNA synthesis → inhibits maturation of erythroblast to reticulocyte → megaloblastic anaemia.

2. Vit. B_{12} → releases THFA → utilized for the conversion of serine to Glycine

3. Generation of thymidylate, an essential constituent of DNA, which is important for the maturation of Pro-Erythroblast to Erythroblast and then to reticulocyte

4. Conversion of Serine to Glycine → methylene THFA, which generate thymidylate.

Dose : Folic acid 5-10 mg/oral, 5 mg/IM.

Clinical uses : 1. In folate deficiency (due to inadequate dietary intake, malabsorption, chronic alcoholism, increased demand as in pregnancy and lactation and in long term use of antiepileptic drugs like Phenytoin, Phenobarbitone, which are enzyme inducers.

2. In Methotrexate toxicity and in high dose of Methotrexate in malignancy: It is given as folinic acid followed by Methotrexate to rescue the normal cell recovery.

3. In megaloblastic anaemia with Vit.B$_{12}$

4. It is also given in pregnancy to prevent neural tube defect in offspring.

ERYTHROPOIETIN

Erythropoietin is essential for normal erythropoiesis

It is produced from the peritubular cells of kidney

Secretion: Anaemia and hypoxia are sensed by kidney cells and induce rapid secretion of Erythropoietin, which acts on erythroid marrow and 1. Stimulates proliferation of colony forming cells of the eryhroid series. 2. Induces haemoglobin formation and erythroblast maturation. 3. Releases reticulocyte in the circulation

It has no effect on RBC life span

Clinical uses :

1. The primary indication is in anaemia with renal failure
2. Anaemia in AIDS patients treated with zidovudin
3. Cancer chemotherapy induced anaemia
4. To increase preoperative blood production for autologous transfusion in surgery

Dose : 2000-4000 IU/IM.

Adverse effects: increased clot formation, hypertensive episodes, serious thrombo-embolic events, flu like symptoms

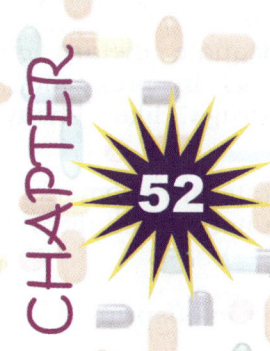

Drugs used in thrombo-embolic disorders- Coagulants, anticoagulants, antiplatelets and fibrinolytic drugs

CHAPTER 52

DRUGS USED IN THROMBO-EMBOLIC DISORDERS

I.   Drugs effective in venous thrombosis (both prophylaxis and treatment)

     ANTICOAGULANTS

II.   Drugs effective in arterial thrombosis (only prophylaxis)

     ANTIPLATELET DRUGS

III.   Drugs effective in both arterial and venous thrombosis (only treatment and not for prophylaxis) THEY DISSOLVE ALREADY FORMED THROMBUS

     FIBRINOLYTIC AGENTS

COAGULANTS

Substances which promote coagulation and are indicated in haemorrhagic states.:

1. Vit.K (K_1, K_2, K_3)-Phytonadione, Menadione
2. Fibrinogen (fresh whole blood or plasma)
3. Antihaemophilic factor (used in haemophilia only)
4. Adrenochrome monosemi carbazone (for epistaxis)
5. Ethamsylate (used in prevention and treatment of capillary bleeding in menorrhagia, after tooth extraction etc.)
6. Local haemostatics (styptics)-for epistaxis like bleeding

    i)   Thrombin

    ii)   Fibrin

    iii)   Gelatin foam

    iv)   Russel viper venom(local application)

    v)   Vasoconstrictors (Adr 1%)

    vi)   Astringents

VITAMIN-K

- It is a fat soluble vitamin

- Essential for the synthesis of clotting factors II(prothrombin), VII, IX AND X IN LIVER

- Deficiency is due to liver diseases, malabsorption syndromes, long term antimicrobial therapy etc.

- Symptoms: HAEMATURIA-FIRST TO OCCUR, other sites of bleeding are in GIT, nose, under the skin

Mechanism of action

- It acts as cofactor → synthesis of coagulation proteins like factors II, VII, IX AND X in LIVER.

Clinical uses:

1. In dietary deficiency- very rare

2. In liver diseases (cirrhosis, viral hepatitis)

3. In obstructive jaundice or malabsorption syndrome

4. In prolonged antimicrobial therapy (bacterial flora in the GIT, synthesise vit.K. If antimicrobial therapy is given for long time → ↓ (inhibit) the bacterial flora and synthesis of Vit.K is reduced.

5. In new born (some cases of haemorrhagic diseases)

6. To reverse the effect of overdose of oral anticoagulants

Adverse effects: fall in BP, flushing, breathlessness etc

Pathophysiology of Thrombo-embolic Disoders

- COAGULATION FACTORS are in balanced with ANTITHROMBIN, PROTEIN-C, FIBRINOLYSIN, ANTITHROMBOPLASTIN (Normally antithrombin side is dominant, and hence blood is in fluid state (free from thrombosis)

- If coagulation factors are activated, intra vascular clot occur → THROMBOSIS

- mainly venous thrombosis (coagulation factors in the venous blood are activated in bedridden or stagnation of blood in the vein and heart for long time and in atrial fibrillation, drug induced (by O.C.P. on long term use, in which Estrogen stimulates the synthesis of some clotting factors) → initiate venous thrombosis (red thrombus) and pulmonary embolism (common). The common symptom of venous thrombosis is pain in the leg and swelling.

- On the contrary, arterial thrombosis (white thrombus) is mainly due to platelet aggregation with fibrin.

- Arterial thrombosis will cause Myocardial Infarction (heart attack), cerebral thrombosis (transient ischaemic attack, stroke)

- Drugs which inactivate the coagulation factors are effective in venous thrombosis (anticoagulants)- both for prophylaxis and treatment
- Drugs which inhibit platelet aggregation are effective in arterial thrombosis (antiplatelet drugs)-prophylaxis only
- Drugs which lyse the already formed thrombi (arterial and venous thrombosis)- Fibrinolytic agents – Treatment only. But not useful for prophylaxis.

ANTICOAGULANTS

Drugs which prevent clot/coagulation of blood

CLASSIFICATION OF ANTICOAGULANTS:

I.   Parenteral (act both in vivo and vitro)

    1. Heparin and LMW (Low Molecular Weight) Heparin

II.   Oral anticoagulants (act only in vivo)
    1. Dicuumarol
    2. Warfarin sodium
    3. Pheninedione

III. Used in vitro only (in vivo, they are highly toxic) Useful for the collection of blood for Lab. test

    i)   Sodium citrate
    ii)   Sodium Oxalate
    iii)   Sodium edetate

HEPARIN

- Medical student, Mc. Lean discovered Heparin
- First, it was found in the mast cells of liver, hence the name
- Later it was found abundant in lungs, intestinal mucosa of Ox and Pig, which are the normal source of Heparin
- Heparin is mucopolysaccharide with high molecular weight (recently it was found that Low Molecular Weight-LMW Heparin more potent).
- It carries strong electro negative charge.
- IT DOES NOT CROSS PLACENTAL BARRIER (HENCE CHOICE IN PREGNANCY)
- IT IS NOT EFFECTIVE ORALLY (BECAUSE OF BIG MOLECULE AND HIGHLY IONIZED). GIVEN by SC/IV INJECTION

Actions: 1. It is an Anticoagulant 2. It is an Antiplatelet drug

Mechanism of action As anticoagulant

- It is a powerful anticoagulant.
- It carries strong electro negative charge
- Site of action of Heparin is in the blood
- Coagulation factors carry strong electro positive charge.
- Heparin forms the complex with coagulation factors and inactivates them

- The very important action is that stimulation of

$$
\text{Heparin} \xrightarrow{\quad\quad} \text{(activates) Antithrombin III} \xrightarrow{\quad\quad}
\begin{array}{c}
\text{Antithrombin III} \\
\text{Activated} \\
\text{thrombin} \\
\text{Ixa, Xa} \\
\downarrow \\
\text{Inactivated} \\
\text{thrombin,} \\
\text{X, IX} \\
\downarrow \\
\text{Anticoagulant} \\
\text{action.}
\end{array}
$$

- It also inhibits the conversion of Fibrinogen to Fibrin
- - The onset of action of Heparin is very quick and short duration. LMW Heparin is long acting.
- It is effective anticoagulant both in vivo and in vitro

Clinical uses :

1.   IN DEEP VEIN THROMBOSIS AND PULMONARY EMBOLISM (BOTH AS PROPHYLAXIS AND TREATMENT)

2.   In MI (inferior to antiplatelet drugs)

3.   Unstable angina (Short term use → reduce the occurance of MI in unstable angina patients

4.   In Rheumatic heart disease, Atrial fibrillation- prevents stroke due to embolism from fibrillating heart

5.   In vascular surgery, prosthetic heart valve, retinal vessels thrombosis, extracorporeal circulation and in haemodialysis with antiplatelet drugs prevents thrombo-embolism

6. In haematoma and thrombophlebitis

Heparinised blood is not suitable for blood count (alters the shape of RBC and WBC), fragility testing and compliment fixation test

Dose: 5,000- 10,000 IU/IV infusion as long as required

LMW Heparin-20-40mg/SC/once daily

MECHANISM OF ACTION OF ANTICOAGULANT DRUGS

EXTRINSIC PATHWAY

Tissue Trauma

(OAC) VII

TF

VII a

Ca++

X ⟶ Xa (H)

INTRINSIC PATHWAY

Contact with damaged endothelial cell

XII ⟶ XIIa (H)

XIa ⟵ XI (OAC)

(H)

Ca++

IXa ⟵ IX (OAC)

(H)

X (OAC)

THROMBOPLASTIN

Ca++

(OAC)

LIVER ⟶╫ **PROTHROMBIN II** ⟶ **THROMBIN II a** (H)

FIBRIN ⟶ **FIBRIN INSOLUBLE**

OAC- Oral Anticoagulant (Inhibit SYNTHESIS of factors) , H- Heparin, 'a ' – activation factors,

(H) – inhibits activated coagulation factors.

Adverse effects: BLEEDING (antidote is Protamine sulphate), reversible alopecia. hypersensitive reaction (not for LMW Heparin)

Advantages of LMW Heparin:

1. It is long acting (SC/once daily)

2. It causes less bleeding (less effect on factor II)

3. It does not affect clotting time (hence no need for lab test for dose control)- given on the basis of body weight

4. It is equally effective as unfractioned Heparin

ORAL ANTICOAGULANTS (O.A.C.) (WARFARIN SODIUM)

Dicumarol, Acenocumarol, warfarin sodium

- They are EFFECTIVE ORALLY
- They are EFFECTIVE ONLY IN VIVO
- The onset of action is slow (the circulating prothrombin should be cleared before it starts acting in 1-2 days)
- The prolonged duration of action for OAC is because of protein bound
- They are mainly used as maintenance therapy after initial therapy with Heparin for 1 or 2 days

Mechanism of action

- Competitive antagonist of Vit.K
- Vit.K acts as cofactor and is essential for the synthesis of factors II (prothrombin), VII, IX and X in the liver. Oral anticoagulants act by competing with Vit.K ↓(inhibit) the synthesis of all the above coagulation factors in the LIVER → Anticoagulant action.

Clinical uses : AS THAT OF HEPARIN

- **Dose** regulation INR – International Normalised Ratio (ratio between the prothrombin time before and after oral anticoagulant therapy). The INR should be kept as 2:3

Adverse effects: Bleeding (antidote is Vit.K). Other adverse effects are similar to Heparin

1. Protein binding: Aspirin displaces Warfarin from protein binding site and increase the toxicity of Warfarin

2. Metronidazole inhibits the metabolism of Warfarin and increases the toxicity of Warfarin

3. Broad spectrum antibiotics inhibit gut flora and inhibit the synthesis of Vit.K → ↑ (enhance) the anticoagulant action of Warfarin

4. With enzyme inducer like Rifampicin, the efficacy of Warfarin is reduced

THE DIFFERENCES BETWEEN HEPARIN AND ORAL ANTICOAGULANTS (WARFARIN)

S.No		Heparin	Oral Anticoagulants
1	Chemistry	Mucopolysaccharide	Coumarin derivatives
2	Source	Hog lungs, pig's intestine	Synthetic
3	R.O.A	Parenteral (SC/IV)	Oral
4	Onset of Action	Immediate	Slow
5	Duration of action	4 - 6 Hours	3 - 7 days
6	Activity	Active both vivo & vitro	Effective only in vivo
7	Mechanism of action	Stimulate Anti-thrombin III & inactivates factor X	Inhibits synthesis of clotting factors in the liver
8	Antagonist	Protamine sulphate	Vitamin K
9	Lab control	Clotting time	Prothrombin time (INR)
10	Drug Interactions	Few	Plenty
11	USES	For initiation therapy in (thromboembolic disorders)	As maintenance therapy

ANTIPLATELET DRUGS (ANTI THROMBOTIC)

- Antiplatelet drugs that interfere with platelet function (inhibit platelet aggregation and adhesion) and prevent the formation of arterial thrombosis further. But they do not affect the already formed thrombus.
- Arterial thrombosis is due to platelet aggregation with Fibrin
- Hence, these drugs are mainly used as prophylactic in arterial thrombosis and not for the treatment.

DRUGS:

1. Low dose Aspirin (Ecosprin) (75mg-350mg/daily). The normal analgesic dose is 500mg/3/daily

2. Clopidogrel

3. Ticlopidine

4. Glycoprotein (GP) IIb / IIIa inhibitors - Absciximab

LOW DOSE ASPIRIN (75 – 350mg)

Mechanism of action (Fig.61)

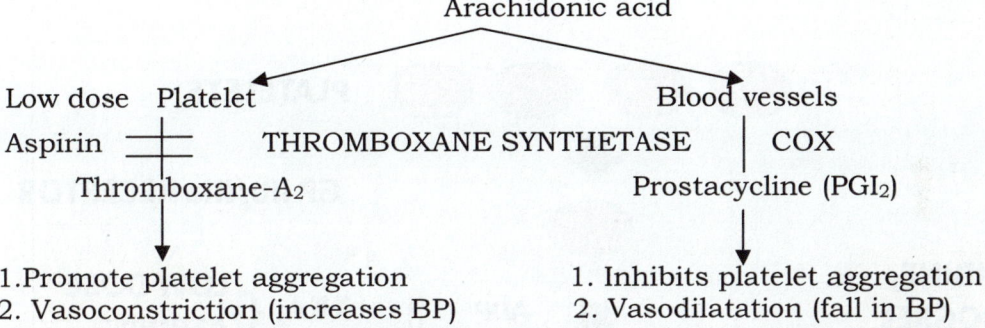

Arachidonic acid

Low dose   Platelet   Blood vessels

Aspirin   ╪   THROMBOXANE SYNTHETASE | COX

Thromboxane-A_2 Prostacycline (PGI_2)

1.Promote platelet aggregation   1. Inhibits platelet aggregation
2. Vasoconstriction (increases BP)   2. Vasodilatation (fall in BP)

The low dose Aspirin specifically inhibits Thromboxane-A_2 synthesis without affecting Prostacycline synthesis. Hence, it is a good antiplatelet, cheap and are having less side effects for long term use.

Clinical uses :

1. In pregnancy induced hypertension

2. In coronary thrombosis (MI), cerebral thrombosis (stroke). It prevents re-infarction and reocclusion after fibrinolytic therapy. It reduces the incidence of coronary and cerebral thrombosis.

3. In unstable angina (reduces the risk of MI)

4. In coronary bypass implant, the patency of the implanted bypass vessels is improved and incidence of reocclusion is reduced. In coronary angioplasty, coronary stent procedure, it reduces the incidence of stent thrombosis.

5.   In prosthetic heart valves, arterio-venous shunt it is given with Heparin/O.A.C., it reduces the formation of microthrombi on artificial heart valve and the incidence of embolism. It also prolongs the patency of chronic arterio-venous shunt implanted for haemodialysis

6.   In colonic cancer and polyps. It is due to increased concentration of Thromboxane-A_2

7. It slows the progression of cataract.

Adverse effects: less than that of in normal dose. But displaces Warfarin from its binding site and increases the toxicity of Warfarin (the dose of Warfarin is reduced)

GP IIb / IIIa receptor inhibitor : ABCIXIMAB

- It is a monoclonal antibody.
- It binds to GP IIb / IIIa receptor and inhibits fibrinogen cross-linking of platelet. It prevents platelet aggregation and the formation of arterial thrombosis (Fig.61)

Fig: 61 Mechanism of action of antiplatelet drugs

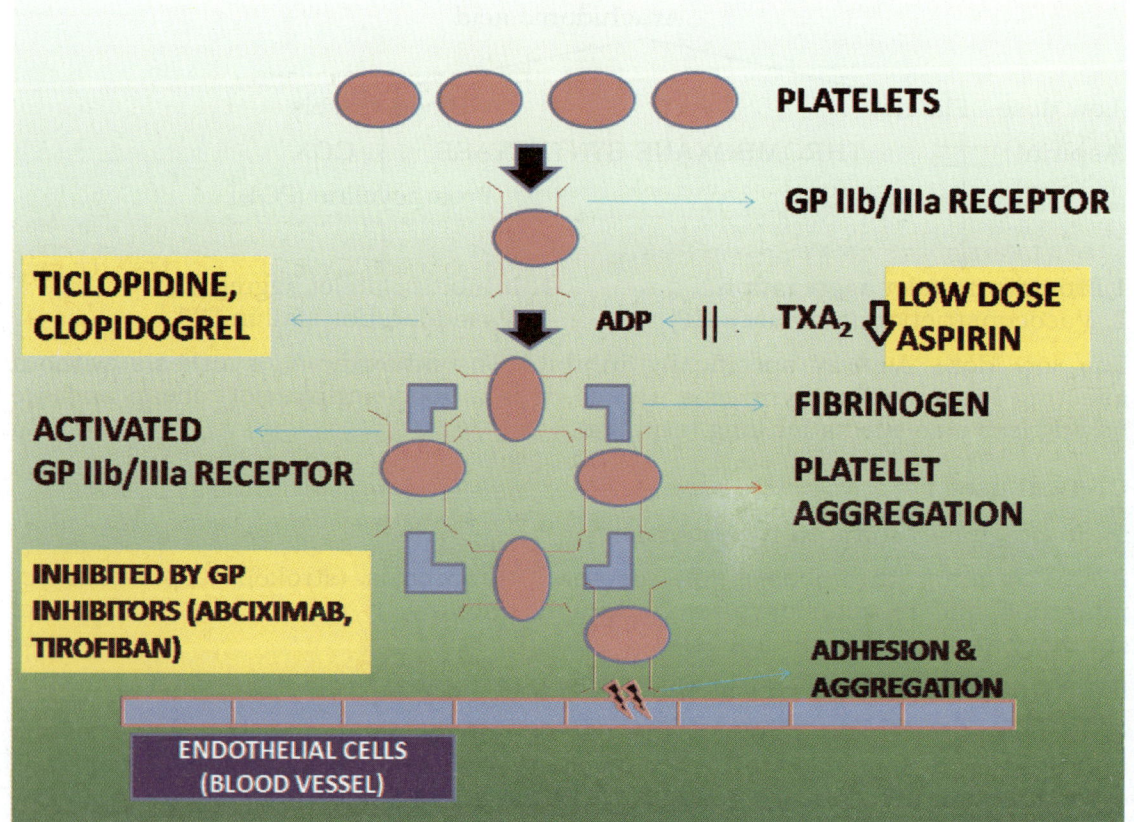

TICLOPIDINE

- It is an antiplatelet drug
- **Mechanism of action** : (Fig.61) Acts on receptors in platelets and inhibits ADP (Adenosine di-phosphate) as well as Fibrinogen induced platelet aggregation (ADP and FIBRINOGEN are powerful platelet aggregator)
- Synergistic action with low dose Aspirin, because of its different sites of action and different mechanism of action

Clinical uses : Same antiplatelet use as that of low dose Aspirin

Adverse effects: occasionally thrombocytopenia

CLOPIDOGREL

- Better tolerated
- Similar mechanism like that of Ticlopidine
- Alternate to low dose Aspirin

FIBRINOLYTIC AGENTS (THROMBOLYTICS)

DRUGS:

1. Streptokinase

2. Urokinase

3. Alteplase (rt PA- recombinant tissue plasminogen activator)

Mechanism of action

They are Plasminogen activators. Plasminogen is converted into plasmin by Plasminogen activator, Plasmin inturn converts the insoluble fibrin (Thrombus) to soluble fibrin (Thrombolytic action)

Mechanism of action of FIBRINOLYTIC AGENT

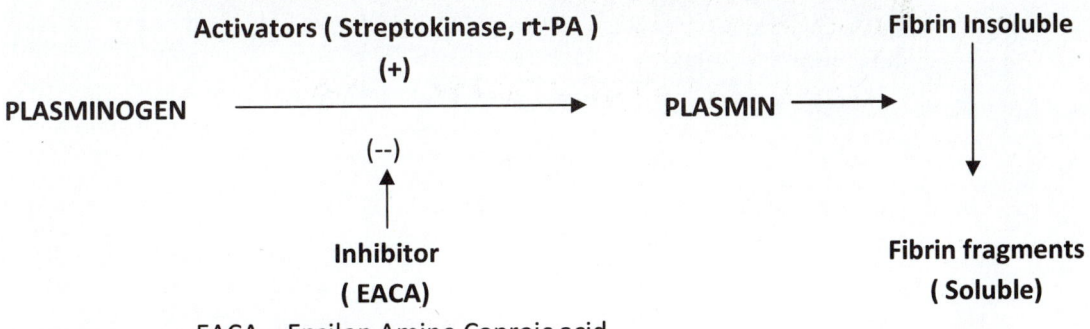

EACA = Epsilon Amino Caproic acid

Clinical uses : IN BOTH VENOUS AND ARTERIAL THROMBOSIS (TREATMENT ONLY AND NOT FOR PROPHYLAXIS)

1. In deep vein thrombosis and pulmonary embolism

2. IN MI (HEART ATTACK)

3. In cerebral thrombosis

Important Note : Fibrinolytic agents will be effective when they are administered within golden hour (4-6 hrs.) If it is delayed they will be less effective.

STREPTOKINASE

- It is an enzyme obtained from Beta haemolytic streptococci. It is not antibiotic
- It is a fibrinolytic agent

Mechanism of action : As above

- **Clinical uses** : As above (**Dose:** 15 lakhs units/IV)
- **Adverse effects**: BLEEDING (Antidote is Epsilon Amino Caproic Acid – antifibrinolytic agent) hypersensitive reactions

  Contraindicated in all situations, where risk of bleeding is increased (surgery)

rt-PA (RECOMBINANT TISSUE PLASMINOGEN ACTIVATOR)

- It is produced by DNA recombinant technology
- It produces more specific action on thrombus. So, there is less bleeding. It is preferred to Streptokinase, but costly.
- POTENT FIBRINILYTIC
- NO HYPERSENSITIVE REACTIONS
- CLINICAL USES, ADVERSE EFFECTS AND ANTIDOTE – SIMILAR TO THAT OF STREPTOKINASE

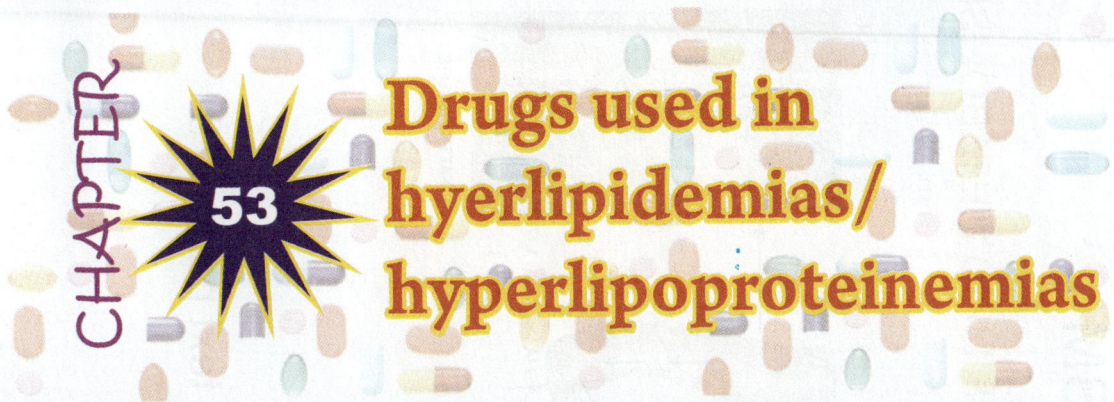

53 Drugs used in hyerlipidemias/ hyperlipoproteinemias

Since lipoproteins play an important role in the transport and metabolism of lipids, whenever there is hyperlipoproteinemia, it is followed by hyperlipidemia.

The causes of hyperlipoproteinemia are nephritic syndrome, diabetes mellitus myxoedema, chronic alcoholism, oral contraceptives, β adrenergic blockers, diuretics, etc.,

Primary cause is genetic.

Atherosclerosis: Inflammatory disorder of high lipid deposit (cholesterol) due to vessels injury → narrowing of blood vessels → thrombosis → Coronary Artery Diseases (CAD) (MI, Angina pectoris), stroke and peripheral vascular diseases.

Main lipids are cholesterol, triglycerides etc.

Increased concentration of low density lipoproteins (LDL), which carry/ transport cholesterol in the body

↓

Higher concentration of cholesterol is deposited in the arterial wall

↓

Atherosclerosis-Atheroma (main cause)

↓

Increases the risk of CAD (Coronary artery diseases like angina)

Source of cholesterol: From dietary intake of meat, dairy products, diets rich in unsaturated fats (reduce hepatic clearance of cholesterol)

Synthesis of cholesterol in the body (in liver):

Acetyl Co-A → Mevalonic acid → Squalene → Lanosteol → cholesterol. The liver is the primary organ for cholesterol synthesis, uptake and degradation

The circulations of Lipids and Lipoproteins:

The lipids present in the body are Cholesterol and Triglycerides. Both Cholesterol and triglycerides are useful to the body. But excess of blood Cholesterol and Triglycerides are harmful effects (atherosclerosis, pancreatitis etc.,)

Fig. 62 LIPID METABOLISM

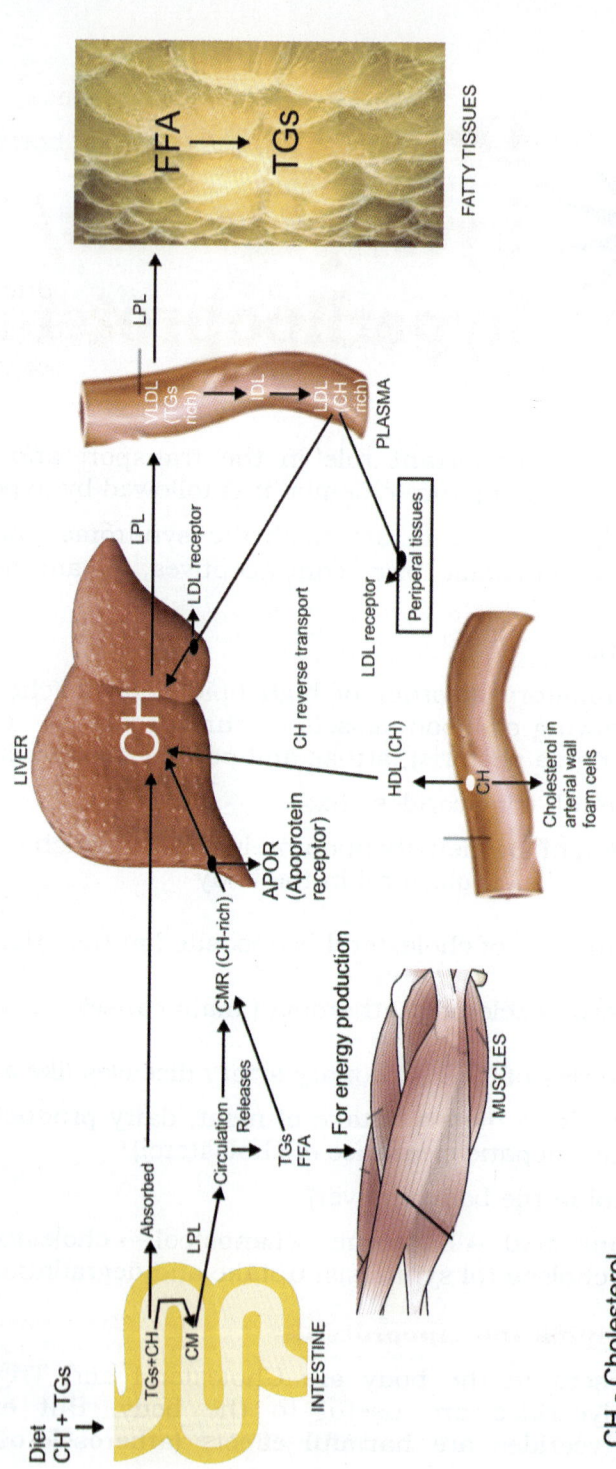

EXOGENOUS LIPID METABOLISM

ENDOGENOUS LIPID METABOLISM

For explanation refer text page 279

CH - Cholesterol
TGs - Triglycerides
CM - Chylomicron
CMR - Chylomicron ramnents
FFA - Free Fatty Acid
VLDL - Very Low Density Lipoprotein
IDL - Intermediate Density Lipoprotein
LDL - Low Density Lipoprotein
HDL - High Density Lipoprotein
LPL - Lipoprotein Lipase

Functions of Cholesterol

(1)   It is necessary for the synthesis of cell membranes.

(2)   It is the precursor for the synthesis of steroidal hormones.

(3)   It is the precursor for the synthesis of bile acid.

Functions of TGs

(1)   It mainly acts as the storage of lipids for fuel production.

The lipids as such cannot be transported in the blood. They have to combine with lipoprotein (lipid+protein complex) for the transport to the various parts in the body.

The Lipoproteins are classified as follows depending upon the molecular size and density.

(1)   Chylomicron

(2)   Chylomicron ramnents

(3)   VLDL (Very Low Density Lipoprotein) TGs rich

(4)   IDL (Intermediate Density Lipoprotein)

(5)   LDL (Low Density Lipoprotein) – CH rich – Bad lipid

(6)   HDL (High Density Lipoprotein) – Good lipid

Exogenous pathway of lipid transport : (Fig.62)

Cholesterol + Fats (TGs) in diet → Part of Cholesterol is absorbed and reaches liver via portal vein.

Part of CH + TGs → incorporated into the core of Chylomicron in the intestine releases TGs and free fatty acid (taken up by the muscles for energy production). The TGs is stored in the fat. Chylomicron, then converted into chylomicron ramnents (CH rich) and transported into liver via portal vein through APOR (Apoprotein receptor).

Endogenous pathway (Fig.62)

CH and TGs are synthesised in the liver VLDL (TGs rich) – circulation IDL → LDL → (releases TGs, FFA)

Occupies LDL receptor in the liver – taken up by the liver back. In this way the plasma Cholesterol is maintained in normal level. (<200 mg/dl)

Cholesterol occupies (LDL receptor) in the peripheral tissues and taken up by the peripheral tissues. That cholesterol is used by the tissues for the synthesis of steroidal hormones, cell membranes.

Reversal Cholesterol transport by HDL

Also HDL, which is synthesized in the liver → circulation → takes up Cholesterol in the arterial wall foam cells → carries back to liver → reduces plasma cholesterol level. Increased HDL is a useful cholesterol.

Levels of plasma lipids

Plasma lipids	desirable(mg%)	Border line high(mg%)	High(mg%)
1. Total cholesterol	125-200	200-239	>240
2. LDL (bad)cholesterol	<100	130-159	160-189
3. Triglycerides	< 150	150-199	200-499
4. HDL(good)cholesterol	>85		

- High LDL cholesterol and low HDL cholesterol increase the risk factor for CAD, Atherosclerosis.
- High trigycerides, partly increase the risk of CAD and pancreatitis

CLASSIFICATION OF ANTIHYPERLIPIDEMIC DRUGS

i.   H.M.G-CoA (3-Hydroxy 3-Methyl Glutaryl C0-enzyme-A) Reductase inhibitors (statins)

      i)   Atorvastatin
      ii)   Rosuvastatin
      iii)   Lovastatin
      iv)   Fluvastatin
      v)   Simvastatin

II.   Fibrates:

      i)   Fenofibrate

      ii)   Gemfibrozil

III.   Bile acid sequestrants:

      i)   Cholestyramine

IV.   Cholesterol absorption inhibitors

      i)   Ezetimibe

V.   Niacin

VI   Omega-3 poly unsaturated fatty acids (Sun flower oil, corn oil, fish oil) – reduce plasma cholestral level

Fig.63 Sites of action of hypolipidemic drugs

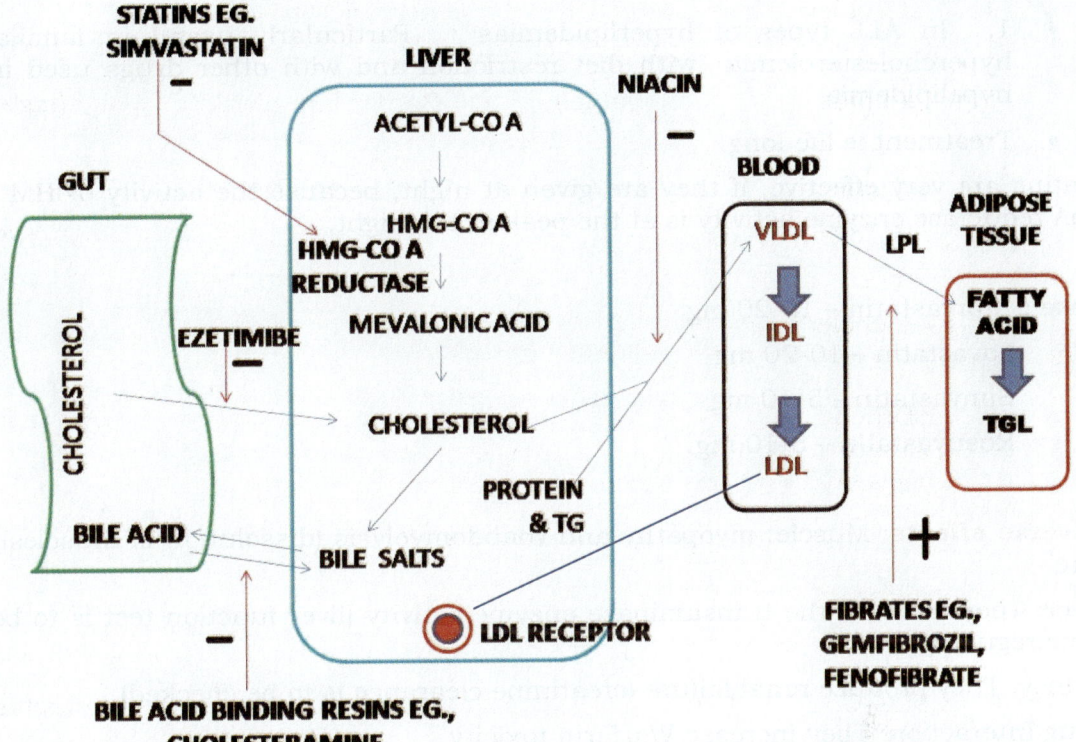

VLDL – Very low density Lipoprotein; LDL – Low density lipoprotein; IDL – Intermediate density lipoprotein; HDL – High density lipoprotein; CH – Cholesterol; TG – Triglyceride; LPL – Lipoprotein Lipase.

STATINS (HMG Co-A reductase inhibitors)

Mechanism of action: (Fig.63)

$$\text{HMG Co – A} \xrightarrow[\text{Reductase}]{\text{HMG Co - A}} \text{Mevalonic acid} \longrightarrow \text{cholesterol}$$

They ↓ (Inhibit) HMG Co A reductase → ↓ (reduce) synthesis of Mevalonic acid → ↓ (reduce) cholesterol synthesis within the liver.

- Low intracellular cholesterol → ↑ (increase) the synthesis of LDL receptors in the liver → promote uptake of cholesterol by the liver from the blood.

Also in some patients → ↑ (they increase) HDL concentration → increase removal of cholesterol from the blood and reduces plasma cholesterol level.

- All the above mechanisms reduce the plasma cholesterol level and reduce the risk of CAD

Clinical uses of STATINS

- 1. In ALL types of hyperlipidemias : Particularly useful in familial hypercholesterolemia with diet restriction and with other drugs used in hypelipidemia.
- Treatment is life long.

Statins are very effective, if they are given at night, because the activity of HMG CoA reductase enzyme activity is at the peak in the night.

Dose : Atorvastatin – 10-20 mg

Lovastatin – 10-20 mg

Simvastatin – 5-10 mg

Rosuvastatin – 5-10 mg.

Adverse effects: Muscle: myopathy and rhabdomyolysis (dissolution of muscles)-rare

Liver: They increase the transaminase enzyme activity (liver function test is to be done regularly)

Kidney: They produce renal failure (creatinine clearance is to be checked)

Drug Interaction: They increase Warfarin toxicity

FIBRATES

- It is an antihyperlipidemic drugs.

Mechanism of action (Fig.63)

- Fibrates activate PPAR-alpha (ParoxisomeProliferatorActivated Receptor-alpha) → ↑ (stimulate) lipoprotein lipase → reduce VLDL and TGs (mainly) level in the plasma.
- They inhibit the conversion of VLDL to LDL → slightly reduce the blood cholesterol level.
- They also fibrinolytic and show antiatherosclerotic effect.

NIACIN

It is a group of Vitamin B-complex..

It is used in hyperlipidemias

Mechanism of action (Fig.63)

Niacin

↓

Inhibits lipolysis in adipose tissues, the primary precursor of ciculating FFA

↓

reduces FFA level in the blood

↓

reduces the TGs synthesis in the liver

↓

reduces VLDL synthesis

↓

reduces plasma LDL concentration

↓

decreases both cholesterol and triglycerides concentration

Also it increases HDL level.

Also it stimulates plasminogen activator → it increases fibrinolytic activity.

Clinical uses :   1. In BOTH hypercholesterolemia and hypertriglyceridemia

Wide spectrum anti hyperlipidemic drug.

Useful in thrombosis associated with hypercholesterolemia.

Adverse effects: cutaneous vasodilatation → cutaneous flush → accompanied by uncomfortable warmth and pruritus (PGs mediated)

Aspirin (PGs synthesis inhibitor) prevents cutaneous flush, abdominal pain, hyperuricemia (precipitates gout), hyperglycemia (precipitates DM)

CHOLESTEROL ABSORPTION INHIBITORS (EZETIMIBE)

They are used in hyperlipidemia

Mechanism of action (Fig.63)

They inhibit the absorption of dietary and biliary cholesterol from the intestine.

- They increase cholesterol synthesis in the liver as compensatory mechanism. (It is inhibited by statins).

- They produce synergistic action with statins

Clinical uses : 1. They are used alone in hypercholesterolemia (if statin is contraindicated). Otherwise they are combined with statin.

BILE ACID SEQUESTRANTS (CHOLESTYRAMINE)

They are antihyperlipidemic drugs.

Mechanism of action (Fig.63)

Bile acid is produced from cholesterol
↓
secreted into the intestine
↓
reabsorbed back to liver with cholesterol.
↓
Bile acid sequestrant complexes with bile acid
↓
prevent reabsorption of cholesteral back to liver.
↓
Those bile acid complexes with cholesterol is excreted into the faeces
↓
reduce plasma cholesterol level.

Clinical use: 1. In hypercholesterolemia (with statin)

Adverse effects: flatulence

The status of hypolipidemic drugs in the treatment of hyperlipoproteinemia:

- It has been found out that raised plasma cholesterol (LDL-CH)/Low HDL/CH is directly proportional to increased risk of cardio vascular diseases.
- To reduce the raised LDL-CH level (Primary hypercholesterolemia), first drug is statins, either alone or with other suitable hypolipidemic drugs.
- To increase HDL-CH level – No single drug is effective. Combination of statins with nicotinic acid / fibrates are useful.
- To reduce plasma TGs: (The increased plasma TGs may lead to the risk of pancreatitis and coronary Artery Diseases) Fibrates & Nicotinic acid are preferred. If needed statin is to be added.

Non-pharmacological measures :

1) Avoid fatty diets 2) Avoid smoking and alcohol, 3) Take reduced cholestral rich diet and saturated fatty acids 4) regular exercise 5) body weight control 6) consume sufficient unsaturated fatty acids.

SECTION

IX

GASTRO INTESTINAL SYSTEM

GASTROINTESTINAL TRACT

Learning objectives

- Able to remember antiulcer drugs with special mention about anti H.pylori drugs

- To enumerate the various antiemetic drugs and their mechanisms of action

- To know about the drugs used in constipation and diarrhea

- To be aware of the management of irritable bowel syndrome (IBS) and inflammatory bowel disease (IBD)

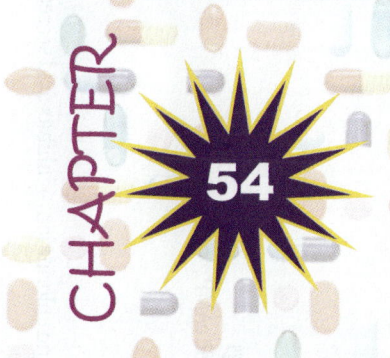

Treatment of peptic ulcer and related disorders

CHAPTER **54**

TREATMENT OF PEPTIC ULCER

Peptic Ulcer means, an erosion of mucus surface in the stomach (Gastric Ulcer) or in the duodenum (Duodenal Ulcer), characterized by burning epigastric pain. 'GASTRIC ACIDITY' means, an increase in acid secretion without ulcer due to many reasons. Gastroesophageal Reflux means, regurgitation of acid into esophagus which causes burning sensation in the throat.

DRUG THERAPY IN PEPTIC ULCER

Peptic ulcer is due to imbalance between the defensive factors (gastric mucus, PGs and innate resistance of the mucosal cells) and aggressive factors (acid, pepsin, bile & H.pylori)

$$\text{pepsinogen} \xrightarrow{\quad \text{HCL} \quad} \text{pepsin}$$

Physiology of gastric acid secretion: (Fig.64)

Gastric acid is needed for the digestion (In the presence of acid, the pepsinogen is converted to pepsin, which is a proteolytic enzyme to digest protein.) But excess gastric acid will lead to gastric mucosal erosion and cause ulcer. The gastric acid is synthesized in the parietal cells of stomach. The enterochromaffin cell like Histaminocytes (which synthesis and release Histamine) are present nearby. Gastrin and muscarinic receptors are present on the Histaminocytes. The stimulation of those receptors release Histamine from the Histaminocytes. There are Histamine, Gastrin, muscarinic, Prostaglandins receptors are present on the parietal cells of stomach. The parietal cells of the stomach are constantly stimulated by Histamine, ACh, Gastrin and the acid secretion is maintained. Among those, Histamine induced acid secretion is maximum. Histamine, ACh and Gastrin stimulate the respective receptors → stimulate c-AMP (The gastric acid

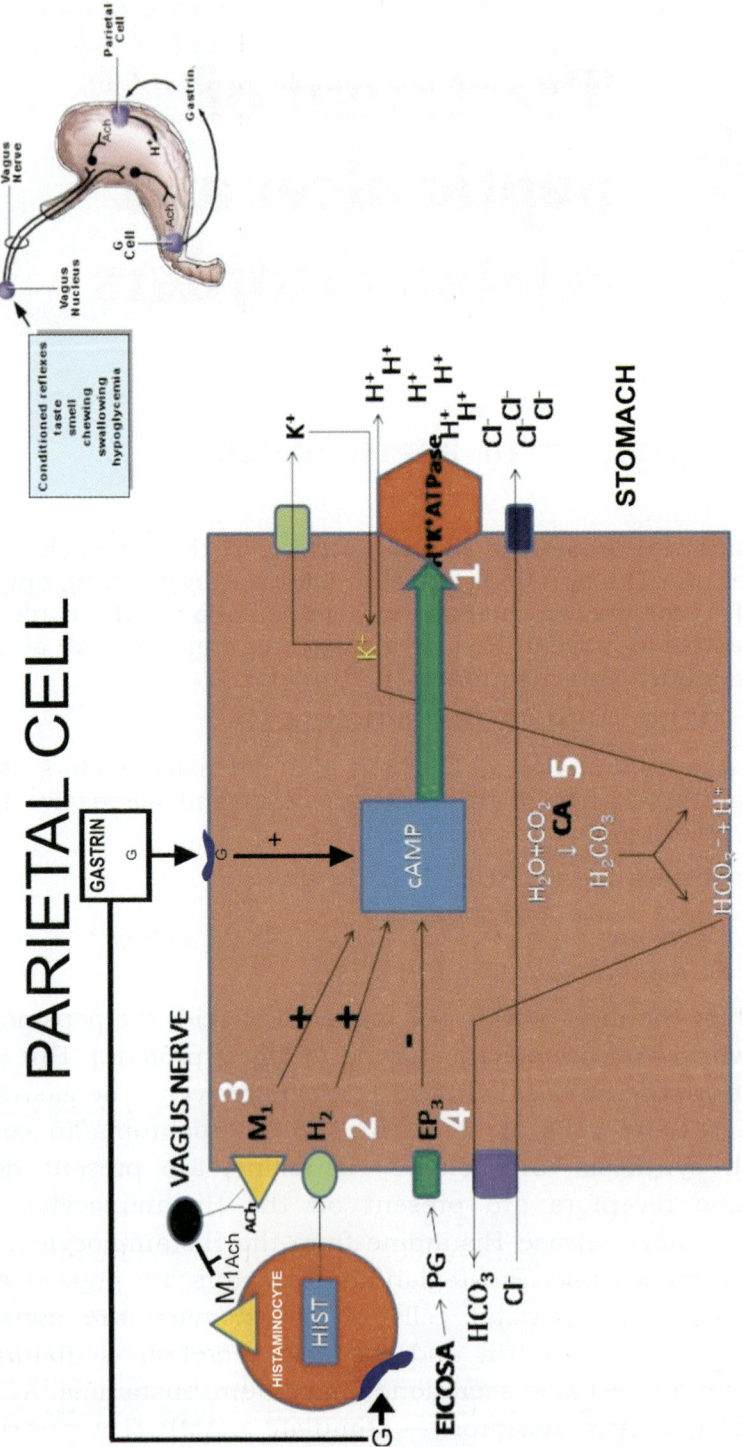

Fig. 64 Secretion of Hydrochloric acid and sites of action of Anti-ulcer drugs

Anti-ulcer drugs inhibits the gastric acid secretion by inhibiting the proton pump directly or through inhibiting the cAMP.

1 - Proton pump inhibitors - inhibit proton pump → inhibit secretion of hydrochloric acid

2 - H_2 Antagonists - Block H_2 receptors → inhibits the cAMP → inhibits acid secretion

3 - Muscarinic Blockers - Block M_1 receptors → inhibits acid secretion

4 - Prostaglandin analogues - stimulates the prostanoid receptors → inhibits the cAMP → inhibits acid secretion

5 - Carbonic anhydrase inhibitors - inhibit the enzyme carbonic anhydrase → non-avilability of bicarbonate ion and chloride ion → inhibits acid secretion

stimulant response of Gastrin and ACh is fully expressed only in the presence of cAMP generated by H_2 activation, hence Histamine induced acid secretion is maximum) → stimulate the proton pump → synthesis of HCl from H+ and Cl- (H+ comes from Carbonic acid by the action of Carbonic anhydrase present in the parietal cells and Cl- comes from the exchange with K+.)→ secreted into the lumen of the stomach. The stimulation of parasympathetic nerve (vagus), which supplies to the parietal cells releases Ach and stimulates the muscarinic receptors in the parietal cells of stomach → secretion of acid into stomach. The tension, excitement will stimulate the acid secretion. The PGs have got gastric mucosa protective action by increasing the mucus production and decreasing acid secretion by inhibiting c-AMP.

Gastric acid secretion (Fig64)

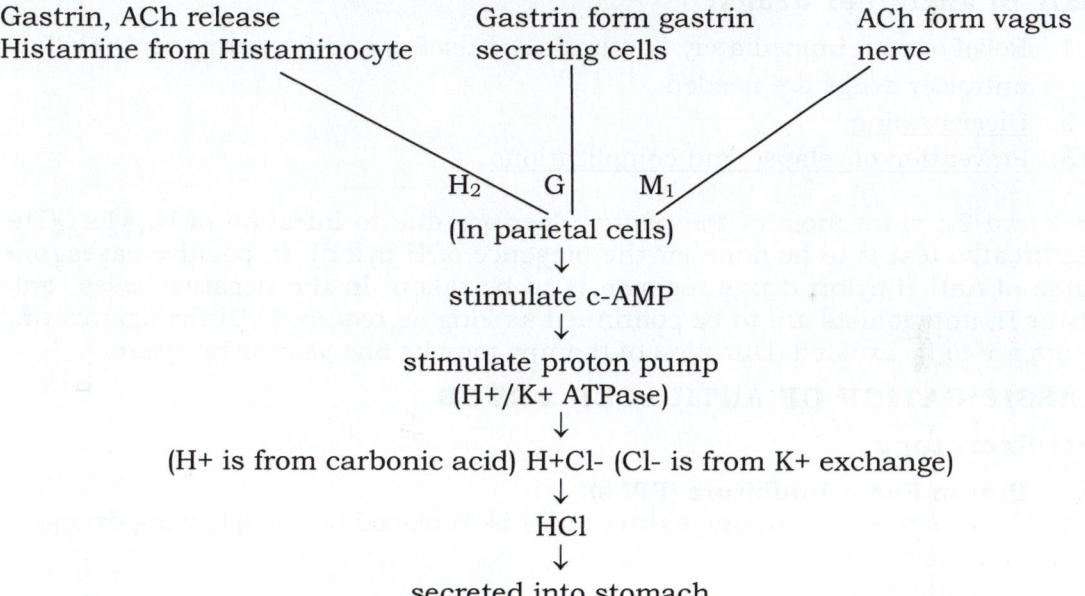

Gastrin, ACh release   Gastrin form gastrin   ACh form vagus
Histamine from Histaminocyte   secreting cells   nerve

H_2 G M_1
(In parietal cells)
↓
stimulate c-AMP
↓
stimulate proton pump
(H+/K+ ATPase)
↓
(H+ is from carbonic acid) H+Cl- (Cl- is from K+ exchange)
↓
HCl
↓
secreted into stomach

Any drug inhibits proton pump directly or indirectly (through cyclic AMP) will act as antiulcer.

Pathophysiology of peptic ulcer:

Peptic ulcer is due to imbalance between the defensive factors(gastric mucus, PGs and innate resistance of the mucosal cells) and the aggressive factors (acid, pepsin, bile and H.pylori). The mechanism of ulcer produced by H.pylori is given under Anti H.pylori drugs later on in this chapter. The main cause of the ulcer is due to excess secretion of gastric acid by H.pylori infection (duodenal ulcer mainly). The acid causes erosion of gastric mucosa and ulcer, if untreated will cause gastric bleeding in severe cases.

Aggravating factors: cigarette smoking, alcohol, frequent and prolonged use of NSAIDs., tension, esxcitement, spices etc.,

Drugs which are contraindicated in peptic ulcer: NSAIDs, Glucocorticoids, cholinergic drugs.

Related conditions: Zollinger-Ellision syndrome→tumour of gastrin secreting glands→ release of excess gastrin → excess secretion of gastric acid → peptic ulcer.

GERD: (Gastro eosophageal reflex disease) is due to the acid eructation from stomach to the eosophagus→ attack of acid on the mucous membrane of eophagus→irritation→ pain and difficult in swallowing.

Aggravating factors: heavy meal in the night, fatty and spicy meal, alcohol and some unknown factors.

Role of drugs in peptic ulcer and related diseases:

Goals of antiulcer drugs:

1. Relief of pain immediately (antacids are useful) and for permanent relief, antiulcer drugs are needed.
2. Ulcer healing.
3. Prevention of relapse and complications.

For 1 and 2 : since most of the peptic ulcer are due to infection of H.pylori (The urea breathe test is to be done for the presence of H.pylori). In positive cases, one course of Anti H.pylori drugs regimen is to be taken. In the negative cases, only PPIs or H_2 antagonists are to be continued as long as required. All the aggravating factors are to be avoided. Duration of therapy may be one year or two years.

CLASSIFICATION OF ANTIULCER DRUGS

Anti Secretory

   I.   **Proton Pump Inhibitors (PPI s)**
     1)   Omeprazole (prototype drug but it is replaced by the following drugs)
     2)   Lansoprazole
     3)   Pantoprazole
     4)   Rabeprazole
  II. **H_2 antagonists**
     1) Ranitidine
     2) Famotidine
     3) Roxatidine
 III. **Anticholinergic (not used)**
     1) Pirenzepine
 IV. **Prostaglandins analogue**
     1) Misopristol
  V. **Mucosal protective**
     1) Sucralfate
     2) Colloidal bismuth subcitrate

VI. **Ulcer healing drug**
1) Carbenoxolone
VII. **Anti – H. Pylori drugs**
1) Amoxicillin
2) Clarithromycin
3) Tetracycline
4) Tinidazole
5) Bismuth subsalicylate
6) With PPIs
VIII. **Acid neutralizing drugs (antacids)**
- They are not useful in peptic ulcer, where the acid secretion should be inhibited round the clock for quick healing. But the antacids are very very short acting. So, it is very difficult to inhibit the acid secretion round the clock by the antacids.
- However, they are very much useful in hyperacidity and for immediate relief in GERD.

Drugs: commonly used drugs in combination are Magnesium salts (diarrhea) and Aluminium salts (constipation) since they neutralize the side effects of each other.

1) Magnesium trisilicate+ Aluminium hydroxide (Digene, Gelusil)

Clinical uses of antacids: 1) Systemic antacid – sodium bicarbonate – uses:

i. In systemic acidosis (oral /IV)
ii. In Phenobarbitone poisoning to alkalinise the urine (I.V)
iii. In GERD – for immediate relief (oral)
iv. To alkalinise the urine (oral) in UTI (to prevent the growth of micro-organisms and potentiates the action of drugs used in UTI.
2) In hyperacidity (digene, gelusil)

PROTON PUMP INHIBITORS (PPIs)

- They are most powerful antiulcer drug with prolonged action
- They are useful in peptic ulcer and related disorders.

Mechanism of action : (Fig.64)

All the PPIs are prodrug and converted into active form 'sulfenamide'cation within the parietal cells of the stomach. The active form of PPIs inhibit the proton pump ($H^+ K^+$ ATPase), which is the final step of acid secretion. Hence they are the most potent antiulcer drugs. They are administered before breakfast for better effect.

- In peptic ulcer there is excess stimulation of $H^+ K^+$ ATP ase (proton pump) which releases both H^+ and Cl^- which then combine to form HCl in the stomach.
- PPIs inhibit directly the final step involved in acid secretion.
- Inhibit directly $H^+ K^+$ ATP ase (proton pump) which secretes acid into stomach.
- The enzyme is present in the parietal cells.

Clinical uses of PPIs:

1) In peptic ulcer (gastric & duodenal ulcer): PPIs are more potent than H_2 antagonist. The ulcers heal rapidly when given along with anti H.pylori drugs for 4 to 6 weeks

2) In bleeding ulcer: They reduce acid secretion, which promote clot formation and stop bleeding.

3) Stress ulcer. They are given by IV route

4) Zolinger – Ellison's syndrome (it is tumour of the gastrin secreting cells → excess gastrin is released → stimulates the proton pump and more acid is secreted into stomach) PPIs are given as long as required (may be 4 to 5 years). If it is not controlled, then surgery is preferred.

5) In GERD – symptomatic relief for longer duration, and for healing of esophageal ulcer, PPIs are given as long as required.

6) In gastritis and hyper secretory states in some special conditions.

7) To control regurgitation of acid in some on prolonged anaesthesia, as preanaesthestic medication.

Dose : Lansoprazole – 15 to 30 mg/OD, Rabeprazole – 10 to 20 mg/OD

Adverse effects: loose motion, abdominal pain, dizziness.

- There may be rebound increase in acid secretion after sudden withdrawal of PPIs . It is better to withdraw gradually.

D/I – Omeprazole is a microsomal enzyme inhibitor →↑(increases the toxicity of warfarin, diazepam etc.,)

(replaced by newer PPIs, which do not possess (eg. Lansoprazole, pantoprazole, rabeprazole) microsomal enzyme inhibitory action.

H_2 ANTAGONISTS

Mechanism of action of H_2 antagonists:

They block selectively H_2 receptors (H_1 receptors are not blocked) in the parietal cells of the stomach and inhibit the Hist induced gastric acid secretion. They inhibit c-AMP and in turn inhibit the proton pump, which is needed for the synthesis and secretion of HCl into stomach. They suppress the basal and food induced acid secretion. They also inhibit the acid secretion by Histamine, which is released from the enterochromaffin cells (Histaminocytes) of parietal cells by gastrin, ACh.

They are less effective than PPIs.

Caution : It has been found recently (September, 2019) that Ranitidine causes cancer. The Manufacturer of Ranitidine had suspended its production.

Clinical uses :

    Same that of PPIs

Dose : Famotidine – 150 mg, Roxatidine (Rotane) – 150 mg.

Anti H.pylori drugs

    The etiologies of peptic ulcer are many. One of them is due to colonization of duodenal mucosa by H.pylori. About 90% of duodenal ulcer, 50-60% of gastric ulcer and probably 50% cases of non-ulcer dyspepsis are responsible for chronic atrophic gastritis. H.pylori is also risk factor for gastric adenocarcinoma and to some extent for non-hodgkin's lymphoma affecting stomach. This bacterium, unlike others produces urease, which hydrolyses urea to ammonia and neutralizes HCl to create neutral protective cloud from the acid environment. H.pylori also produces proteolytic enzyme, causes mucosal erosion and chronic inflammation, which will lead to ulcers. H.pylori infection can be detected by urea breathe test before taking the PPIs. In absence of acid, H.pylori becomes less virulent. And also they develop resistance very rapidly to anti H.pylori drug. The combination of anti H.pylori drugs with PPIs are more efficacious in eradicating H.pylori. Many combination regimens are followed. The common regimen is triple drugs therapy (for 14 days) and followed by PPIs for another 4 weeks or 6 weeks for complete healing of ulcer.

- Commensal in 20-70% of normal individual.
- Faster ulcer healing with PPIs/ H$_2$ antagonists.
- 90% of the peptic ulcer patients show H. pylori positive.
- If it is not treated in time → it will lead to peptic ulcer, gastritis, carcinoma, dyspepsia etc.,
- H.pylori develops resistance fast, if a single drug is given.
- That is why, 3 or 4 drugs combinations is required for the treatment of H. pylori associated peptic ulcer, to prevent development of resistance by H.pyroli.

Combination regimen: thrice daily for 1-2 weeks.

1) omeprazole 80mg or (Lansoprazole 30mg) + clarithromycin 500mg/BD + Amoxicillin 1G/BD + Metronidazole 500mg/BD (Heligo combi pack/Helibact combi pack)
1) Amoxicillin + Tinidazole + Lansoprazole
2) Amoxicillin + Clarithromycin + Lansoprazole
3) Clarithromycin + Tinidazole + Lansoprazole

GASTRO ESOPHAGEAL REFLUX DISEASE(GERD)

It is a very common problem presenting as burning sensation in throat due to acid regurgitation & aggravated by heavy meal or lying flat immediately after taking food.

- Repeated reflux of acid gastric contents into esophagus causes esophagitis, erosion , ulcer, pain on swallowing and increase the risk of esophageal carcinoma and disturbance in sleep.
- The primary barrier to reflux is tone of LES (Lower Esophageal Sphimcter) → gastrin, fatty diet, alcohol, coffee and smoking → relaxes LES → ↑ (increase) reflux → also delayed gastric motility → easy regurgitation of acid. Progesterone decreases reflux (reflux is common in pregnancy)

DRUGS:

i. Proton pump inhibitors
ii. H_2 Antagonists
iii. Antacids
iv. Sodium alginate
v. Prokinetic agents

PPIs& H_2 Antagonists inhibit acid secretion and give relief for longer period.

III) Antacids – for quick relief only.

iv) Sodium alginate – it forms a thick frothy layer , which float on the gastric contents and prevent the contact of acid with esophageal mucosa

v) Prokinetic agents - increase esophageal sphincter tone and promote the gastric emptying and bring relief.

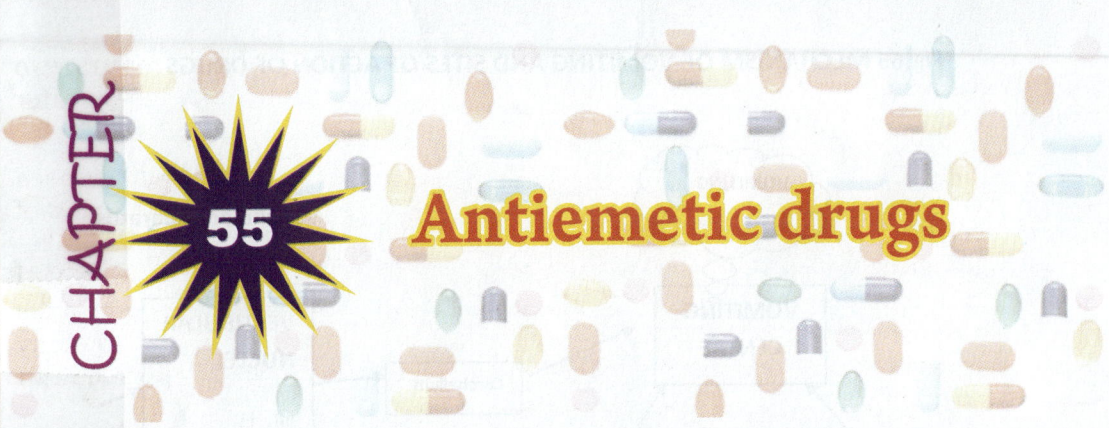

CHAPTER
55 **Antiemetic drugs**

ANTIEMETICS

Those drugs which are used to suppress or to prevent vomiting

Drugs are classified on the basis of actions on their receptors

I. Dopamine antagonists.
    1) Prokinetic agents:
    i)   Metoclopramide
    ii) Domperidone (commonly used)
    iii) Mosapride
II. 5 HT_3 antagonist
    1)   Ondansetron
    2)   Granisetron
III. M_3 receptor antagonists(anticholinergic)
    1) Hyoscine
    2) Dicyclomine
IV. H_1 antagonists
    1) Promethazine
V.   misc
    1) Pyridoxine

Types of vomiting

1) Drugs (Including anticancer drugs) induced vomiting
2) Disease induced vomiting (uremia, Acute Myocardial Infarction)
3) Pregnancy Induced Vomiting (Morning Sickness)
4) Motion Sickness: Vomiting occurs in susceptible individuals, when they travel in angular motion, circular motion(while travelling in hilly area),ups and downs motion (during ship journey, flight journey)
5) Post – operative vomiting (general anaesthetics induced vomiting)
6) Radiation induced vomiting

Fig.65 MECHANISM OF VOMITING AND SITES OF ACTION OF DRUGS

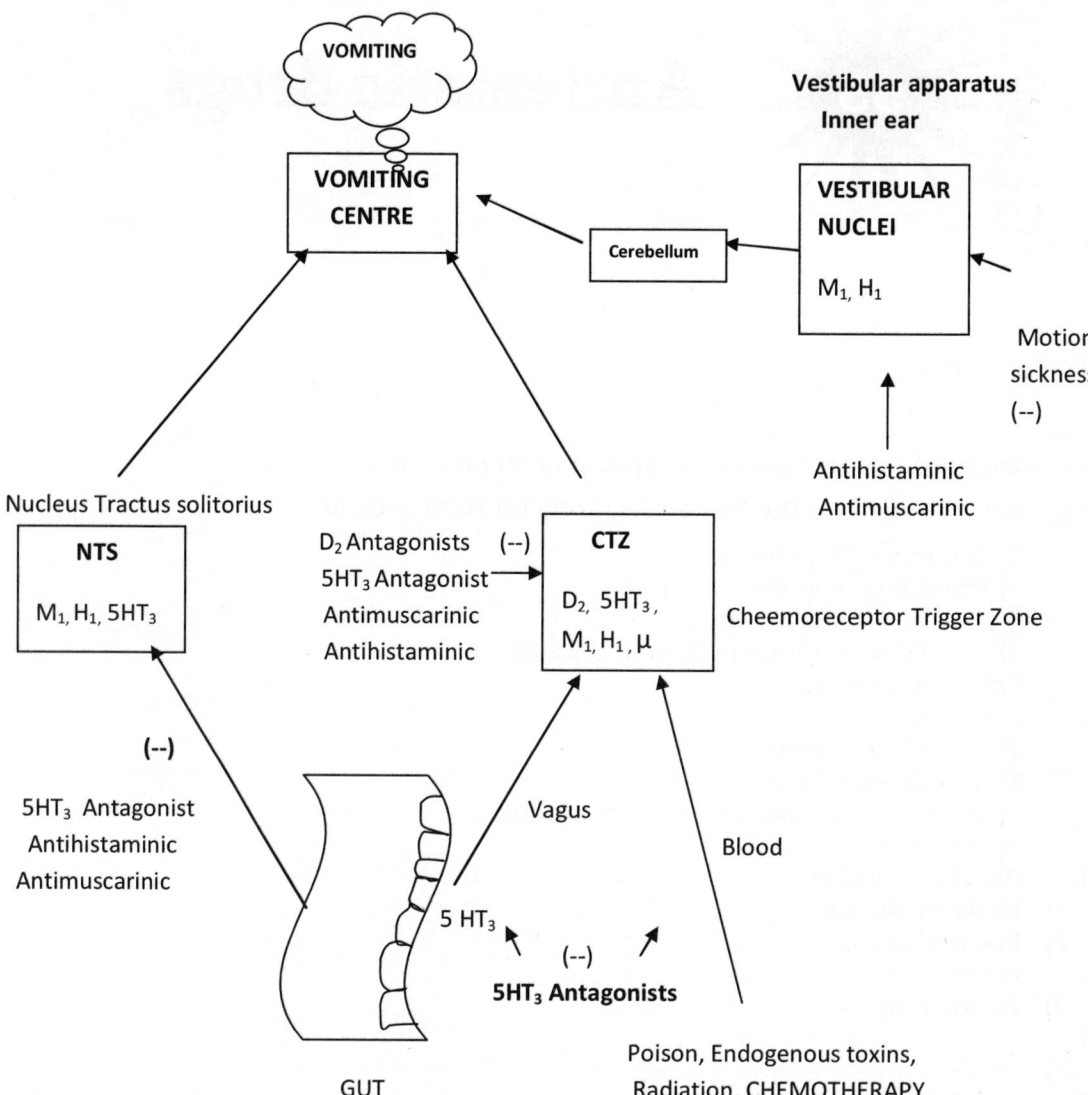

Relay stations

1) Chemoreceptor trigger zone (CTZ)
2) Nucleus Tractus Solitorius (NTS)

All the vomiting impulses from the periphery go via relay stations to vomiting centre except from motion sickness.

Receptors of vomiting are present in the relay stations and afferent vagus from GIT

1) DA_2
2) $5HT_3$
3) H_1
4) M_1
5) μ(mu)

PROKINETIC AGENTS

METOCLOPRAMIDE (not used now a days)

- Prokinetic agents means, increase the G.I.T motility (promotes gastric emptying)

Mechanism of action (Fig.65)

1) Dopamine is inhibitory transmitter in GIT. Metoclopramide ↓(inhibits) DA_2 Receptors in the nerve ending of G.I.T →↑(increases) release of ACh into the stomach → increases gastric motility.
   → Increases peristaltic movement of G.I.T and gastric emptying
   → If there is no food in the stomach → There won't be any vomiting
2) Inhibits $5HT_3$ receptor in ENS (Enteric Nervous System) →↑(increases) release of ACh→↑(stimulates) G.I.T motility(by stimulating M_3 receptors) → gastric emptying →prokinetic action
3) ↑ (stimulates)$5HT_4$ receptors →↑(stimulates) release of ACh →prokinetic action
4) They also inhibit DA_2 receptors in CTZ, NTS and act as antiemetic

Clinical uses of prokinetic agents:

I.   As prokinetic (metoclopramide 10mg/oral/IM)
  1) In diabetic gastroparesis and in post vagotomy
  2) For emergency evacuation of bowel just before general anaesthetic, if food is taken before 4 hrs
  3) To facilitate duodenal endoscopy
II. As Antiemetic
  1) In all types of vomiting except motion sickness
III. In GERD (Gastroesophageal reflux disease) in some (obese) the regurgitation of acid into esophagus,→ pain & ulcer. Here prokinetic agents → gastric emptying → no regurgitation → relieve burning sensation of throat in GERD, useful in mild cases. Otherwise antiulcer drugs are very much useful
IV. In dyspepsia
V.   In persistent hiccup

Adverse effects:

- Metoclopramide crosses BBB → it inhibits DA_2 receptor in EPS (Extra Pyramidal System) produces parkisonism like adverse effects. Hence it is not preferred to prevent vomiting due to L-Dopa (Domperidone is preferred since it does not produce parkinsonism side effects, since it does not cross BBB).
- It inhibits prolactin release inhibitory hormone and stimulates milk secrection and produces galactorrhoea
- It produces loose motion due to increased intestinal motility

DOMPERIDONE

- First line drugs in that group as antiemetic

Mechanism of action : (Fig.65)

- Broad spectrum antiemetic
- It inhibits DA_2 receptors in GIT → stimulates the release of ACh → stimulates smooth muscles contraction of GIT → gastric emptying → prokinetic action (Antiemetic action)
- It does not cross BBB. But reaches CTZ (which is not covered by BBB) and inhibits DA_2 receptor in CTZ. Hence → Antiemetic action. (since it doesn't cross BBB except CTZ). It inhibits DA_2 receptors present only in CTZ (not any where else), → no parkinsonism and galactorrhoea adverse effects. It is very much useful in L-Dopa induced vomiting without affecting the antiparkinsonism action of L-Dopa.

Clinical uses :

I. As prokinetic (same like metoclopramide)
II. As antiemetic – in all types of vomiting except motion sickness, morning sickness and it is particularly useful in L-Dopa induced vomiting.

Dose : Domperidone (Domstal) – 10 mg.

Adverse effects: loose motion

MOSAPRIDE

- It has got only prokinetic action. (no DA_2 inhibition action) $5HT_4$ agonist action on GIT
- No anti emetic action. No EP side effects. No galactorrhoea.
- More potent action on intestinal motility.
- It is mainly used in constipation, particularly in children.

Clinical uses :

1) As prokinetics USES
2) In constipation

Adverse effects: Abdominal cramp, Diarrhea

ONDANSETRON

- Broad spectrum antiemetic except in motion sickness and in morning sickness.

Mechanism of action : (Fig.65)

Anticancer drugs, radiation → in the intestine →disintegrate enterochromaffin cells and release 5HT → occupy $5HT_3$ receptor in the vagus afferent nerve→carry vomiting impulse to CTZ, NTS → ↑ (stimulate) $5 HT_3$ receptors in CTZ and NTS → carry vomiting impulse to vomiting centre and produce vomiting.

- Ondanesetron is a $5HT_3$ antagonist. It blocks all the $5HT_3$ receptors in vagal afferent nerve, CTZ and NTS → prevent vomiting due to drugs and radiation.

Clinical uses :

1) In anticancer drugs induced vomiting (drug of choice)
2) In post – operative vomiting
3) In radiation sickness
4) In drug induced vomiting

Dose : 4-8 mg/oral or IV

ANTICHOLINERGIC
Hyoscine

- It is very effective only in motion sickness which occurs due to angular motion (bus travel in the hill)or ups and downs motion (ship travel) → stimulates labrynthine →↑ (stimulates) semicircular canal → ↑ (stimulates) M_1 receptors→ carry vomiting impulse to vomiting centre → vomiting .
- Hyoscine ↓(inhibits) M_1 receptors in Semicircular canal, CTZ/NTS→ antiemetic action.

Dose :

One tab. is taken ½ hr before the proposed journey by susceptible individuals .

- In pregnancy induced vomiting (morning sickness), Dicyclomine, cyclizine+vit B_6 are preferred.

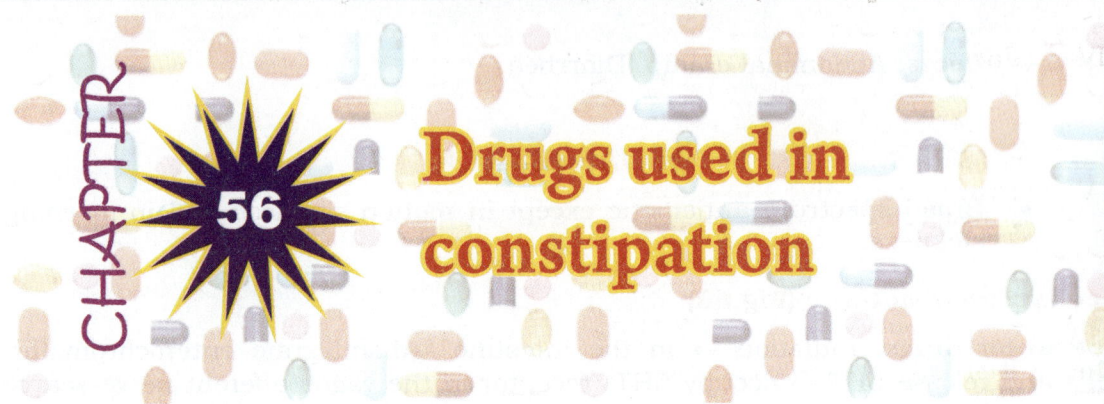

CHAPTER 56

Drugs used in constipation

- Constipation is the condition in which it is difficult (with straining) to empty the bowel.
- Purgatives are drugs which empty the bowel easily as watery stool.
- Laxatives are mild purgative makes the stool soft and semisolid.
- Purgatives and laxative are used in constipation.

Drugs :

I. Bulk – forming laxative: wheat bran, ispaghula

Mechanism of action : WATER is absorbed and bulk of the intestinal content is increased→↑ **(stimulate)** peristaltic movement refluxly→ evacuation of bowel as soft & semi solid stool.   Site→ large intestine → slow onset of action.

II. Osmotic purgative → Lactulose
Water is retained by osmosis in the intestine and the volume of intestinal contents increased →↑(stimulates) intestinal motility → evacuation of bowel with watery in nature
It is also used in hepatic encephalopathy, which is due to accumulation of NH_3 in the colon. Lactulose converts NH_3 to NH_4 salts and then excreted
Adverse effects: Flatulence

III. Lubricant laxative – liquid paraffin, phenolphthalein
- It is pharmacologically inert mineral oil
- It lubricates the faecal matter .
- Easy evacuation of bowel.

Adverse effects :

- It is not palatable , soil the cloth by leaking through anus

Clinical uses :

It is mainly used in the conditions in which straining to be avoided (haemorrhoids or cardio vascular disease) and in bed ridden patients.

IV. Faecal softener or surfactant laxative: Docusate sodium
- Decrases the surface tension of food in the bowel.
- Mild laxative – softens the stool.
- Slow onset of action and it is given at bed time.

V. Irritant purgative – senna, Bisacodyl
- They irriate small intestine/colon, stimulate peristaltic movement → evacuation of bowel with watery stool.
- Onset of action is quick and they are administered early in the morning.
- Bisacodyl is commonly used.

Dose : Bisacodyl (Dulcolax) – 5 mg tab

Clinical uses of Irritant purgative:

1) In constipation
2) Before and after anorectal surgery
3) In bed ridden patients
4) Before and after anthelmintic drugs

Adverse effects : Flatulence, abdominal cramp

VI. Enema – soap solution is administered with pressure through rectum and used to evacuate bowel (watery stool)
1) Used in emergency evacuation of bowel before surgery.
2) In chronic constipation.

   Disadvantage: self medication is difficult, embrassment to the individual.

General uses of purgatives:

1) In constipation (irritant purgatives)
2) In bed ridden patient (liquid paraffin)
3) To avoid undue straining during defaecation (in haemorrhoids & cardio vascular diseases)-liquid paraffin, faecal softener (Docusate sodium)
4) Before and after any anorectal surgery (Bisacodyl)
5) Before and after anthelmintics (Bisacodyl)

Common Adverse effects : Flatulence, Abdominal cramp

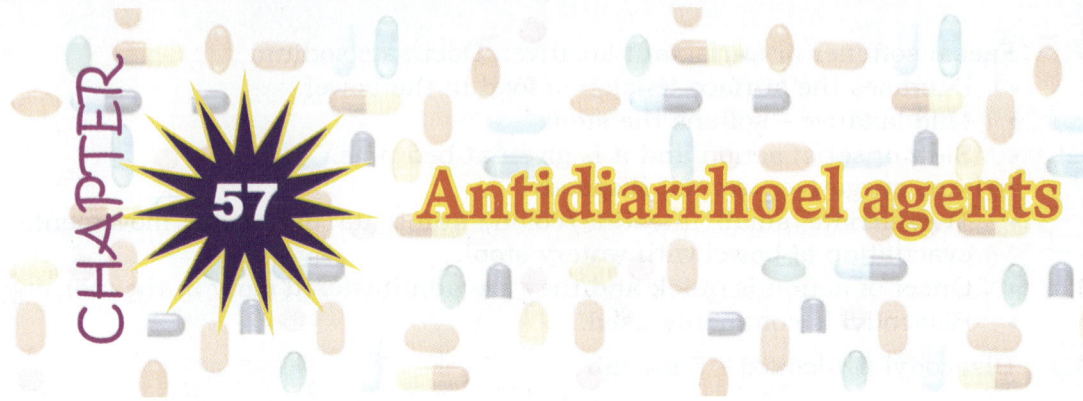

CHAPTER 57 — Antidiarrhoel agents

Diarrhea is abnormally frequent evacuation of watery stool.

Infectious diarrhea caused by E.Coli and Salmonella is common among travellers.

Dysentery is any of disorders marked by inflammation of the intestine especially of the colon with abdominal pain, painful straining at stool, tenesmus and frequent stools containing blood and mucus normally due to infection.

Eg: - Bacillary Dysentery By Shigella Sp-Treated by Norfloxacin

- Amoebic dysentery – Caused By Protozoa E. histolytica – Treated By Tinidazole
  Here, we discuss the drugs used only in non-specific (non – infectious) diarrheas.
  Nonspecific diarrheas are mainly due to increased intestinal motility or increased intestinal secrection (secretory diarrhea)

Drugs:

I. Anti motility & anti secretory
1) Opioid analogues
Loperamide – It is commonly used

– It is an Opioid analogue. It does not cross BBB (no analgesic, no vomiting, no respiratory depression action, no addiction liability)

- Lopermide stimulates 'μ' receptors in the G.I.T. → Relaxation of smooth muscles and constrictions of sphincters. → Food contents accumulate in the intestine. → Facilitates water absorption. → The stool will become solid. → Constipative effects.

Dose : Loperamide (Lopamid) – 2 mg.

C/I – In infectious diarrhea, in children below 2 years.

2) Racecadotril

- It also doesn't cross BBB.
- It is an opioid Analogue.

- It inhibits enkephalinase – prevents degradation of enkephalin→ increases local concentration of enkephalin at intestinal mucosa and then action is similar to Loperamide.

II. Anticholinergics:
They are Muscarinic blockers at intestine →relaxation of intestinal smooth muscle → ↓ (inhibit) intestinal motility→constipative action – useful in diarrhea (atropine substitute is preferred – Dicyclomine)

III. Adsorbent: kaolin, bismuth subsalicylats → adsorbs irritants & toxins and excrete them.

IV. Misc. Lactobacillus sporogens
  - Replace useful bacterial flora that is lost during acute diarrhea.
  - As adjuvant in non – specific & specific diarrheas.

V. Non- pharmacological measure:
ORT (Oral Rehydration Therapy)

ORT (Oral Rehydration Therapy)

It contains all the necessary electrolytes (Na+K+) + glucose (for energy replacement) which might have been lost in severe diarrhea.

- As replacement therapy, it is mainly needed in severe diarrhea (if the fluid loss is more than 10% of body weight). An ORS (Oral rehydration solution) equivalent to fluid loss is infused over 2-4 hours.
- In mild to moderate diarrhea – 2 -3 L/day of any one of the ORS (Oral rehydration solution)
- Coffee, tea, soft drinks, hypertonic juices are to be avoided, since they make diarrhea worst
- The cereal based ORS is also available (with precooked rice flour)

Precooked rice flour →RELEASES AMINOACOIDS THAT TOO STIMULATE Na+/water absoption from the colon and glucose also stimulates sodium / water absorption from the colon.

New formula as per WHO – ORS (2002)

WHO RELEASED NEW FORMULA WITH LOW Na+, LOW GLUCOSE ORS

CONTENT S

Nacl – 2.6g

Kcl – 1.5g

Trisodium citrate–2.9g

Glucose-13.5g

Water-1L

Total osmolarity is 245mols/L

PROBIOTIC

Intestinal flora contains many useful nonpathogenic micro-organisms. They are protective to our body. They kill pathogenic micro-organisms in the intestine.

In infectious diarrhea, those useful micro-organisms are washed away and the infectious diarrhea will be aggravated.

Examples: Lacotbacillus, Bifida bacterium, Sacchraromyces boulardil are some of the probiotics.

The probiotics are very much useful in the following conditions:

Clinical uses:

1. In acute infectious diarrhea, where the protective micro-organisms present in the intestinal microflora are washed away and infectious diarrhea will be aggravated
2. In broad spectrum antibiotics induced diarrhea (in which the most of the useful intestinal flora is destroyed by broad spectrum antibiotics)
3. In ulcerative colitis
4. In irritable bowel syndrome (where diarrhea might have washed away the intestinal flora)

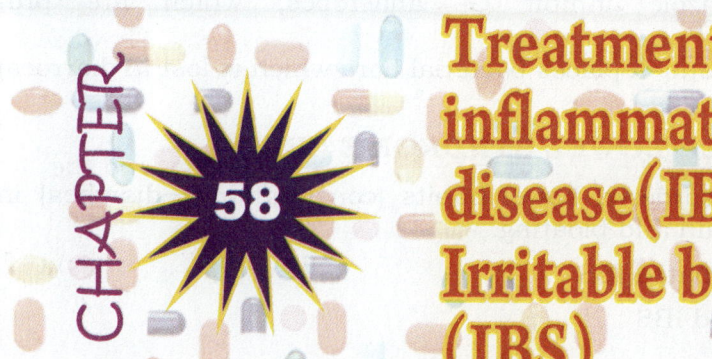

Treatment of inflammatory bowel disease(IBD), Irritable bowel syndrome (IBS)

CHAPTER 58

TREATMENT OF INFLAMMATORY BOWEL DISEASE (IBD)

Two important inflamatory bowel diseases are

I.   Ulcerative colitis
II. Crohn's disease

The pathogenesis of these two diseases involve immune mechanism and may be due to imbalance between the pro-inflammatory and anti-inflammatory factors. Drugs used in ulcerative colitis are

1) ASA (acetyl salicylic acid)containing drugs
    i.   Sulfasalazine
    ii. Mesalamine and enteric coated ASA which release ASA and better tolerated
    iii. Balsalazine

Mechanism of action

- They are anti-inflammatory like salicylate inhibit PG Synthesis. PGs are inflammatory producing substances.
- They inhibit the production of pro–inflammatory cytokines.

Other USES: As Disease Modifying Anti Rheumatic Drugs (DMARDs)

2) Immunosuppressive Agents – It is believed that – IBD may be due to immune disorder
    i.   Glucocorticoids – Prednisolone, Dexomethasone
    ii. Cyclosporine – induces remission
        - Effective in patients who are not responding to GC
    iii. Antimetabolites anticancer drugs (immunosuppressives – Azathioprine, Methotrexate)

3) Anti TNF α (In crohn's disease only)
    i)   Infliximab
    ii) Adalimumab
    - Increased TNFα is found in the faeces of crohn's patients

4) Antimicrobial agents

- Only in crohn's disease
- Norfloxacin, Tinidazole inhibit G- anaerobes, which are pro-inflammatory.
- Lactobacillus (probiotic=replaces bacterial flora which is lost in diarroea)

IRRITABLE BOWEL SYNDROME (IBS)

IBS – is characterized by disordered bowel habits (constipation / diarrhea) in association with abdominal pain and bloating.

Two types - constipation dominated IBS

-diarrhea dominated IBS

Aim: To relieve abdominal pain

To correct the disorders of bowel habit

Treatment in diarrhea dominated IBS

- Anti diarrheal – antispasmodic
1) Opioid – fedotozine (new drugs)
2) Dicyclomine (atropine substitute- antispasmodic & antidiarrheal)
3) Antidepressant – to relieve abdominal pain
4) $5 HT_3$ Receptor antagonist in GIT – Alosetron

It inhibits intestinal hypermotility and relieves abdominal pain

Treatment in constipation dominated IBS

1) Chloride Channel Activator
   It increases Intestinal Secretion and peristaltic movement leads to purgative action

2) Clonidine - ↓(inhibits) abdominal pain

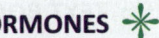
SECTION

X

HORMONES

HORMONES

Learning objectives

- To enumerate the hormones and their sites of release
- To know about the functions of anterior pituitary hormones and their clinical uses
- To know about posterior pituitary hormones and their functions
- To be aware of thyroid hormone synthesis and their functions
- Able to remember anti-thyroid drugs with their mechanisms of action and management of thyrotoxicosis
- To enumerate antidiabetic drugs with their mechanisms of action and management of diabetes mellitus
- To know about corticosteroids and their clinical uses
- Able to remember various contraceptives and their mechanisms of action
- To enumerate the sex hormones and their antagonists with their clinical uses
- To be aware of the drugs affecting calcium metabolism and their clinical uses

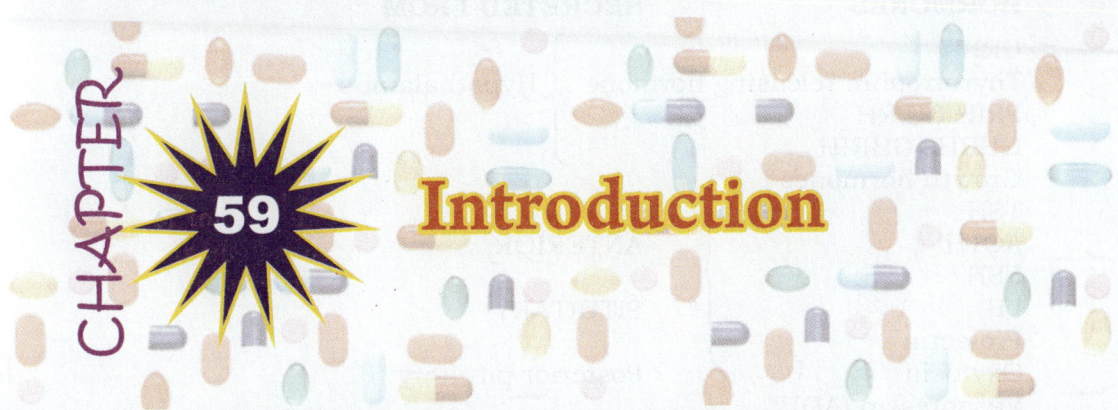

CHAPTER 59

Introduction

Hormones are chemical substances secreted form endocrine glands (ductless glands) and act throughout the body.

Differ from autacoids = local hormones, which act only at the site of release.

The master endocrine gland is 'anterior pituitary gland', which release anterior pituitary hormones. Hormones act either on the cell membrane receptors or on the receptors present in the nucleus. Every hormone has got its own specific receptors through which it activates specific physiological function.

Factor means, its chemical nature is not established.

The Hormones secreted from Hypothalamus and Anterior Pituitary Gland

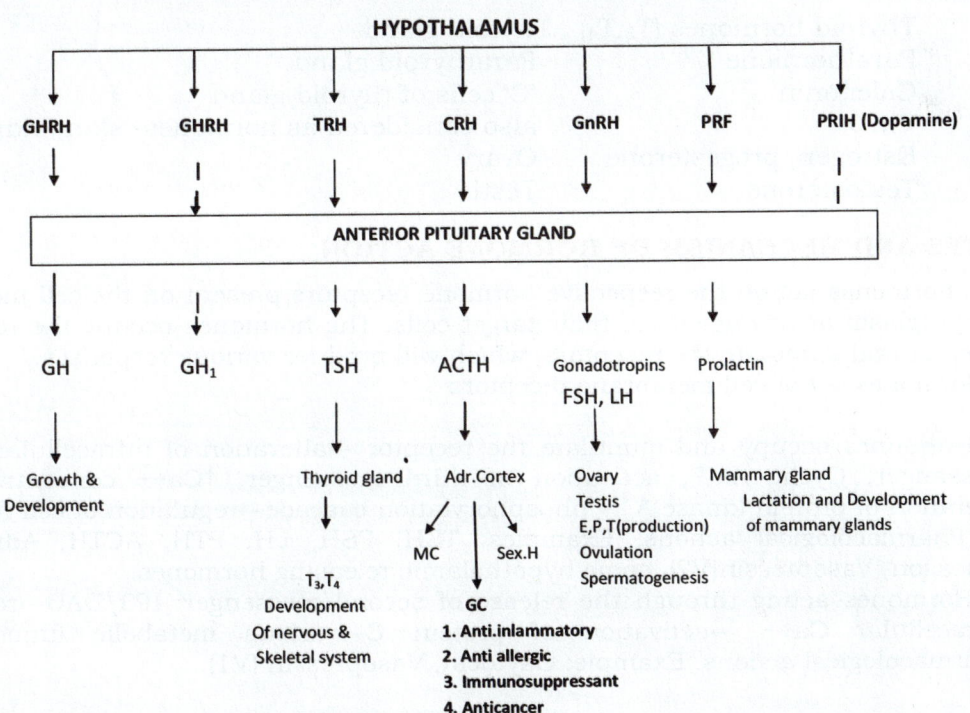

HORMONES	SECRETED FROM
CRH	
Thyrotrophin releasing hormone	Hypothalamus
PRIH & PRH	
GHRH&GHRIH	
Growth hormones	
TSH	
ACTH	ANTERIOR
FSH	
LH	PITUITARY
Prolactin	
Oxytocin	Posterior pituitary
Vasopressin (ADH)	
Glucocorticoids	Adrenal cortex
Mineralocorticoids	
Adrenaline	Adrenal medulla
Nor adrenaline	
Renin	JGA in the kidney
Insulin	β cells of pancreas
Glucogon	α cells of pancreas
Thyroid hormones (T_3, T_4)	Thyroid gland
Parathormone	Parathyroid gland
Calcitonin	'C' cells of thyroid gland
Vit.D	also considered as hormones- skin, kidney
Estrogen, progesterone	Ovary
Testosterone	Testis

SITES AND MECHANISM OF HORMONE ACTION

The hormones act on the respective hormone receptors present on the cell membrane at cytoplasm or at nucleus of their target cells. The hormones occupy the respective receptor and stimulate the receptors, which will produce various responses.
I. Hormones act at cell membrane receptors

1. Hormones occupy and stimulate the receptor →alteration of intracellular second messanger, Cyclic AMP, activation of third messenger, ↑Ca++ concentration → alteration of protein kinase A → phosphorylation cascade→regulation of cell functions → Pharmacological actions. Examples: TSH, FSH, LH, PTH, ACTH, Adrenaline, Glucagon, Vasopressin(V2), some hypothalamic releasing hormones.
2. Hormones acting through the release of second messenger: IP3/DAG→release of intracellular Ca++ →activation of protein C→various metabolic functions → Pharmacological actions. Example: Oxytocin, Vasopressin (V1).

3. Direct activation of Protein Kinase A→phosphorylation cascade→regulation of various enzymes → Pharmacological actions. Example: Insulin, Growth Hormone, Prolactin.

II. Hormones act at cytoplasmic receptors: Hormones penetrate the cell membrane → reach cytoplasmic receptor → stimulate the receptors → migrate to nucleus and bind to specific genes → DNA mediated RNA synthesis → synthesis of functional proteins → Pharmacological actions. Examples: Steroidal Hormones, (Glucocorticoids, Mineralocorticoids, Sex Hormones)

III. Hormones act at nuclear receptors:

The hormones penetrate cell membrane → reach cytoplasm → penetrate the nucleus combines with its receptor → DNA-RNA mediated protein synthesis → Pharmacological actions. Examples: Thyroid Hormones.

Feed Back Mechanism

Secretion of Hormones: The secretion of many hormones (end hormones) is subjected to feed back mechanism involving the hypothalamus, Anteriror pituitary and end hormones. The end hormones are which act on the end organ tissues. They are

(1)   Thyroid hormones (T_3 and T_4)
(2)   Sex hormones (Estrogen, Progesterone and Testosterone)
(3)   Glucocorticoids
(4)   Growth hormone

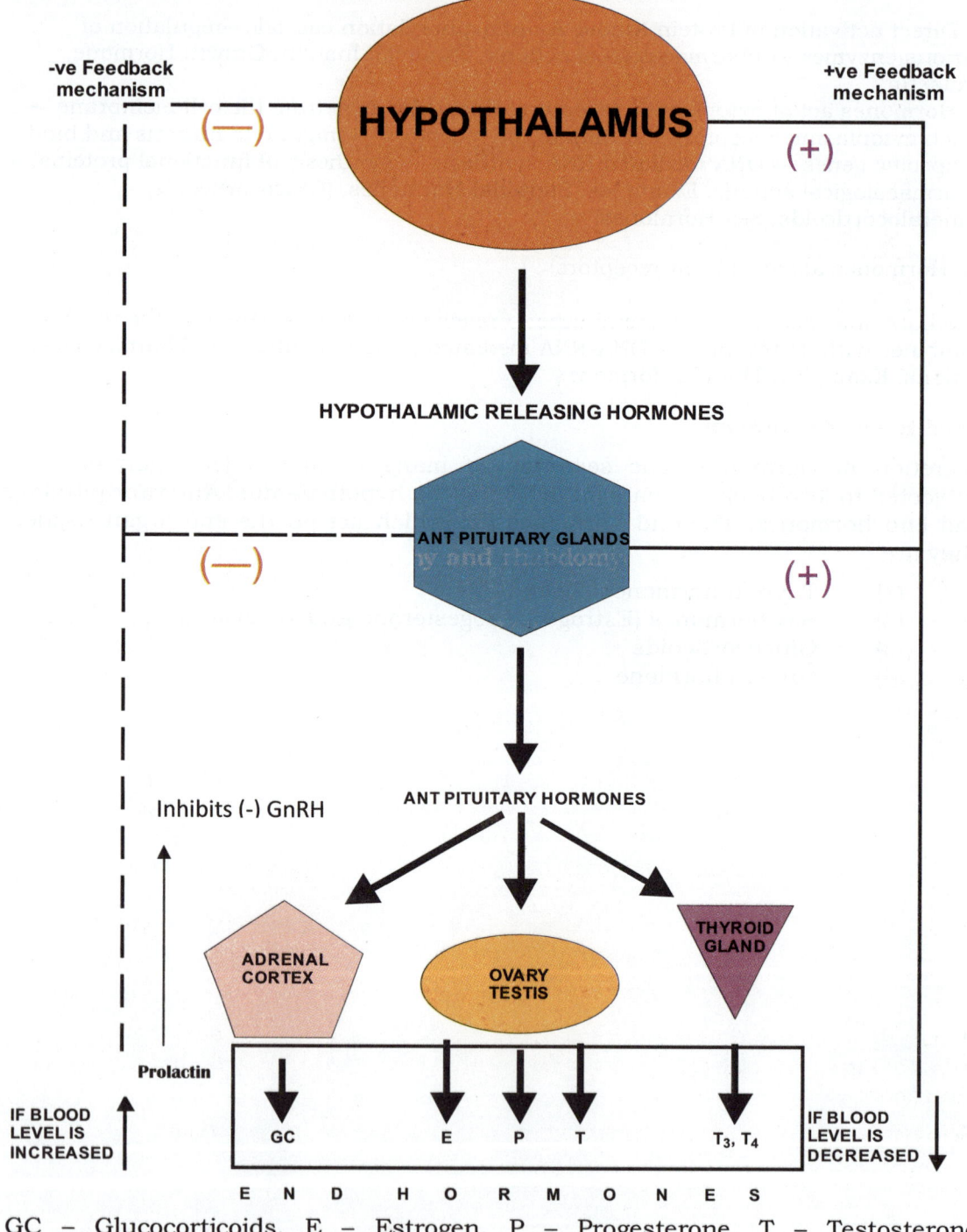

GC – Glucocorticoids, E – Estrogen, P – Progesterone, T – Testosterone, T₃ – Triiodothyronine, T4 – Thyroxine

Fig. 66 Feed Back Mechanism of end hormones

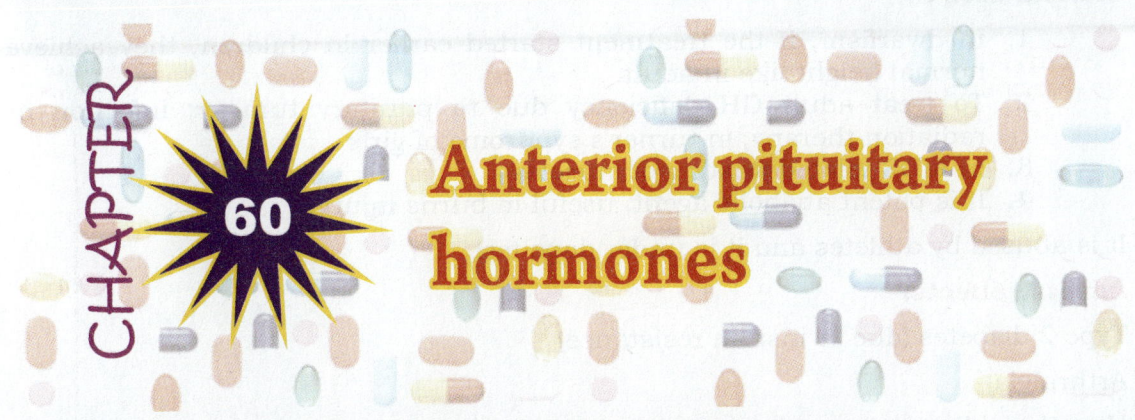

SOMATOSTATIN & OCTREOTIDE (GH inhibitors)

Somatostatin is a GHRIH →inhibits the secretion of GH

It inhibits secretion of TSH from anterior pituitory, inhibits insulin from pancreas and of gastrin from G.I.T.

Use is restricted because of short duration and lack of specificity for inhibiting only GH and of rebound increase in GH secretion after stopping it.

OCTREOTIDE

Somatostatin analogue.
Instead of somatostatin , octreotide is used for inhibiting GH secretion
Less inhibition of insulin → less hyperglycemia.

Clinical uses

1. In acromegaly, particularly in GH secreting anterior pituitary tumour.
2. It also controls symptoms of VIP secreting tumour associated with diabetes, diarrhoea
3. It is useful in bleeding esophageal varices, since it decreases mucosal blood flow.
4. In the treatment of AIDS associated with diarrhoea, breast cancer.
5. In Cushing's syndrome.

GROWTH HORMONE (GH)

It is an hormone secreted from anterior pituitary gland and controlled by hypothalamic hormone, GHRH. The secretion is inhibited by the use of Glucocorticoids, hyperglycemia.

Secretion is also increased by deep sleep, hypoglycemia and exercise.

Actions of growth hormone:

- It increases protein synthesis
- It increases body weight and growth
- The excess causes gigantism in child and acromegaly in adult
- The deficiency of GH causes dwarfism (short stature)

Clinical uses :

1. In dwarfism, if the treatment started earlier in children, they achieve normal height like in adult.
2. To treat adult GH deficiency due to pituitary tumour, infection or radiation therapy, in turner's syndrome of girls.
3. In AIDS related wasting of muscles
4. It is potent anabolic agent, useful in burns injury.

It is abused by athletes and it is under dope test.

Adverse effects:

Type 2 diabetes (due to insulin resistance)

Arthralgia

Hypothyroidism

Headache (due to increased intracranial tension)

PROLACTIN

- It is not useful clinically because of its short duration of action and given parenteral administration.
- It is secreted from anterior pituitary gland
- It is under the control of hypothalamic PRF & PRIH
- PRIH is dopamine in nature
- Dopamine inhibits prolactin secretion by acting on DA_2 receptor in anteriror pituitary gland and DA antagonist like metoclopramide, increases milk secretion.
- Main stimulus for prolactin secretion is by suckling of breast nipples and dopamine antagonist increases milk secretion.
- There is progressive increase of prolactin secretion during pregnancy and maximum at the time of delivery till breast feeding is stopped.

Functions of Prolactin

- Prolactin with Estrogen and Progesterone causes development of breast during pregnancy
- It promotes proliferation of ductal as well as acinar cells in the breast
- It induces synthesis of milk proteins and lactose
- High prolactin blood level inhibits Ganadotropic hormones→ inhibits ovulation, natural contraceptive during lactation period (lactational amenorrhoea) → pregnancy does not occurs.
- Hyperprolactinemia causes Galactorrhoea, amenorrhoea, infertility in women and sterility, impotence and gynaecomastia in men. Hyperprolactinemia is treated by Bromocriptine (Ref. Page No.246)

GONADOTROPINS (GN)

- Are FSH (Follicular Stimulating Hormone) and LH (Leutinizing Hormone)
- Controlled by GnRH (FSH/LH RH) from hypothalamus.

- Secreted from anterior pituitary.
- Subjected to negative feed back mechanism.

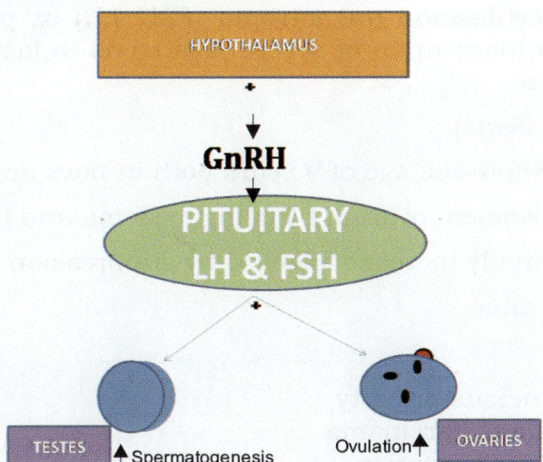

Fig.67 Actions of Gonadotropins

Action of FSH: (Fig.67)

In females

- It induces Follicular growth
- It induces development of Ovum
- It induces production of estrogen

males

it supports spermatogenesis

Action of LH: (Fig.67)

- It Induces full development of graafian follicle and trigers ovulation,
- Maintenance of corpus luteum
- Progesterone production from corpus luteum

It stimulates Testosterone production

from leydig cells of testis

Clinical uses of gonadotropins (FSH, LH)

Preparations:

- Menotropins (FSH+LH) preparation obtained from urine of menopausal women
- Urofollitropin (pure FSH)
- **HCG (FSH+LH) (human chorionic gonadotropins** is derived from from urine of pregnant women

1. In amenorrhoea and infertility, when clomiphen citrate failed or when non ovulation is due to polycystic ovaries→ it induces ovulation (HCG is given)

2. Hypogonadotrophic hypogonadism in males (HCG). It may be due to deficient of testosterone and manifested by delayed puberty, defective spermatogenesis and male sterility.

3.   Cryptorchism (undescended testis in children) can cause infertility. HCG is tried in children between 1-7 years old. The descent of testis can be achieved after 4-6 weeks of treatment. If there is no descent of testis it is better to go for surgery.

4.   To aid in vitro fertilization (menotropin (FSH+LH) or pure FSH) are used to induce simultaneous maturation of several ova so as to facilitate their harvesting for in vitro fertilization.

Excess Gn (Adverse effects)

Precocious puberty before the age of 9 years both in boys and girls

Polycystic ovaries in women, ovarian bleeding, oedema and headache

Gn RH analogues initially increase followed by suppression of Gn

i. Leuprolid   ii. Goserline

USES:

1.   In precocious puberty
2.   In prostatic carcinoma
3.   In polycystic ovaries

DRUGS ACTING ON UTERUS

Drugs may be either uterine stimulant or uterine relaxant

Uterine stimulants (ECBOLIC/OXYTOCIC)	uterine relaxants (TOCOLYTIC)↓ inhibit uterine motility (I.V. infusion)
Oxytocin Prostaglandins Methylergonovine	β₂ agonists (IV infusion) i.Salbutamol ii.Isoxuprine iii.Ritodrine
USES Oxytocin (IV infusion) for induction of labour PGs to induce abortion (cervical priming) vaginal tablet Methylergonovin – In PPH (Post Partum Haemorrhage) (IV)	Calcium Channel Blockers (IV infusion) decrease tone of myometrium Nifedipine Felodipine
	Magnesium sulphate IV infusion Oxytocin antibody (atosiban)
	Clinical uses To delay or postpone labour To arrest threatened abortion In dysmenorrhoea

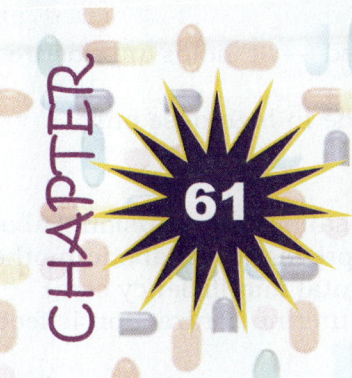

CHAPTER
61

Posterior pituitary hormones and drugs acting on uterus

OXYTOCIN

It is a posterior pituitary hormone secreted along with ADH (Anti Diuretic Hormone)

Main actions:

- uterine stimulant
- milk ejection

ORALLY NOT EFFECTIVE, SHORT DURATION OF ACTION, GIVEN BY I.V INFUSION

Stimuli for oxytocin secretion:

- dilatation of vagina, cervix
- suckling of baby at the breast
- Estrogen
- ovarian polypeptide, relaxin causes oxytocin releases

Mechanism of action: Oxytocin acts through G-protein coupled Oxytocin receptors → stimulates second messenger IP_3 (inositol triphophate), stimulates the release of $Ca++$→ contraction of uterus.

Actions:

1. **On uterus:** AT TERM it increases frequency and force of contraction of uterus
   - Estrogen sensitizes the uterus before oxytocin to act
   - Uterine sensitivity to oxytocin is increased last 9 weeks of pregnancy
   - And also oxytocin receptors are increased.

It induces stronger contraction on body and fundus with relaxation of lower segment for safe induction of labour (unlike Ergonovine, which contracts all segments at a time → foetal asphyxia → not suitable for induction of labour)

Oxytocin causes rupture of uterus in high dose.

2. On breast
- Milk ejection reflux (suckling) → suckling releases oxytocin and increases milk secretion

- Milk production is not increased (that depends on prolactin secretion)
  Other actions:
  - Umblical vessels → markedly constricted → it helps in closure of that at birth
  - It stimulate slightly Anti Diuretic Hormone in high dose only

Clinical uses

1. For induction of labour oxytocin : 5 IU/ saline/ IV infusion (labour needs to be induced in case of toxemia of pregnancy, diabetic mother, erythroblastosis, ruptured membrane, placental insufficiency etc.,)
2. In uterine inertia (Oxytocin is needed when uterine contraction is feeble and labour is not progressive satisfactorily).
3. In PPH (Post Partum Haemorrhage) (methyl ergonovine is preferred)
4. In breast engorgement → intranasal spray, if ejection of milk is not sufficient

Adverse effects: rupture of uterus, water intoxication (due to ADH action, avoided in renal insufficiency).

ANTIDIURETIC HORMONE (ADH)
VASOPRESSIN

ADH is secreted from posterior pituitary along with Oxytocin

Secretion of ADH is controlled by body hydration: Body dehydration→ increases ADH release → ↑ (increases) plasma osmolarity and concentration of Extra Cellular Fluid volume.

Drugs affecting ADH secretion

1) ADH secretion is enhanced by angiotensin II, Morphine, PGs, Histamine
2) ADH secretion is inhibited by Atrial natriuretic peptile, Alcohol

Mechanism of action :

Vasopressin receptors are V_1 and V_2

Stimulation of V_1 receptor causes vasoconstriction

Stimulation of V_2 receptor causes stimulation of smooth muscle and stimulate receptors in CD (Collecting Duct) and DT (Distal Tubule) to increase water permeabity

(antidiuretic action is by releasing ADH at DT and CD)

Pharmacological actions

1. On kidney (V_2) ↑ increase permeability of water in DT and CD →↑ reabsorption of water→ anti diuretic action. Deficiency of ADH →diabetes insipidus is characterised by polyuria, polydypsia

2. On blood vessels (V_1)→ vasoconstriction (particularly mesenteric blood vessels →useful in oesophageal varices → also causes clot in this area.
3. On other smooth muscles (V_2) stimulates uterus (oxytocic like action), stimulates Gastrointestinal peristalsis → evacuation of bowel and expulsion of gases from GIT.
4. It releases coagulation factor VIII & Van willebrand's factor→ useful in haemophilia and Von Willebrand's diseases→ check bleeding in these condtions.

Clinical uses of ADH/VASOPRESSIN/DESMOPRESSIN

- Vasoprossin → stimulates both V_1 and V_2 receptors
- Desmopressin potent V_2 agonist (no V_1 action)
- Based on V_2 actions, desmpressin (intranasal spray, oral, parenteral etc.,) is used
- Based on V_1 action (Vasopressin- Lyperssin) is used. ORALLY NOT EFFECTIVE. GIVEN BY I/M inj.

I. Based on V_2 actions (Desmopressin)

1. In diabetes inspidus (DI) only in neurogenic type (not effective in nephrogenic type)
   i. Neurogenic DI (depending on ADH secretion)
   ii. Nephrogenic DI- kidney is unresponsive to ADH
2. Bed wetting in children and nocturia in adults (antidiuretic action along with water intake restriction)
3. Haemophilia, Von willebrand's disease → check bleeding by releasing coagulation factors.

II. Based on V_1 receptors (vasopressin)

4. In bleeding oesophogeal varices → constriction of mesenteric blood vessels → reduce blood flow through liver to the varices→ clot is also formed, useful action to stop bleeding.

Adverse effects: parenteral → rise in B.P, constricts coronary blood vessels (precipitates angina). C/I in ischaemic heart diseases, hypertension. Belching, abdominal cramp and diarrhea.

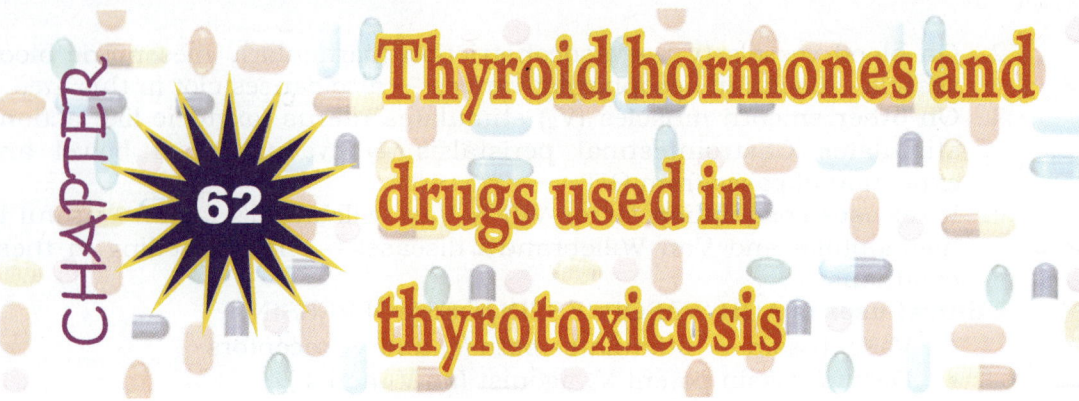

THYROID HORMONE

Secretion is under the control of TSH (Thyroid Stimulating Hormon) from Anterior pituitary

Hypothalamus

↓

TRH (Thyrotropic Release Hormone)

↓

Anterior pituitary

↓ TSH

Thyroid gland

↓

Thyroid hormones

- Thyroid hormones are two: T_3 and T_4
- T_4 (Thyroxine), T_3 (Triodothyronine)
- T_3 is more active

Synthesis of thyroid hormones

1. Iodide uptake: iodide is trapped by thyroid gland by active transport and getting concentrated in thyroid gland.
2. Oxidation and iodination : oxidized to iodine by thyroid peroxidase enzyme and then iodinating to monoiodotyrosine (MIT) and diodotyrosine (DIT)
3. Coupling : combination of 2 molecules of DIT form T_4 and combination of one molecule of MIT and one molecule of DIT form T_3
4. Storage and release : stored in thyroglobulin→ broken by proteolytic enzyme → release of T_3 and T_4 into circulation.
5. Peripheral conversing of $T_4 \rightarrow T_3$, which is more active and less amount is secreted.

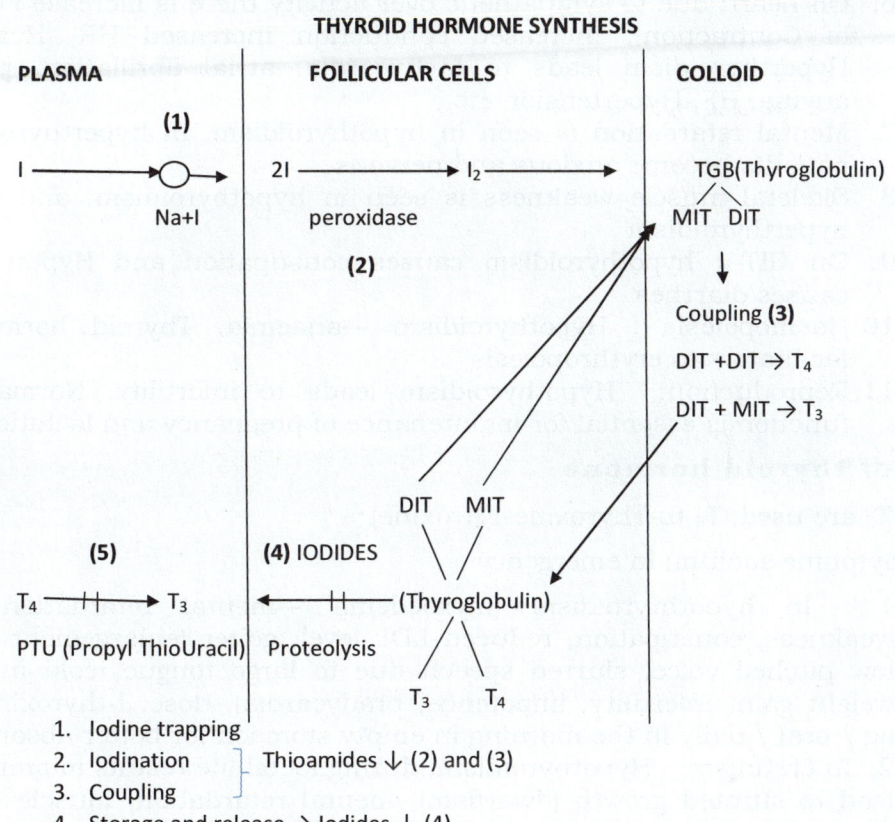

THYROID HORMONE SYNTHESIS

PLASMA FOLLICULAR CELLS COLLOID

(1)

I ──────▶〇──────── 2I ──────────▶ I₂ ──────────▶ TGB(Thyroglobulin)

Na+I peroxidase MIT DIT

(2) ↓

Coupling (3)

DIT +DIT → T₄

DIT + MIT → T₃

DIT   MIT

(5) (4) IODIDES

T₄ ──╫──▶ T₃ ◀──╫── (Thyroglobulin)

PTU (Propyl ThioUracil) Proteolysis

T₃   T₄

1. Iodine trapping
2. Iodination ⎤ Thioamides ↓ (2) and (3)
3. Coupling ⎦
4. Storage and release → Iodides ↓ (4)
5. Inhibits the conversion of T₄ to T₃

Actions of thyroid hormones

1. Growth and development: thyroid hormones are essential for normal growth and development. Essential for mental growth by improving myelination of the nervous system. Hypothyroidsm leads to impairment of myelination

2. Plasma FFA (Free Fatty Acid) level is increased →lipogenesis and cholesterol synthesis is decreased. Hypothyroidism→ increases LDL concentration → hypercholesterolemia.

3. Carbohydrate metabolism also increased → hyperglycemia. Hyperthyroidism→ insulin resistance Type 2 DM like.

4. Protein metabolism →catabolic. Hyperthyroidism →muscle wasting, weight loss. Hypothyroidism→ myxoedema → increase mucoprotein synthesis and accumulation.

5. Calorigenic: they increase BMR (Basal Metabolic Rate) → increase cellular metabolism → increase body temperature. In hypothyroidism there is cold intolerance. In hyperthyroidism there is heat intolerance.

6. On heart: due to sympathetic over activity there is increase FOC (Force of Contraction), increased conduction increased HR (Heart Rate). Hyperthyroidism leads to tachycardia, atrial fibrillation, precipitate angina, HF, Hypertension etc.,

7. Mental retardation is seen in hypothyroidism. In hyperthyroidism the patients become anxious and nervous.

8. Skeletal muscle weakness is seen in hypothyroidism, and tremor in hyperthyroidism

9. On GIT : hypothyroidism causes constipation and Hyperthyroidism causes diarrhea

10. Haemopoiesis : Hypothyroidism →anaemia. Thyroid hormones are facilitators to erythropoiesis

11. Reproduction: Hypothyroidism leads to infertility. Normal thyroid function is essential for maintenance of pregnancy and lactation.

USES of thyroid hormone

T_4 and T_3 are used, T_4 (L-Thyroxine-Eltroxine)

T_3 (liothyronine sodium) in emergency

1. In hypothryroidism (myxoedema →mental retardation, muscle weakness, constipation, reduced LDL level, goiter (enlargement of gland), low pitched voice, slurred speech due to large tongue, cold intolerance, weight gain, infertility, impotence, bradycardia). dose: l-thyroxine 50-100 µg / oral / daily in the morning in empty stomach for better absorption.

2. In cretinism: Hypothyroidism, during foetal life results in cretinism will lead to stunted growth (dwarfism), mental retardation, muscle dystrophy etc., It may be due to iodine deficiency in food and drinking water. Iodized salts are useful.

3. In Hypothyroidism during pregnancy, in endemic area → to prevent foetal mental retardation →levothroxine/ daily is given with iodine intake

4. In endemic goitre, which occurs in person consuming daily the Iodine deficient water, food. Iodine is given with levothyroxine till euthyroid sate is reached.

5. In Non toxic goitre (enlargement of thyroid gland)- defect in thyroid hormone synthesis. There is increased TSH level stimulates thyroid gland → enlargement of thyroid gland → goitre → more Thyroid hormones are released. Only T_4 is given as replacement therapy. T_4 inhibits TSH (Fig.68)

6. In thyroid nodules: TSH is more. T_4 , reduces TSH secretion by negative feed back mechanism, benign functioning nodules regress. (Fig.68)

7. Myxoedema coma: There is progressive mental deterioration. It is an emergency condition

8. After Radio active Iodine: to treat post radiation hypothyroidism

9. In refractory oedema, infertility, menstrual irregularities

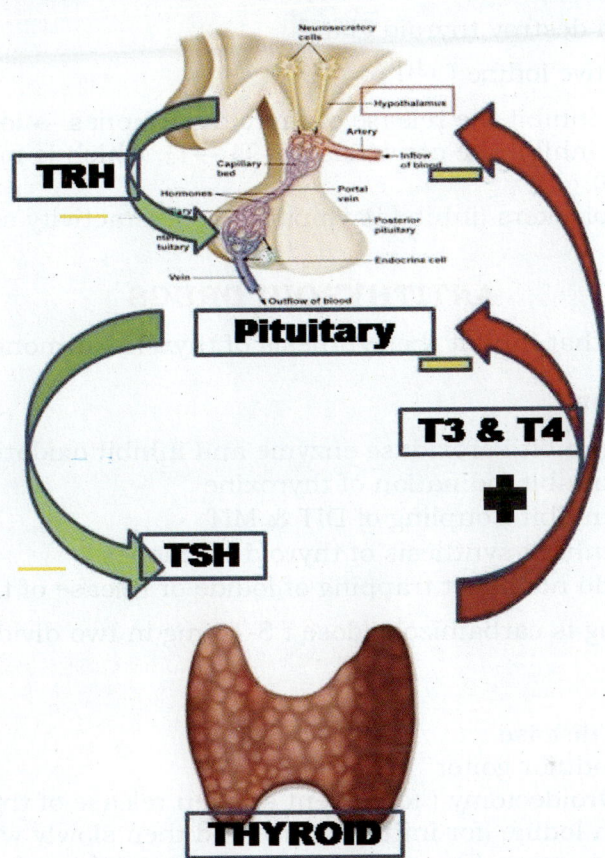

Fig.68 Negative feedback mechanism of T₃, T₄

Adv.effects: tachycardia, palpitation, tremor, weight loss, diarrhoea, heat intolerance, profuse sweating even in mild sunlight, insomnia, precipitate angina.

THE DRUGS USED IN HYPERTHYROIDISM OR THYROTOXICOSIS

THYROTOXICOSIS

(Grave's disease in adult) is due to hyperthyroidism and is characterised by heat intolerance even in slight sun exposure, profuse sweating, tachycardia, palpitation, increased FOC, increased O_2 consumption, high output failure, diarrhoea, reduced LDL level etc.,

DRUGS

  I. Antithyroid drugs: inhibit synthesis of thyroid hormones

    i)Carbamizole

ii)Propylthiouracil→ uselful in pregnancy

II.Drugs which destroy thyroid gland

i)Radioactive iodine (^{131}I)

III. Drugs which inhibit the release of thyroid hormones → iodides (pot/sod)
IV. Drugs which inhibit the conversion of T_4 →T_3, which is more potent
(Propylthiouracil).
V. β adrenergic blockers (inhibits sympathetic orveractivity seen in
thyrotoxicosis)

ANTITHYROID DRUGS

Drugs that inhibit the synthesis of thyroid hormones

Mechanism of action :

- They inhibit Peroxidase enzyme and inhibit oxidation of iodides
- They inhibit Iodination of thyroxine
- They inhibit Coupling of DIT & MIT
- They inhibit synthesis of thyroid hormones
- They do not affect trapping of iodide or release of thyroid hormones.

Commonly used drug is carbamizole (dose : 5-10 mg in two divided doses)

Clinical uses :

1. In grave's disease
2. In toxic nodular goiter
3. Before thyroidectomy (to prevent sudden release of thyroid hormones)
4. Along with Iodine (for initial control and then slowly withdrawn}
5. In thyroid storm (Propylthiouracil which inhibits the conversion of T_4 →T_3 with propranolol are better combination)

Advantages	Disadvantages
1) Well tolerated	1) **Adverse effects**: Hypothyroidism, agranulocytosis, loss of hair
2) Safe in children and pregnancy (propylthiouracil)	2) Prolonged (sometime life long) treatment is needed
3) No surgical scar or damage to parathyroid gland and recurrent laryngeal nerve	3) Poor Patient's compliance and expensive treatment
4) If hypothyroidism, it is reversible	4) Relapse is common
	5) Slow onset

RADIOACTIVE IODINE (^{131}I)

Used in thyrotoxicosis

Mechanism of action :

It is taken orally (5-10 millicurie/single dose) and is concentrated in thyroid gland → it emits β rays → penetrates only upto 3-5 mm in the soft tissue and DESTROYS thyroid gland. (Parathyroid gland is not affected) → fibrosis (medical thyroidectomy) and also emits γ rays used for dose regulations.

Clinical uses :

1. In Grave's disease
2. In toxic nodular goitre

ADVANTAGES	DISADVANTAGES
1.very convenient	1.not recommended for children & pregnant women
2.patient's compliance is good	2.thyroid carcinoma – rare
3.no relapse	3.slow onset of action
4.no surgery (no scar, no damage to laryngeal nerve)	4.prolonged observation for permanent hypothyroidism
5.Inexpensive	5.special facilities for handling the radioactive materials are necessary

SODIUM/POTASSIUM IODIDE

Oldest drug used in hyperthyroidism (high dose) as well as in hypothyroidism (low dose)

Mechanism of action

Quick onset of action

Inhibit the release of thyroid hormones

Maximum benefit occurs only for 2 weeks (once the gland is saturated because of the inhibition of release of thyroid hormones) → spills out / leaks out hormones → thyroid hormones level are increased in the blood and hence not effective in hyperthyroidism, which needs more than 2 weeks treatment.

Also decrease TSH secretion

Reduce blood supply to the thyroid gland and reduce bleeding during thyroidectomy

The gland becomes firm (easy for the surgeon to handle the gland)

Clinical uses :

1. Before thyroidectomy (it is given 2 weeks before thyroidectomy)

2. For prevention of endemic goiter (available as iodized salt)

3. To rapid control of hyperthyroidism/ thyrotoxic crisis.

4. Non endocrine USES: i) As antiseptic (Povidone-iodine) ii) KI- as expectorant

Adverse effects: swelling of eye lids, lip, larynx in sensitive individuals, salivation, lacrimation, rhinorrhoea. Avoided in pregnancy.

THYROID STORM:

- Excess thyroid hormones activity
- Extreme hyper metabolism may occur
- After thyroidectomy in an inadequately prepared patients (excess, sudden release of thyroid hormones (surgical storm)
- In the presence of infection, injury to thyroid gland, there is excess release thyroid hormones (medical storm)
- Manifestations: hyperpyrexia, dehydration, marked tachycardia, extreme irritability, delirium, increased sympathetic activity etc.,

Treatment:

1. Hospitalization and treatment of coma

2. Large dose of antythyroid drug (propylthiouracil), since it has additional action of inhibiting the peripheral conversion of $T_4 \rightarrow T_3$

3. Sodium Iodide (IV infusion) inhibit quickly the release of thyroid hormones

4. Propranolol IV 10mg/ 4 hrly inhibit sympathetic overactivity

5. Hydrocortisone (100mg/IV) – Sodium / water retention to counteract the dehydration

6. Oxygen

7. IV fluids and Glucose (to prevent dehydration)

8. Paracetamol (for hyperpyrexia)

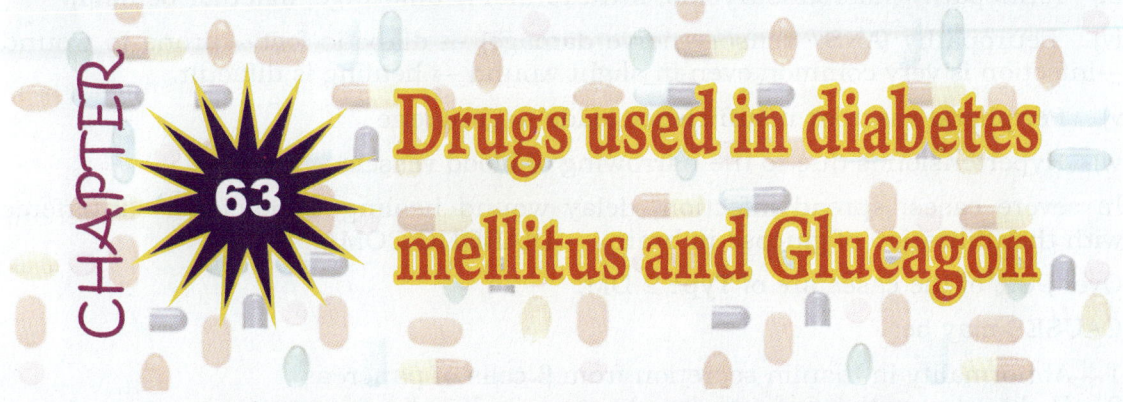

Drugs used in diabetes mellitus and Glucagon

CHAPTER 63

DRUGS USED IN DIABETES MELLITUS (DM)

DM is the most common endocrine disorder and is caused by a decrease in the concentration of circulating Insulin and/ or decrease in the responsiveness of the peripheral tissues to Insulin (Insulin resistance)

It is metabolic disorder involving not only carbohydrate but also protein and lipid.

It is characterized by heperglycemia, glucosuria, hyperlipidemia, negative nitrogen balance and ketonemia.

Common clinical manifestations are:

1. polyuria
2. polydipsia (thirst)
3. Polyphagia
4. weakness, fatigue
5. recurrent blurring vision
6. vulvovaginitis, pruritus, balanitis (inflammation of glans penis)

Complications of DM:

Sometime it may be asymptomatic (or unnoticed by the patients) till the patients present one or more diabetic complications

Untreated or poorly treated DM can lead to complications (prolonged hyperglycemia) such as

1. prolonged exposure of hyperglycemia → accumulations of GLYCOSYLATED END PRODUCTS (SORBITOL, GLYCEROL) IN THE BLOOD VESSELS → THICKENING OF CAPILLARY BASEMENT MEMBRANES → ↑ VESSEL WALL MATRIX AND CELLULAR PROLIFERATION →PREMATURE ATHEROSCLEROSIS (NARROWING OF THE LUMEN) → REDUCED BLOOD FLOW TO ALL THE ORGANS

i) diabetic nephropathy- sclerosis of glomerular capillaries → renal failure
ii) coronary artery diseases

iii)   retinopathy (microaneurysms, intra retinal heamorrage, macular oedima)

iv)   neuropathy (ANS/ sensory nerve damage) → diabetic foot→ prone to wound →infection is very common even in slight wound → healing is difficult.

v)   Peripheral vascular insufficiency leads to gangrene

vi)   Hypertension is due to the narrowing of blood vessels

In severe cases: spread infection, delay wound healing, ketoacidosis (interferes with the utilization of glucose in brain) → DIABETIC COMA.

Over 90% of the cases are of Type 2 DM.

CAUSES may be:

1.   Abnormality in Insulin secretion from β cells of pancreas
2.   Reduced sensitivity of peripheral tissues to Insulin
3.   Reduction in the number of Insulin receptors
4.   Exhibits Insulin resistance
5.   Excessive of hyperglycemic hormones (Glucagon, Glucocorticoids)
6.   Obesity

CLASSIFICATION OF ANTIDIABETIC DRUGS

I,   Injectable: INSULIN (HUMAN INSULINS):

(prepared by DNA recombinant technology)

1. Human actrapid (Human regular Insulin→ short acting)

2. Human monotard (Human lente Insulin→ intermediate acting)

3. Human Insulatard (Human isophane Insulin→ intermediate acting)

4. Human mixtard (Human soluble Insulin-30% + isophane Insulin-70%) long acting

II.   Insulin analogues:

   1. Insulin glargine (Long acting)
   2. Insulin Aspart (short acting)

III.   Oral antidiabetic agents:

1.   Sulphonyl ureas:

   i)   Glibenclamide

   ii)   Glipizide

   iii)   Gliclazide

   iv)   Glimepiride

2.   Biguanide: METFORMIN

3.   Meglitinide: Repaglinide

4.   Glitazones: Pioglitazone

5.   α-glucosidase inhibitors: ACARBOSE, Miglitol

6. DPP IV (Dipeptidyl Peptidase-IV) inhibitors: Sitagliptin, Vidagliptin, Teneligliptin

7. Newer drugs: Sodium Glucose Co-Transporter-2 (SGLT-2) inhibitors: Dapaglifozin, Remoglifozin, Sotaglifozin

Diagnosis of DM

- If fasting blood sugar is more than 125mg/dl
- If post prandial blood sugar is more than 200mg/dl
- If HbA$_1$C is more than 6.4%
- The Hb becomes glcosylated and form HbA$_1$C and its concentration indicates severity and duration of hyperglycemic state
- Prediabetic;
  If PPBS is between 140mg/dl and 199mg/dl
  If FBS is between 100mg/dl and 124mg/dl

Major types of DM : Type 1 and Type 2

Type 1	Type 2
1. Juvenile onset (upto 20 yrs)	1. Adult onset (maturity onset-over 40 yrs)
2. Autoimmune disease	2. High degree of genetic predisposition
3. Circulating Insulin is ABSENT	3. Circulating Insulin is low or normal
	4. Reduced responsiveness of peripheral tissues to Insulin
4. Treatment is only by Insulin	5. Oral antidiabetic agents are effective and sufficient

INSULIN

It is an injectable antidiabetic agent.

Secreted from β cells of pancreas

Control:

1. blood glucose level: glucose receptors are present on the β cells of pancreas → increase blood glucose → Act on glucose receptors in the β cells of pancreas → increase release of Insulin → reduce blood glucose.

2. Hormonal: Glucagon → increase Blood sugar level → Increase Insulin release

3. Stimulation of β$_2$ receptors → inhibits Insulin release → Hyperglycemia

Glucose is very important for storage of fuel and energy production

But at the same time, excess glucose → DM and dangerous.

Insulin reduces excess blood glucose and produces hypoglycemia

Deficiency of Insulin → hyperglycemia → DM

Mechanism of action (Ref: Mechanism and site of action of Hormones)

Insulin receptors are present everywhere, particularly in LIVER, ADIPOSE TISSUES AND SKELETAL MUSCLES (highly sensitive)

Insuline promotes the entry of glucose into cells and also uptake of glucose by cells through Glucose Transporters (GLUT) by active transport.

Muscle activity (exercises)→ increase glucose entry into muscles → Insulin sparing effect.

Actions of Insulin: Reduce blood glucose level

It acts on 3 important organs: LIVER, ADIPOSE TISSUES AND SKELETAL MUSCLES

LIVER	MUSCLE	ADIPOSE TISSUES
1. Increase glucose uptake & glycogen synthesis	1. Increase glucose uptake & utilization	1. Increase glucose uptake and storage as fat and glycogen
2. Inhibits glycogenolysis → reduces glucose output	2. Stimulates AA(Amino Acids) entry → increase protein synthesis	2. Stimulates Lipogenesis
3. Inhibits gluconeogenesis (conversion of non carbohydrates → glucose)	3. inibits proteolysis → reduces release of AA → inhibits gluconeogenesis in liver	3. Inhibits lipolysis & inhibits the release of FFA + glycerol → inhibits gluconeogenesis in the liver
↓	↓	↓
reduce blood glucose	**reduce blood glucose**	**reduce blood glucose**
Insulin deficiency causes increase in blood glucose	Insulin deficiency causes Increase in blood glucose - catabolism	Insulin deficiency causes Increased production of ketone bodies Ketonuria Ketoacidosis (diabetic coma)

Dose of Insulin= 0.3 – 0.7 U/kg/daily/SC (approximately 20-50 U/ day)

usually given in two divided doses, 2/3 of dose is given at pre-breakfast and the rest is given at pre-supper/ pre-lunch

INSULIN DEFICIENCY:

1. Hyperglycemia
2. Ketoacidosis (interferes with glucose utilization by brain) → diabetic coma
3. Catabolism
4. Fat is broken down→ FFA and glycerol in the blood →to liver with Acetyl Co A → diverted to produce ketone bodies (acetone, acetoacetate) →keto acidosis and ketonuria
5. Leads to increased LDL level

Clinical uses :

1. In Type1 DM

2. In Type2 DM

i) not responding to diet, exercise and oral antidiabetic agents

ii) DM associated with pregnancy, infection, trauma- to tide over anxiety temporarily in those patients

iii) In diabetic ketoacidosis

3. Non diabetic USES: i) In hyperkaelemia (Insulin+glucose drip) ii)In burns (Insulin+glucose drip) to reduce Na+ and K+ loss.

Adverse effects:

I.   Hypoglycemia
   - mild
   - severe
   - due to inj.of large dose of Insulin
   - missing a meal
   - performing vigorous exercise
   - mild : symptoms are due to sympathetic over activity → PALPITATION, anxiety, tremor, sweating etc., (glucose oral → in the form of sweet candy is sufficient)
   - severe : if blood glucose goes below 40mg/dl → neuro glucopenic syndrome → due to deprivation of brain nutrients (glucose) → dizziness, behavioral change, confusion, visual disturbances, fall in B.P, fatigue, weakness, seizure → COMA (IV glucose therapy)

CLASSIFICATION OF ORAL ANTIDIABETIC AGENTS

I. ↑ (stimulate) insulin release – sulphonyl ureas

   1) first generation – chlorpropamide (not used) →replaced by 2nd generation
   2) second generation
      i.   Glibenclamide
      ii.   Glipizide
      iii. Gliclazide
      iv.   Glimepiride

II.   Meglitinide Analogues

      i.   Repaglinide
      ii.   Nateglinide

III. Newer drugs → DPP IV (Dipeptidyl Peptidase IV) inhibitors

      i) Sitagliptin

      ii) Vidagliptin

      iii) incretin mimetic →Exenatide

IV. Insulin sensitizers: (to overcome insulin resistance →insulin sensitizers → potentiates the actions of insulin). They do not release insulin.

    i.   Biguanide → METFORMIN

    ii.   GLITAZONE → i) Rosiglitazone
                    ii) Pioglitazone

    iii.   Amylin mimetic drug → Pramlintide

    iv.   Sodium Glucose Co-Transporter-2 (SGLT-2) inhibitor → Dapaglifozin

    v.   α glucosidase inhibitor → Acarbose, Miglitol

Oral antidiabetic agents are useful only in Type 2 DM (not effective in Type 1)

Characteristic feature of Type 2 DM:

1) maturity onset → 40 years

2) most common type 85-90 %

3) strong genetic predisposition

4) insulin resistance (reduced sensitivity of peripheral tissues to Insulin) → may be due to down regulation of Insulin receptors)→less GLUT (Glucose Transporter protein) also

5) circulating insulin less/ normal

6) only 10% of Type 2 DM, may require Insulin (when Insulin requirement is > 40 units per day → in surgery, trauma, stress, obese etc)

Approach to Drug therapy in Type 2 DM

Improve Insulin availability (insulin releasers)	overcome Insulin resistance → potentiates Insulin action (Insulin sensitizers)
• Sulphonyl ureas	- Metformin
• Meglitinide analogues	α Glucosidase inhibitor,SGLT – 2 inhibitor
• DPP IV inhibitors	- Pioglitazone

SULPHONYL UREAS

• Only second generation sulphonyl ureas are used

• they are oral hypoglycemic agents

• all the drugs are similar except some pharmacokinetic properties

ACTION: reduce the blood glucose (Hypoglycemia)

Adverse effects:

        HYPOGLYCEMIA, weight gain, flatulence, to be avoided in pregnancy, liver diseases

Mechanism of action of Sulphonyl ureas:

Sulphonyl ureas

↓

Stimulate sulphonyl urea receptors present in β cells of pancreas

↓

closure of K⁺ channel

↓

Depolarization

↓

Increase Ca⁺⁺ influx

↓

Degranulation

↓

release of Insulin from β cells of pancreas

↓

Insulin acts on Liver, adipose tissue, sk.muscle

↓

hypoglycemia

- also slightly decrease glucagon release
- 30-40% functional β cells should be available for its effective action
- not effective in Type 1 DM
- extrapancreatic action →increase insulin receptors in the target tissues

Clinical uses :

1) in Type 2 DM (best in not complicated, if blood sugar is < 200mg/dL & Insulin requirement is < 40 units/day)

- Gliclizide → inhibits platelet aggregation →useful in DM associated with Cardio vascular disease
- Glimepride →rapid onset, long acting, less hypoglycemia
- Chlorpropamide → useful in diabetes insipidus

Doses:

Glibenclamide – 6 to 20 mg / 2 doses / before breakfast and meal

Glimepiride – 1 to 4 mg/ daily

Gliclazide – 80 to 240 mg/daily

MEGLITINIDE ANALOGUE

- Oral hypoglycemic agent used in Type 2 DM
- Example: Repaglinide, Nateglinide

Mechanism of action: like that of sulphonyl urea

- rapid onset and short duration of action
- effective in early release of Insulin after meal

Clinical uses :

1. in Type 2 DM → in combination with other oral antidiabetic agent (not with sulphonyl ureas)

Adverse effects: HYPOGLYCEMIA

BIGUANIDE - METFORMIN

- one of the most important oral antidiabetic drugs in the treatment of Type 2 DM
- It does not produce hypoglycemia

Mechanism of action:

- It reduces blood glucose
- It does not release Insulin
- It is Insulin sensitizer
- It increases responsiveness of target cells to Insulin
- Circulating Insulin is essential for its action

    1) It stimulates $GLUT_1$ (Glucose transporter), which increase Glucose uptake by peripheral tissue → independent action → reduces Insulin resistance

    2) It inhibits hepatic gluconeogenesis → main action

    3) It inhibits Glucagon output

    4) It increases glucose uptake & peripheral utilization

    5) It increases the sensitivity of peripheral tissues to Insulin (reduces Insulin resistance)

    6) It reduces Glucose absorption

    7) It reduces LDL & VLDL level

    8) It potentiates all the actions of Insulin.

- It produces ANOREXIA → reduces body weight

Clinical uses :

1. In Type 2 DM

2. In polycystic ovary disease (menstrual irregularities, infertility) occur due to increased Anti insulin hormone → Insulin resistance → Metformin reduces Insulin resistance and hence useful in that condition → stimulates ovulation → pregnancy occurs

Dose: 2-4 gm/ daily at breakfast & at night with evening meal

Adverse effects: LACTIC ACIDIOSIS (rare), (more in alcoholic), METALLIC TASTE, ANOREXIA ($\downarrow$ body weight)

- It does not produce hypoglycemiam, abdominal discomfort, diarrhoea
- C/I in kidney and liver diseases

GLITAZONE - PIOGLITAZONE

- oral antidiabetic drug

Mechanism of action:

Pioglitazone

$\downarrow$

stimulates PPAR γ (Peroxism Proliferator Activated Receptor GAMMA)

$\downarrow$

stimulates $GLUT_4$ (Glucose transporter)

$\downarrow$

increases the entry of glucose into peripheral tissues

$\downarrow$

reverse Insulin resistance

$\downarrow$

Insulin sensitizing action

$\downarrow$

Reduces blood glucose level (but not hypoglycaemia) and reduces HbA_1C

- It also inhibits hepatic gluconeogenesis
- It reduces blood glucose & reduces HbA_1C

Clinical uses:

first line drug in Type 2 DM (alone or with other antidiabetic agents)

Adverse effects:

Fluid retention, (aggravate HF) → oedema, anaemia, weight gain

- with O.C.P (oral contraceptive pill) → failure of contraception

α GLUCOSIDASE INHIBITORS

ACARBOSE. Miglitol

- oral antidiabetic agent
- used in Type 2 DM

Mechanism of action:

- drug is taken at the beginning of the meals

- inhibits α glucosidase → inhibit hydrolysis of oligosaccharides to glucose and other sugars → delays the absorption and digestion of carbohydrate and thereby lower post-prandial glucose level
- It does not increase Insulin release
- It does not potentiate Insulin action

Clinical use: In Type 2 DM (particularly useful in post prandial hyperglycemia)

Adverse effects: Flatulence, abdominal cramp, diarrhea

DIPEPTIDYL PEPTIDASE (DPP) IV INHIBITORS

Example : Sitagliptin

- oral antidiabetic agent
- no hypoglycaemia

Mechanism of action:

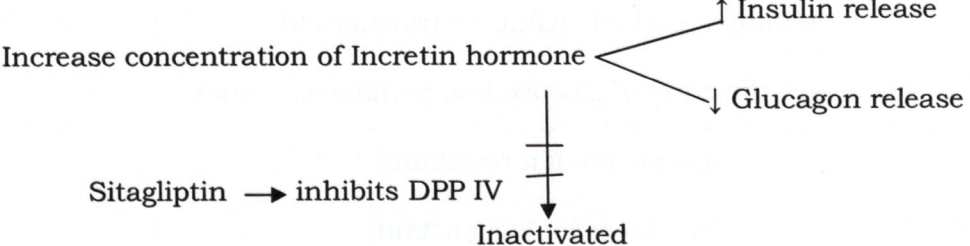

Sitagliptin inhibits enzyme DPP-IV → increase the concetration of incretin in GIT → release insulin in response to meal and inhibit inappropriate release of glucagon.

SGLT2 inhibitor (Sodium glucose transporter-2 inhibitor)

Example : Dapaglifozin

- Oral antidiabetic agent

Mechanism of action :

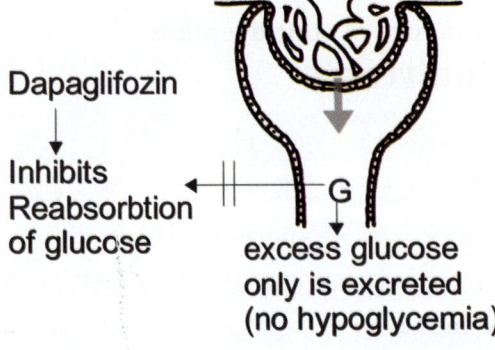

Dapaglifozin → in the U.T → inhibits reabsorption of excess glucose →only excess glucose is excreted. (Normal glucose reabsorption will be going on) → reduce blood glucose level in DM without producing hypoglycemia.

Drawbacks

1) Susceptibility to UTI (because of glucose in the urine, the organisms causing UTI will grow fast)

2) Loss of electrolytes K+ - hypokaelemia

INCRETINOMIMETIC Exenatide

Mechanism of action :

- Similar to incretin

↑ Insulin release

↓ Glucagon release

- Reduce blood glucose

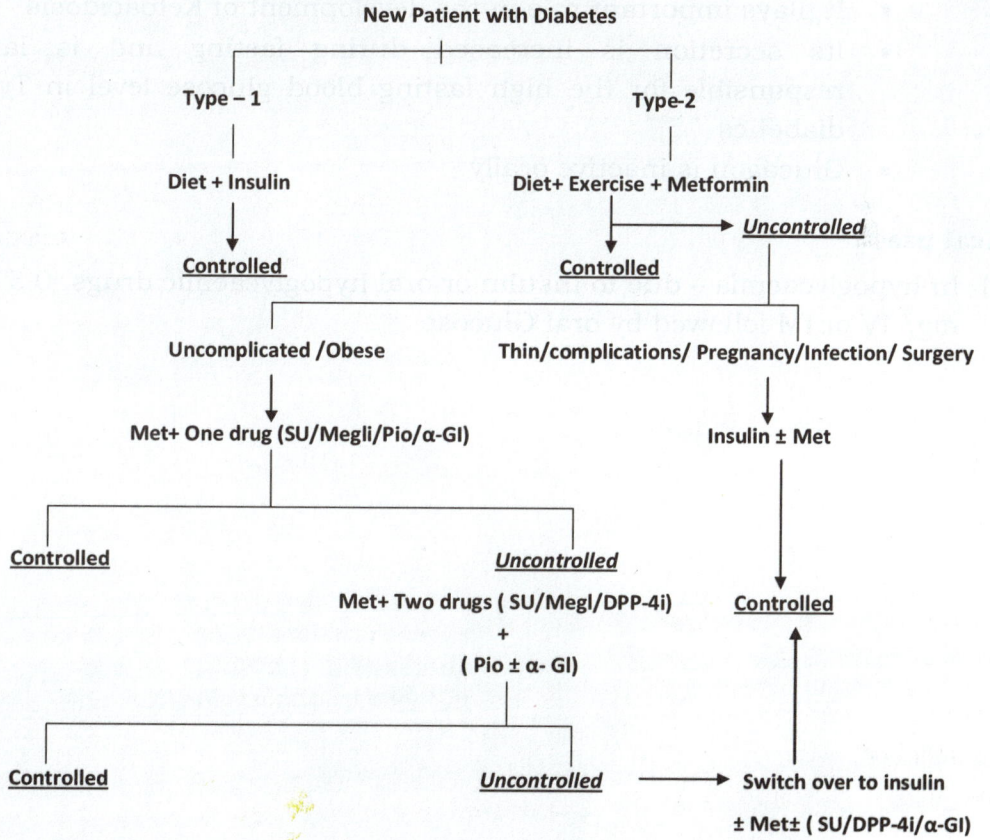

MANAGEMENT OF DIABETES MELLITUS

New Patient with Diabetes

Type – 1

Diet + Insulin

↓

Controlled

Type-2

Diet+ Exercise + Metformin

↓ → *Uncontrolled*

Controlled

Uncomplicated /Obese

↓

Met+ One drug (SU/Megli/Pio/α-GI)

Controlled

Uncontrolled

Met+ Two drugs (SU/Megl/DPP-4i)
+
(Pio ± α- GI)

Controlled

Uncontrolled ⟶ Switch over to insulin
± Met± (SU/DPP-4i/α-GI)

Thin/complications/ Pregnancy/Infection/ Surgery

↓

Insulin ± Met

↓

Controlled

GLUCAGON

Control of secretion – Incretin GLP – I - ↓ (inhibits) Glucagon secretion

- High Glucose level - ↓ (reduces) Glucagon secretion
- Insulin – stimulates Glucagon secretion
- Sympathetic ↑ → ↑ (stimulates) Glucagon release

Actions of Glucagon :

- It is hyperglycemic
- Glucagon causes hyperglycemia by enhancing glycogenolysis and gluconeogenesis
- It is hormone of fuel mobilisation
- It plays important role in the development of Ketoacidosis
- Its secretion is increased during fasting and is largely responsible for the high fasting blood glucose level in Type-2 diabetics
- Glucagon is inactive orally.

Clinical uses :

1) In hypoglycaemia – due to Insulin or oral hypoglycaemic drugs. 0.5 – 1 mg/ IV or IM followed by oral Glucose

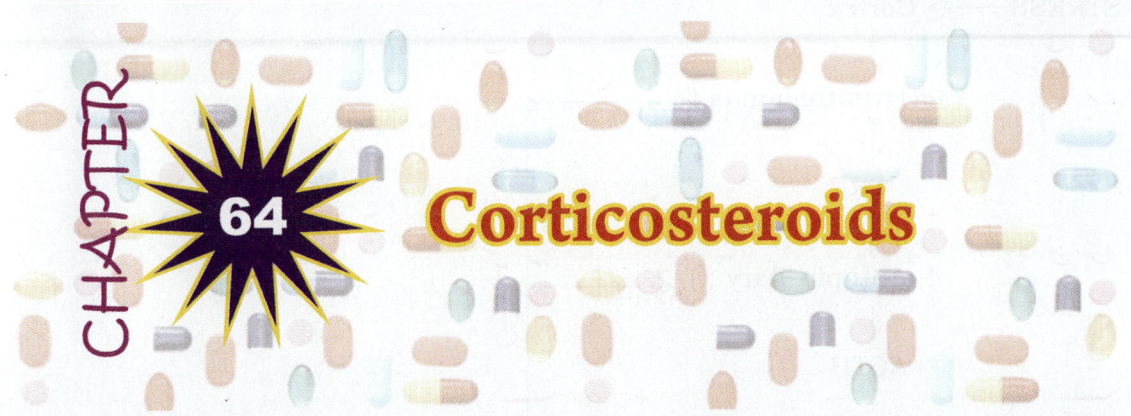

Corticosteroids

Why the name corticosteroids →since these hormones secreted from Adrenal 'cortex' and are having 'steroid' structure.

Mainly two types of corticosteroids

1. Glucocorticoid (Hydrocortisone) → since prominent action on glucose metabolism.
2. Mineralocorticoids (Aldosterone) → prominent action on minerals (Na^+/ K^+)

Control of secretion → by ACTH (Adrenocortico Trophic Hormone) from anterior pituitary.

Negative feedback mechanism

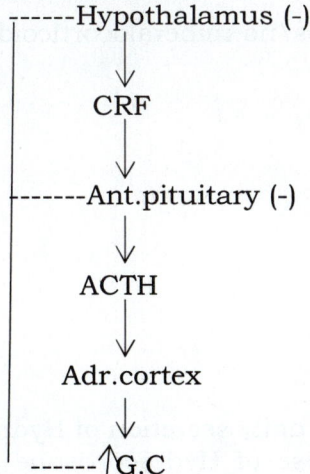

```
------Hypothalamus (-)
            ↓
          CRF
            ↓
------Ant.pituitary (-)
            ↓
          ACTH
            ↓
        Adr.cortex
            ↓
------↑G.C
```

Negative – feed back mechanism

Stress & GC (Glucocorticoids)

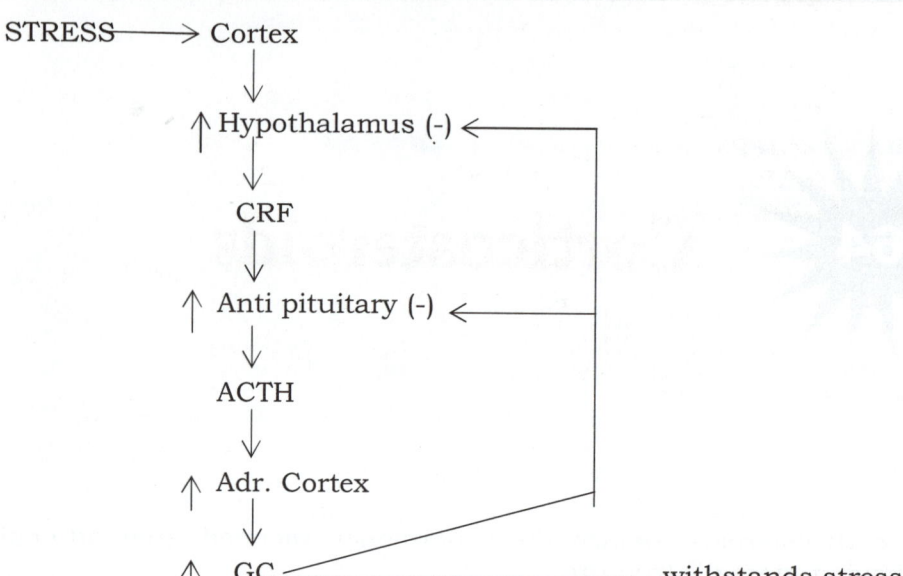

Circadian rhythm of secretion

The hydrocortisone secretion is maximum in the early morning. Daily secretion →
20 to 25 mg Clinical significance is that Hydrocortisone dose should be maximum
in the morning, while given for deficiency conditions.

CLASSIFICATION OF GLUCOCORTICOIDS

   I.   Natural → Hydrocortisone
  II. Synthetic GC : (potent G.C activity, less/no mineralocorticoid activity side
       effects)
      1. Short acting
         i)   Prednisolone
         ii)   Prednisone
      2. Intermediate and long acting
         i)   Triamcinolone
         ii)   Betamethasone
         iii)   Dexamethasone
      3. Topical GC (ref : Topical GC)

ACTIONS OF GC

Physiological actions (due to normal daily secretion of Hydrocortisone)
Pharmacological actions (Higher dose of Hydrocortisone is needed →
side effects will be more → hence synthetic GC is used, which are
having more potent GC activity and less/no mineralocorticoid side
effects). For pharmacological actions (for which **Clinical uses**) synthetic
GCs are preferred.

I Pharmacological actions

1. **ANTI INFLAMMATORY**
2. **IMMUNOSUPPRESSIVE**
3. **ANTI ALLERGIC / ANTI HYPERSENSITIVE ACTION**
4. **ANTI CANCER ACTION**

Mechanism of action:

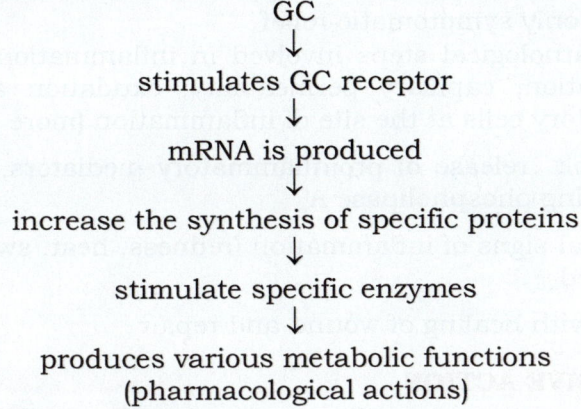

GC
↓
stimulates GC receptor
↓
mRNA is produced
↓
increase the synthesis of specific proteins
↓
stimulate specific enzymes
↓
produces various metabolic functions
(pharmacological actions)

ANTI INFLAMMATORY ACTION

The endogenous GCs prevent an excessive response of the body's powerful defence mechanism during stress, infection and inflammation which otherwise would have been hazardous. The anti inflammatory actions are due to,

1) In macrophages, monocytes → they inhibit the enzyme phospholipase A_2, which in turn inhibit the production of arachidonic acid, leads to reduction in the synthesis and release of PAF, PGs, LTs, which are important mediators of inflammation.

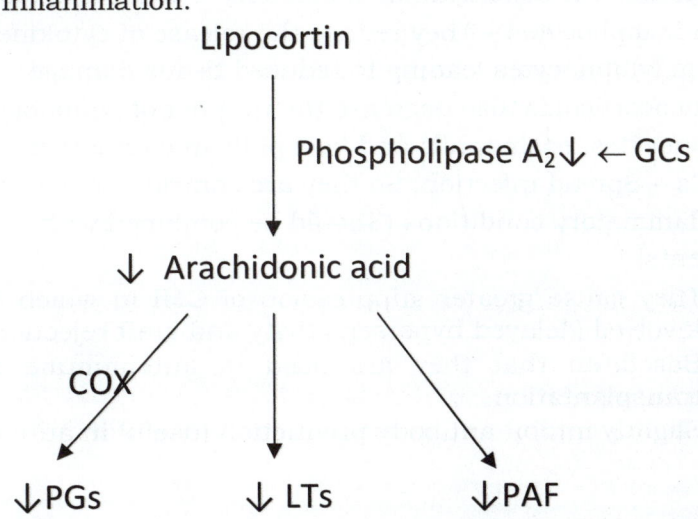

Lipocortin

Phospholipase A_2 ↓ ← GCs

↓ Arachidonic acid

COX

↓PGs   ↓ LTs   ↓PAF

They also inhibit the production of cytokines, TNF – α , which will lead to reduction in T-cell activation and suppression of fibro blast proliferation →reduce inflammation and cell mediated immunity.

Prevent the recruitment of lekocytes to the site of inflammation.

- Do not affect the cause of inflammation
- Potent antiinflammatory for all types of inflammation
- They give only symptomatic relief
- All the pathological steps involved in inflammation are inhibited, i.e., vasodilatation, capillary permeability, exudation and recruitment of inflammatory cells at the site of inflammation (more susceptible).

- Also inhibit release of proinflammatory mediators, (PGs, PAF, LTs) → by inhibiting phospholipase A_2

- All cardinal signs of inflammation (redness, heat, swelling and pain) are suppressed

- Interfere with healing of wound and repair

IMMUNOSUPPRESSIVE ACTION

- Suppress the cell mediated immunity. They act by inhibiting genes that code for the cytokines IL-1, IL-2, IL-3, IL-4, IL-5, IL-6 & IL-8 and interferon - □ (IFN - γ).The lesser cytokines production, reduces the T-cell proliferation.
- Glucocorticoids also suppress the humoral immunity by dimishing IL-2, inhibit the proliferation of B-Lymphocytes and hence inhibit the antibody production.
- Decrease the sensitization of cytotoxic T-Lymphocytes.
- On Lymphocytes – They reduce the release of cytokines (IL-1, IL-2, IL-4) from lymphocytes leading to reduced tissue damage.
- Glucocorticoids also decrease the number of lymphocytes (B and T-cells), monocytes, eosinophils and basophils in circulation.
- GCs - Spread infection. So they are contraindicated in infectious inflammatory conditions (Should be combined with suitable antimicrobial agents).
  - They cause greater suppression of CMI in which T-cells are primarily involved (delayed hypersensitivity and graft rejection)
  - Based on that they are used in autoimmune diseases and organ transplantation
  - Slightly inhibit antibody production (useful in autoimmune diseases)

ANTIALLERGIC OR ANTIHYPERSENSITIVE ACTION

- GCs suppress all types of hypersensitization and allergic phenomenon. They are effective in Type I hypersensitivity reaction (Anaphylactic shock)
- They inhibit B-lymphocytes → inhibit antibody production
- The antigen-antibody reaction is suppressed (useful in anaphylactic shock)
- They are effective in allergic conditions

ANTICANCER ACTION

- They inhibit lymphoid tissues
- In normal individual they are very less effective on lymphoid tissue
- But in lymphoma → they have got very prominent action
- There is increased destruction of lymphoid cells in lymphomas
- Hence these drugs are useful in lymphomas

II. **Physiological actions**

1. Carbohydrate metabolism. They produce anti insulin effect →resistance to insulin → hyperglycemia → caution in DM
2. Protein metabolism : They induce breakdown of proteins → muscle wasting → negative nitrogen balance → catabolism → loss of osteoid from bone
3. Fat metabolism: They stimulate lipolysis. Mobilization of fat and fat is deposited in face (moon face) neck (buffalo hump), stomach (pot belly), fish mouth
4. Calcium metabolism: They cause Hypocalcemia
- They inhibit intestinal absorption Ca $^{++}$
- They increase excretion of Ca^{++}
- They increase bone resorption
- They reduce bone formation → Spongy bones (vertebrae, neck of femur, ribs) and prone to fracture → osteosporosis
5. Water excretion
    Due to their slight mineralocorticoid activity
    They produce Na$^+$/ water retention causes oedema
    and there will be water intoxication after I.V infusion of GC
6. CVS : They cause vasoconstriction and rise in BP, they also increase the pressor action of Adrenaline & Noradrenaline
7. Sk. Muscles → muscle weakness (both in hypocorticism and hypercorticism)
8. CNS → they produce mild euphoria (feeling of well being) → they lower threshold to seizure. Caution in epilepsy
9. Stomach: They increase acid secretion and aggravate peptic ulcer (caution in peptic ulcer)

Clinical uses OF GCs (> 100 USES → no other drug has got so many Clinical uses). Anterior pituitary gland is called as "Master gland". Like that GCs can be called as "Master drug".

I.   **Endocrine uses** (replacement therapy) → (Hydrocortisone is preferred)

II. **Non endocrine uses** (Synthetic GCs are prefared)

I. Endocrine uses

1. Chronic adrenal insufficiency (Addison's disease) Hydrocortisone (oral)

2. Acute adrenal insufficiency

- It is an emergency condition
- May be due to sudden withdrawal of GC
- Hydrocortisone (IV) is given

3. Congenital adrenal hyperplasia (Adreno – genital syndrome)

- Due to genetic deficiency of the enzyme, 21-hydroxylase → GCs synthesis will fall → stimulate hypothalamus and ant.pituitary (due to negative feed back mechanism) → stimulate adr.cortex → GC synthesis will not be there due to the deficiency of 21-hydroxylase. But the synthesis and secretion of Androgen (excessive amount) will go on → virilisation, precocious sexual development. (Hydrocortisone (IV) is given)

II. Non endocrine uses due to their following pharmacological actions

1. Anti-inflammatory action
2. Immunosuppressive action
3. Antiallergic/ antihypersensitivity action
4. Anticancer action

1) Uses are due to anti-inflammatory action and antiallergic action. The systemic as well as topical GCs have one of the widest spectrum of medicinal USES for their anti-inflammatory property. GCs are powerful anti-inflammatory drugs→'itis' means 'inflammation'. Any condition ending in 'itis', GCs are used. (except infectious)

i)   In rheumatoid arthritis (only in severe cases → intra articular injection) –First→ NSAIDs (Non steroidal anti inflammatory drugs are tried) → then DMARDs (Disease modifying anti rheumatic drugs are tried) → lastly knee replacement may be tried.

ii) In osteoarthritis (only in acute exacerbation – intra-articular injection (otherwise NSAIDs are sufficient)

iii) In collagen's diseases → systemic lupus erythematosus (SLE), polyarteritis, nephrotic syndrome, glomerulonephritis

iv) In eye diseases – allergic conjunctivitis, iritis, iridocyclitis, keratitis etc (topical), retinitis, optic neuritis, uveitis (systemic therapy)

v)   In skin diseases (ref topical GCs under miscellaneous)

vi) In intestinal diseases – ulcerative colitis, crohn's disease (Inflamatory Bowel Disease)

vii) In cerebral oedema

viii) In neurocysticercosis (along with Albendazole)

ix) In anaphylactic shock, septic shock

x) In tuberculous meningitis (inflammation prevents the access of the antitubercular drugs to reach the site of action. The inflammation is to be removed in meninges→ so that the antitubercular drugs can effectively reach meninges). GCs are anti-inflammatory and useful in this condition.

xi) In bronchial asthma (inhalational beclomethasone is used as prophylactic)

2) Immunosuppressive uses

i) Because Glucocorticoids inhibit antibody protection (useful in auto immune diseases → myasthenia gravis, haemolytic anaemia, chronic hepatitis, thrombocytopenic purpura)

ii) Glucocorticoids suppress cell mediated immunity (CMI) and hence useful to prevent graft rejection in organ transplantation → GC is given prior to transplantation and continued as long as required.

3) In malignancy, (specific cancer)

1) In acute lymphatic leukemia, Hodgkin's and other lymphomas

2) GC is one of the components in various combinations used as anticancer

III. In ARDS (Acute Respiratory Distress Syndrome) is due to immature lung in foetus. GC is given to mother just prior to delivery. Hydrocortisone governs lung maturation in foetus. If defficiency of hydrocortisone leads to ARDS.

Adverse effects: (Cushing's syndromes)

G Glaucoma, Growth retardation

L Lipolysis

U Ulcerogenic ($\uparrow$ acid secretion)

C Cushing's syndrome

O Osteoporosis

C Cataract, catabolic

O Oedema (Na^+ / water retention)

R Rise in B.P ($\uparrow$ B.P) – vasoconstriction

T Thinning of skin, striae

I Infection is spread (fungal, viral, tuberculosis)

C Cleft palate in the offspring (if given to pregnant women)

O   Osteoid loss

I   Insulin antagonism – Hyperglycemia

D   Delayed wound healing

Doses: Prednisolone 5mg/daily

Betamethasone 2-4 mg/daily

Dexamethasone 2-4 mg/daily

Hydrocortisone 20-25 mg/IV

Contraindications (relative)

1) DM
2) Hypertension
3) Infection (AMA (Anti Microbial Agents) cover should be there) – (viral, fungal, TB)
4) Peptic ulcer
5) Osteoporosis
6) Epilepsy
7) HF
8) Renal failure

Precautions while prescribing GCs

1) Patients should be warned about the toxic effects due to sudden withdrawal of GC → acute adrenal insufficiency → sometime fatal). The patients should be advised to withdraw GC gradually, if used for more than 2 weeks
2) To avoid that complication – the GC is prescribed for alternative day and less potent GC with less dose
3) Hydrocortisone is given maximum dose in the morning (to simulate circardian rhythm)

MINERALOCORTICOIDS – Produce Na+/water retention → increase blood volume, oedema and increase B.P.

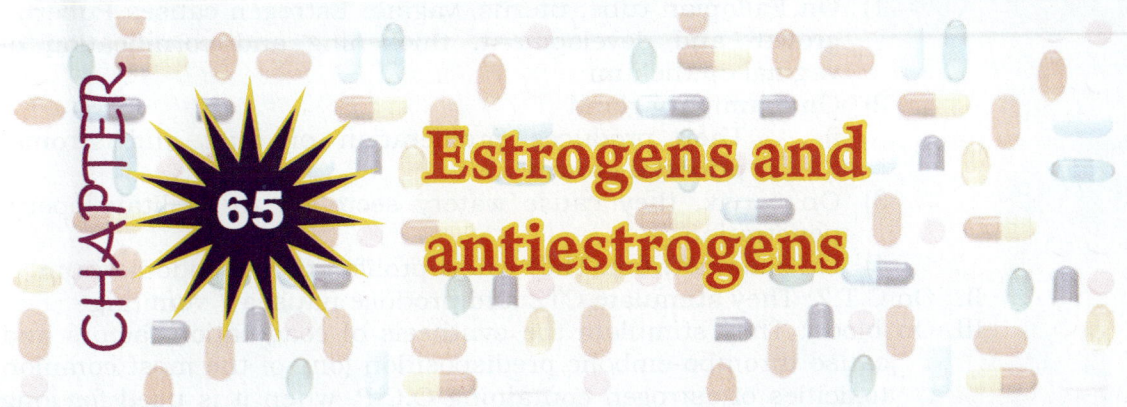

CHAPTER 65

Estrogens and antiestrogens

ESTROGENS

They are female sex hormones (the another one is Progesterone)

I. Natural estrogen
    i)   ESTRADIOL
    ii) Estrone
    iii) Estriol
    They are steroidal hormones. ORALLY NOT EFFECTIVE
II. Synthetic Estrogens (ORALLY EFFECTIVE) – they are commonly used)
    i)   ETHINYL ESTRADIOL
    ii) Mestranol (prodrug for ethinyl estradiol)
    iii) Quinesterol
III. Synthetic non-steroidal estrogen
    i)   Diethylstilbesterol (oral)

Control of secretion:

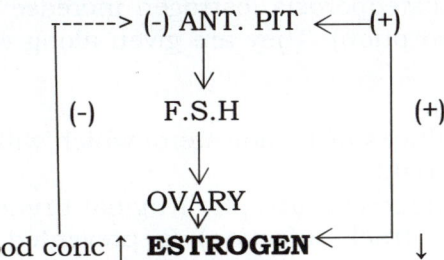

Blood conc ↑ **ESTROGEN**

(feed back mechanism)

- Blood concentration of Estrogen is subjected to 'feed back mechanism'
- Increased Estrogen level in plasma leads to inhibition of FSH secretion
- Reduced Estrogen level in plasma leads to increase FSH secretion

ACTIONS (PHYSIOLOGICAL FUNCTIONS) OF ESTROGENS

- They play important role in menstruation and in pregnancy (with LH & Progesterone)
    I. On female reproductive system:

1) On Fallopian tube, uterus, vagina: Estrogen causes Pubertal growth and development, thickening and cornification of vaginal epithelium

2) On mammary gland
   i) They produces proliferation of duct and stroma, pubertal growth

3) On cervix, they cause watery secretion to facilitate sperm penetration

4) On endometrium: They cause proliferation of endometrium

II. On C.T.Z: They stimulate CTZ and produce nausea / vomiting

III. On blood: They stimulate the synthesis of coagulation factors and cause thrombo-embolic predisposition (one of the most common toxicities of estrogen containing O.C.P, when it is used for long term)

IV. Lipid profile: They reduce LDL level and increase HDL level

V. Metabolic effects: They cause anabolic effect, hyperglycemia and Na^+/ water retention → oedema. They inhibit bone resorption and increase bone mass. They are useful as HRT (Harmone Replacement Therapy) in osteoporosis.

VI) Secondary sex characters :

- They produce growth of hair as female pattern
- The distribution of fat will be as female contour
- They cause pigmentation around nipples
- Estrogens will be responsible for the development of breast
- They produce high pitched voice in female

Clinical uses of ESTEROGENS (ETHINYL ESTRADIOL)

I) In post – menopausal syndromes: As Hormone Replacement Therapy (HRT) with progesterone → prevent osteoporosis (estrogen increase the bone formation and inhibit bone resorption). They are given along with calcium and vit. D.

- Inhibit vasomotor symptoms (hot flush)
- Reduce cardio vascular symptoms (It reduces LDL cholesterol which will be useful in preventing the cardio vascular risk).
- Post menopausal osteoporosis causes urogenital atrophy (vaginal dryness, vaginitis, urinary urgency and urinary track infection) is prevented by estrogens (topical)
- Estrogens lessen CNS symptoms – insomnia, fatigue, which may be due to estrogen deficiency.

II) Estrogen is used as oral contraceptive with progesterone

III) In primary ovarian failure. They induce ovulation.

IV) In dysfunctional uterine bleeding as adjuvant with Progesterone

V) In dysmenorrhoea (NSAID is preferred). Estrogen with progesterone are also beneficial

VI) In acne and hirsutism in female. Acne & hirsutism are due to increase in the concentration of androgens in the blood (Antibiotic, tretinoin are preferred)

VII) Carcinoma of prostate
1) Carcinoma of prostate is androgen dependent
2) Estrogen is anti-androgen and they are useful in this condition

Adverse effects:

In male → gynaecomastia, ↓ decrease libido, feminization, when treated in carcinoma of prostate

In female →Breast tenderness, migraine, nausea, vomiting, withdrawal bleeding, risk of breast cancer, carcinoma of endometrium and cervix, teratogenic (avoided in pregnancy)

Both in male & female → Gall stone, predisposition of thrombo – embolic disorders, hyperglycemia, oedema.

ANTIESTROGENS

I) Selective estrogens receptors modulator (SERM)
  i) Clomiphene citrate
  ii) Tamoxifen, doloxifene
II) Estrogen synthesis inhibitors
  i) Anastrozole
  ii) Letrozole

CLOMIPHENE CITRATE

- SERM
- Both agonist & antagonistic to estrogen

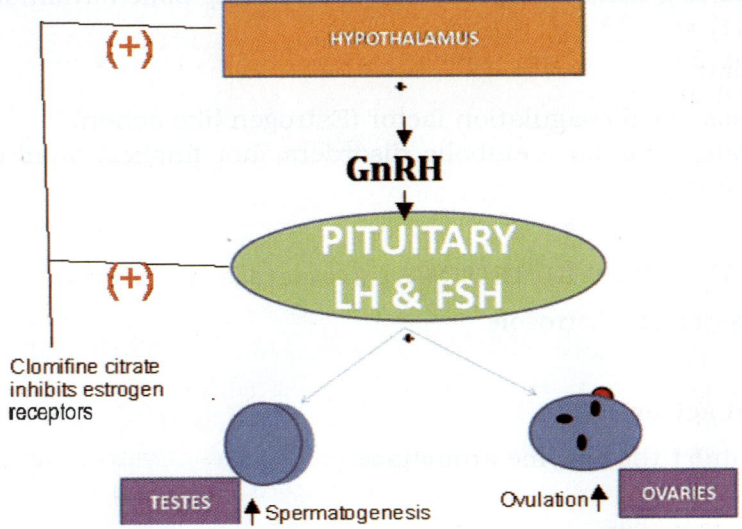

Fig.69 Mechanism of action of Clomiphene citrate

Mechanism of action : (Fig.69)

It inhibits estrogen receptors in the periphery. → due to negative feed back mechanism, it increases the release of Gn RH → increases FSH, and LH release → promotes ovulation (in female) & spermatogenesis (in male).

Clinical uses :

1) In male and female infertility
2) To facilitate in vitro-fertilization (harvesting good & maximum ova)

Adverse effects of clomiphene citrate:

- Multiple pregnancy
- Ovarian enlargement, polycystic ovaries
- Hot flushes, weight gain, alopecia, vertigo

TAMOXIFEN (Raloxifene)

- Potent Estrogen antagonist & agonist

Clinical uses AND Mechanism of action :

1) In breast cancer (estrogen dependent) – Due to its ER (estrogen receptor) antagonistic action, it is used in breast cancer. It is very effective and 1st choice drug.
2) In osteoporosis – Due to ER agonistic action (estrogen like action) on bone by inhibiting bone resorption & by stimulating bone formation.

Adverse effects:

- Increases blood coagulation factor (Estrogen like action)
- Aggravate thrombo – embolic disorders, hot flushes, vomiting, menstrual irregularities.

ESTROGEN SYNTHESIS INHIBITORS (Aromatase inhibitors)

Example : Anastrozole, Letrozole

Mechanism of action :

They inhibit the enzyme aromatase

Testosterone

Anastrozole → inhibits ⊨ Aromatase

Inhibits the conversion of testosterone to estrogen

Reduces Estrogen concentration

Clinical uses :

1) In breast cancer (estrogen dependent) – first line drug in resistant cases to tamoxifen
2) In precocious puberty in female

Adverse effects:

Hot flushes, thrombo – embolic disorders (long term use), joint pain

Drugs used in breast cancer

1) Tamoxifen
2) Estrogen synthesis inhibitors

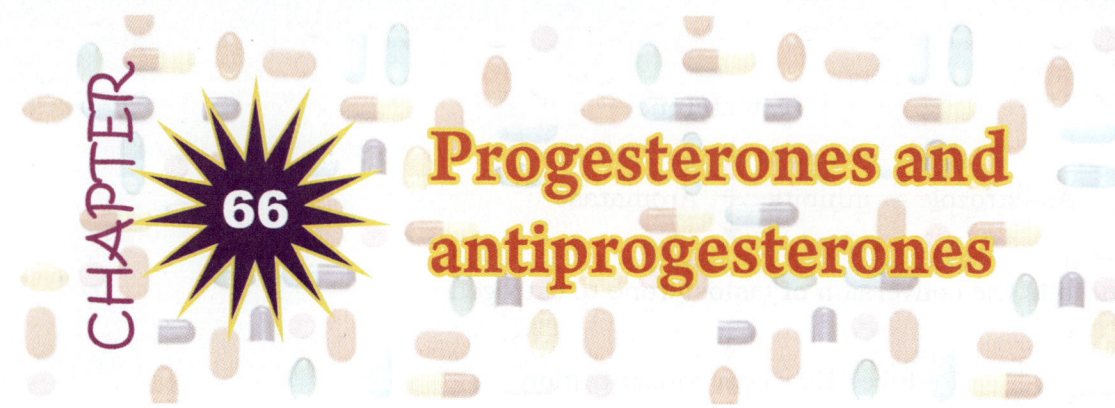

PROGESTERONE

- Progesterone favours pregnancy
- Pro-gest → maintenance of pregnancy – hence the name
- It is female sex hormone (steroidal)

Secretion: Corpus luteum, placenta-mainly

Actions:

1) In non-pregnant women of reproducing age, progesterone is produced by corpus luteum. If no pregnancy occurs in 14 days of coitus → corpus luteum totally degenerate and reduces progesterone concentration in the blood → menstruation occurs

2) If successful coitus → fertilization occurs → blastocyte implanted into the endometrium → immediately starts secreting HCG → LH like action → stimulate corpus luteum → it does not degenerate → corpus luteum of pregnancy stays for about 14 weeks → secrets progesterone continuously.

3) Placenta grows (3rd month) and starts secreting huge amount of progesterone → corpus luteum wanes → placenta keeps the pregnancy going (abortion is common due to progesterone deficiency in 3rd month)

Progestins:

I) Natural – progesterone (parenteral, not preferred)
II) Synthetic (orally effective) – commonly used
    1) Medroxy progesterone acetate
    2) Nor ethindrone
    3) Norgestrel
    4) Lynestrenol
    5) Hydroxy progesterone caproate – I M inj/weekly

Actions:

1) On genital tract:

> Progesterone can produce its effect only after the tissues have been primed by Estrogen → which increases the number of Progesterone receptors at target tissues.

i)   On uterus (already primed by estrogen)
- Stoppage of proliferative stage
- Beginning of luteal or secretory phase → hyperemia, tortuocity of glands & stimulate secretion
- They inhibit uterine contraction

ii)   On Cervix :
- They cause Mucosal plug, plugging of cervical canal of the uterus, mucus becomes thick & viscous → it is impossible for sperm to penetrate

2) On breast : The aleveoli grow with estrogen. They prepare breast for lactation after delivery. They decrease progesterone concentration and increase prolactin secretion.

3) On extra genital effects :
- They cause sedation
- They increase basal body temperature

4) If plasma level of Progesterone is increased → decrease LH secretion from the anterior pitutary → inhibits ovulation (as long as high blood Progesterone → no ovulation occurs) → no pregnancy occurs despite coitus.
- After delivery there is decrease in Progesterone level and increase in Prolactin secretion which starts milk secretion. There is no further pregnancy occurs during this period.

5) They decrease HDL level and produce pro atherogenic effect

6) On mood they cause depression

Clinical uses

Progesterone (high first pass metabolism). **It is not effective orally,** hence it is given by IM inj, which is not preferred by most of the patient.

- The synthetic progesterones **are effective orally** and so clinically used.

1) As oral contraceptive with estrogen (refer oral contraceptive page 356)

2) As Hormone Replacement Therapy (HRT) (refer pages 348 and 369)

> i)   In post menopausal osteoporosis with estrogen

3) Dysfunctional Uterine Bleeding (DUB)

> (excessive menstrual blood flow → extends to 7 – 8 days with large clot and anaemia are common. It is probably due to excess Estrogen/less Progesterone)

- Progesterone has got antiestrogenic activity and is useful in this condition

- Progesterone is started on 5th day of menstrual cycle and continued for 2 weeks and then Progesterone is withdrawn → menstruation occurs → 3 such cycles may be repeated.

4) In endometriosis (dysmenorrhoea, infertility, painful pelvic swelling) → reduce Gn release → inhibit menstruation and reduce bleeding & atrophy of ectopic masses

5) In dysmenorrhoea

6) In pre menstrual syndrome (headache, irritability, breast tenderness)

- Progesterones - inhibit ovulation (they are given with estrogen) → relieve all the symptoms

7) In renal cell carcinoma and in extensive metastasis of endometrial carcinoma

8) In habitual/ threatened abortion due to Progesterone deficiency only.

Adverse effects :

- Breast enlargements, increase body temperature, oedema, mood change, acne, proatherogenic (with estrogen this side effect is antagonized), irregular bleeding, Hyperglycemia (ppt DM)
- If given in early pregnancy → masculinization of female fetus & other congenital abnormalities

ANTIPROGESTIN

(MIFEPRISTONE)

- It is an antiprogestin, antiglucocorticoid and antiandrogenic.

Actions

I)   It is an antiprogestin

- If it is given during follicular phase it attenuates mid cycle Gn surge from anterior pituitary and delay/ failure of ovulation
- If it is given during luteal phase, it prevents secretary changes
- If it is given later in the cycle – it blocks Progesterone support to the endometrium leads to unrestrains release of PGs from it. PGs stimulate uterine contraction and produce abortion
- Mifepristone also sensitizes myometrium to PGs and induces menstruation
- If implantation occurs → it blocks decidualization → conceptus is dislodged → Abortion takes place
- Cervix is softened and it is useful in inducing abortion

II)   Antiglucocorticoids activity is useful in cushing's syndrome

Clinical uses :

1) To induce abortion (termination of pregnancy upto 7 weeks) with PGs
2) For cervical ripening it softens the cervix and facilitates abortion
3) Postcoital (emergency) contraceptive (Mifepristone is given 600 mg/orally/ within 72 hrs of coitus (Interferes with implantation)
4) To expel intrauterine death foetus, (Oxytocin is preferred)
5) It is used as antidepressant
6) In cushing's syndrome (due to its antiglucocorticoids activity)

Adverse effects:

Tiredness, uterine cramp, abnormal discomfort, loose motion etc

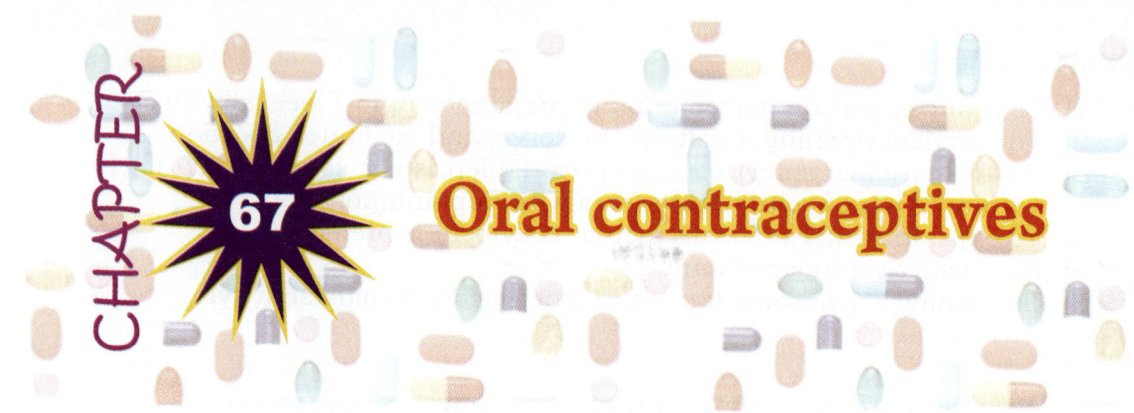

HORMONAL CONTRACEPTIVES

These are the hormonal preparations used for reversible suppression of fertility / or to prevent pregnancy as long as desired.

TYPES OF CONTRACEPTIVES

I)   ORAL
1) Combined Pill (E+P) (Monophase – E and P are in fixed dose combination throughout the course of treatment – Commonly used)
2) Phased Regimens – Biphasic, Triphasic (Estrogen is constant dose and Progesterone dose is gradually increased)
3) Mini pill (Progestin only – Less popular)
4) Post coital (emergency) contraceptive pill (morning after pill)
    i)   High dose of Progestin
    ii)   Mifepristone (Ref: mifepristone)
II)   Injectable (not popular)
1) Implant (S.C) – Progestin only (No estrogen side effect)
2) Long acting Progestin + Long acting estrogen inj once a month

ORAL

1) Combined pill (E+P) – mono phasic (same dose for both throughout the cycle – fixed dose)

	P	E
i)	Norgestral 0.5 mg	Ethenyl estradiol (30 µg) – ovral - G
ii)	Levogestral 0.15 mg	Ethenyl estradiol (30 µg) – ovral – L

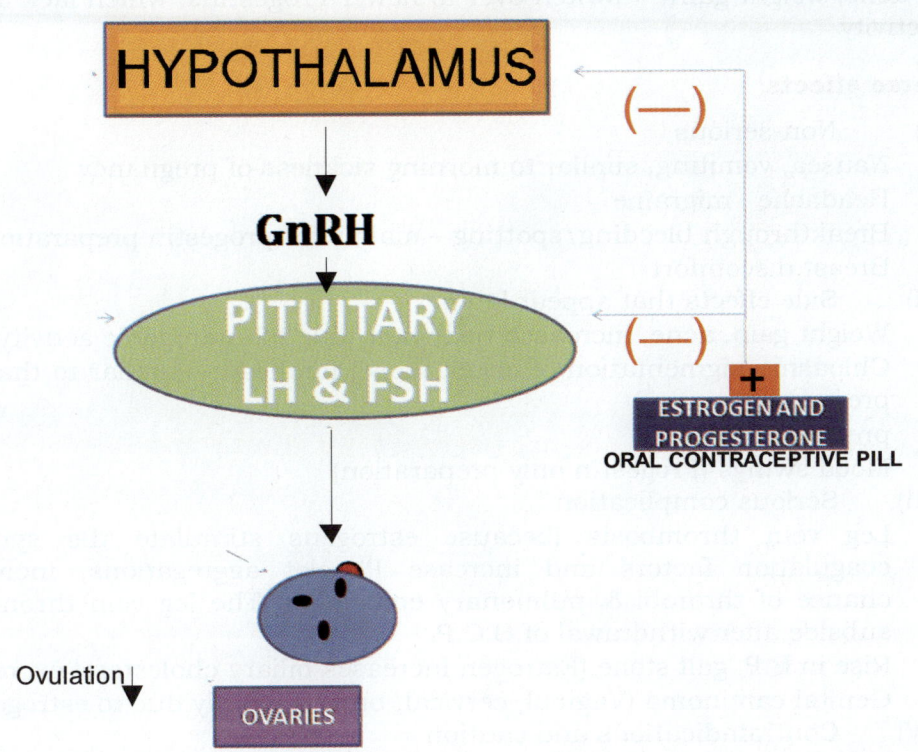

Fig.70 Mechanism of action of Oral contraceptives

Mechanism of action of oral contraceptive (combined pills) : (Fig.70)

1. increased Concentration of E+P in plasma inhibit Gonadotropins (FSH, LH) secretion through feedback mechanism which inhibits ovulation.

2. Progestin – makes the cervical mucus more thick and viscid it becomes very difficult for the sperm to penetrate

Method of administration

1 tab/daily is started on 5th day of menstruation and continued for 21 days, then menstruation occurs. After 7 days gap, the next course is started.

Practical consideration :

- After discontinuation of the tablet, the fertility is returned 1-2 months
- If one tablet is missed → then the 2 tablets are to be taken on the next day
- If tablets are missed more than 2 days, the course is discontinued completely and other methods of contraception to be followed
- If pregnancy occurs during the course, it is to be terminated. Otherwise there will be fetal abnormality.
- If breakthrough bleeding/ spotting occurs. It is better to switch over for pill containing higher dose of Estrogen.

If acne, weight gain → switch over to newer Progestins, which lack androgenic activity

Adverse effects:

I)   Non-serious
- Nausea, vomiting, similar to morning sickness of pregnancy
- Headache , migraine
- Breakthrough bleeding/spotting – mainly for progestin preparation only
- Breast discomfort

II)   Side effects that appear later
- Weight gain, acne, increased body hair (due to androgenic activity)
- Chloasma pigmentation of cheek, nose, forehead →similar to that occur in pregnancy
- precipitate DM
- Mood swings (Progestin only preparation)

III)   Serious complication
- Leg vein thrombosis (because estrogens stimulate the synthesis of coagulation factors and increase Platelet aggregations, increases the chance of thrombi & pulmonary embolism). The leg vein thrombosis will subside after withdrawal of O.C.P.
- Rise in B.P, gall stone (Estrogen increases biliary cholesterol excretion)
- Genital carcinoma (Vaginal, cervical, breast) mainly due to estrogen

IV)   Contraindications and caution
1) Thrombo-embolic disorders
2) Severe hypertension
3) Malignancy of genitals & breast
4) Impending major surgery (to avoid post-operative thrombo-embolism)

V)   Relative contraindication (Caution is required)
- DM
- Obesity
- Smoking
- Mentally ill
- Mild hypertension
- Migraine
- Gall bladder diseases

Drug Interaction

1) With enzyme inducers like Rifampicin, Phenytoin leads to contraceptive failure
2) With Amplicillin & Tetracycline → failure of contraception (due to the suppression of intestinal flora) Ref – Drug interaction

Health benefits of O.C.P:

(Mainly due to the combination of progestin + estrogen)

1) Lower incidence of endometrial/ ovarian carcinoma
2) There is reduced blood loss and reduced anaemia
3) If cycle is irregular, it becomes regular
4) Pre-menstrual tension, dysmenorrhoea are ameliorated
5) Reduced incidence of endometriosis, ovarian cyst and fibrocystic breast diseases (All are due to long term use of estrogen containing O.C.P)
6) Progestin is atherogenic (increases LDL level) and estrogen is anti atherogenic (reduces LDL level)

II POST COITAL (EMERGENCY) CONTRACEPTIVE PILL:

I)   O.C.P (Combined pill) – 2 tablets are given immediately and 2 tablets after 12 hours.

1) It should be administered within 48-72 hours of unprotected intercourse

2) Vomiting is common and it is given with antiemetic

II)   Progestin alone (levonorgestral 0.75mg tablet) → one tablet is given immediately (within 72 hrs of intercourse) and one tablet after 12 hrs
1) It produces less vomiting

III)   MIFEPRISTONE (commonly used)

It is an antiprogestin.

It induces abortion (Ref: mifepristone) 1 tablet (600 mg) is given within 72 hrs of unprotected intercourse.

Side effects are minimal

Mechanism of action :

1)   The endometrium becomes hyperproliferative, hypersecretory, atrophic → blastocyte fail to implant
2)   The uterine and tubular contractions may be modified → disfavours fertilization
3)   It may dislodge a just implanted blastocyte and interfere with fertilization/ implantation

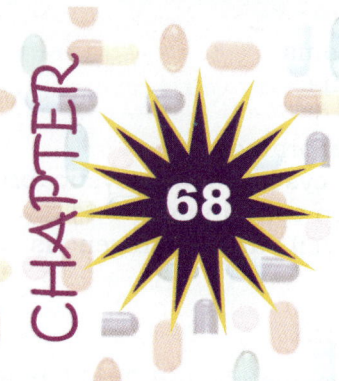

CHAPTER **68**

Testosterones, antiandrogens, anabolic steroids and drugs used in erectile dysfunction

TESTOSTERONE

1) It is a male sex hormone
2) Secreted from testis mainly
3) Natural hormone, testosterone is converted to active dihydrotesterone in the peripheral tissues by the enzyme 5α-reductase

Drugs

I)   Natural: Testosterone (undergoes high first pass metabolism) and it is **not effective orally.** It is given by IM inj

II)   Synthetic androgen **(orally effective)**
   1) Methyl testosterone
   2) Fluoxymesterone

ACTIONS:

I)   On sex organs and secondary sex characters → testosterone is responsible for all the changes that occur in a boy at puberty. The following changes are observed:
   i)   Growth of genitals →penis, prostate, scrotum, seminal vesicles
   ii)   Growth of hair →pubic, axillary, beard, moustache, body hair and male pattern of its distribution
   iii)   Increased activity of sebaceous gland at the face may cause acne
   iv)   Larynx grows. Voice deepens
   v)   Behavioural effects: There is aggressiveness, increased physical vigour and penile erection

II)   On testis: There is maturation of spermatozoa and stimulation of spermatogenesis

III)   Skeleton and skeletal muscles (anabolic effect). The following changes are observed:
   i)   Pubertal spurt of growth (thickness and length)
   ii)   Improvement of bone mineralization
   iii)   It promotes muscle building and body weight increases rapidly
   iv)   Appetite increases

v) Na+/water retention lead to oedema
vi) On Erythropoiesis: It accelerates erythropoiesis by increasing erythropoietin production.

Clinical uses :

1) Testicular failure – delayed puberly in boys (testosterone / dihydrotesterone/IM inj.)
2) AIDS related muscle wasting
3) Hypopituitarism → hypogonadism (delayed feburty, impotence) is one of the features of hypopituitarism.

ANABOLIC STEROIDS

These are synthetic androgens with more anabolic activity and least androgenic activity

Drugs

1) Methandienone (oral)
2) Oxymetholone (oral)
3) Stanozolol(oral)
Combination of anabolic steroid with any other drug is banned in India
The anabolic steroids are subjected to 'dope' test in athletes

Clinical uses :

1) In catabolic states due to its anabolic action (in acute illness, severe trauma, major surgery). There is a feeling of wellbeing, improvement in appetite
2) To enhance physical ability in athletes (discouraged)
3) In malignancy associated anaemia
4) In sub optimal growth in boys.
5) In osteoporosis

ANTIANDROGENS

Drugs that have been used clinically to modify androgen action are

I) **DANAZOL** (orally active)

Mechanism of action

Danazol →binds androgen receptors and inhibits → increases Gonadotropin release (negative feed back mechanism) → increase testosterone release from testis

It also stimulates testosterone synthesis directly

Clinical uses :

1) In endometriosis → relief of dysmenorrhoea is prompt → (because of androgenic side effects, its use is declined)
2) In menorrhagia it reduces menstrual blood loss

3) In fibrocystic breast diseases (chronic cystic mastitis). There is improvement by decreasing pain and engorgement

Adverse effects:

Androgenic side effects →acne, hirsutism, decreased breast size, deepening of voice, oedema, hot flushes, muscle cramp, G.1 upset etc.,

FINASTERIDE

It is a 5α reductase inhibitor

It is an antiandrogen

Mechanism of action

It inhibits the enzyme 5α – reductase and inhibits the conversion of testosterone to active dihydrotestosterone.

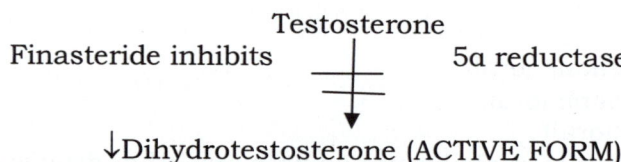

Testosterone

Finasteride inhibits   5α reductase

↓Dihydrotestosterone (ACTIVE FORM)

Clinical uses :

1) In prostate cancer

It decreases prostate size and improves urine flow in prostatic cancer. It is given with α_1 receptor blocker (Prazosin) for better effect.

DRUGS USED IN ERECTILE DYSFUNCTION

Erectile Dysfunction (ED) refers to the inability of men to attain and maintain erect penis with sufficient rigidity to perform sexual intercourse.

DRUGS

I. SILDENAFIL (Oral)

Mechanism of action

NO (Nitric Oxide) is a smooth muscle relaxant (including blood vessels).

Sildenafil

↓

inhibits Phosphodiesterase – 5 (PDE – 5)

↓

potentiates the action of NO, particularly in corpus cavernosum blood vessels

↓

Vasodilatation

↓

penile erection is improved during sexual arousal.

In the absence of sexual activity, there is no erection of penis.

There is no priapism

Dose : 50 mg/ oral / 1 hr before intercourse

USE :

1) In Erectile Dysfunction including in diabetic neuropathy
- It is not effective in men who have lost libido
2) In pulmonary hypertension: It is commonly used. It dilates the pulmonary artery → reduce pulmonary arterial pressure → improve arterial oxygenation in pulmonary hypertension.

Adverse effects :

Due to vasodilatation → headache, nasal congestion, flushing & fall in B.P

- Impairment of colour vision – in some patients
  C/I - in coronary artery disease, with Nitrates → fall in BP → danger in MI
  D/I – The toxicity of Sildenafil is increased with enzyme inhibitors.

II. ANDROGENS :

If ED is due to androgen deficiency, then only androgens are effective.

III. PGs – Inj. into corpus cavernosum (erectile tissue) causes vasodilatation and erection

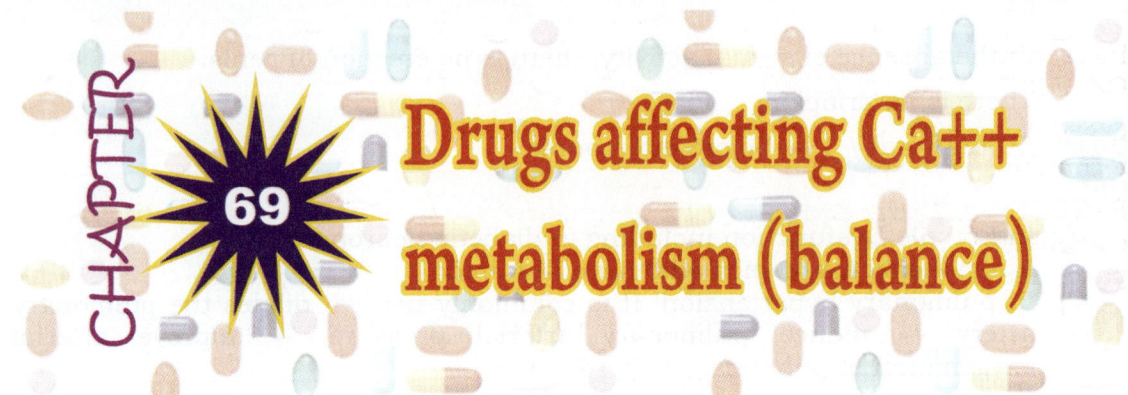

CHAPTER 69

Drugs affecting Ca++ metabolism (balance)

DRUGS AFFECTING CALCIUM METABOLISM (BALANCE)

There are THREE hormones (including Vit.D, which is considered as hormone) affect Ca++ metabolism.

1. Parathormone (from parathyroid gland)

2. Calcitonin (from parafollicular 'C' cells of parathyroid, thyroid glands)

3. Vit.D is synthesized by the skin and kidney from sunlight (UV rays)

Physiological role of Calcium:

1. Ca++ controls excitability of nerves and muscles. It also maintains the integrity of cell membrane.

2. Ca++ is essential for excitation-contraction coupling in all types of muscles.

3. Ca++ is essential for excitation-secretion coupling in exocrine and endocrine glands

4. Ca++ is also responsible for the release of neurotransmitter from the nerve endings

5. Ca++ acts as intracellular messenger for hormones, autacoids etc.

6. Ca++ is necessary for impulse generation in heart (automaticity)

7. Ca++ is necessary for coagulation of blood (small concentration is sufficient)

8. Ca++ has got important role in STRUCTURAL FUNCTION OF BONE AND TEETH.

Remodelling of bone:

Opposite processes of bone resorption and new bone formation are going on. First the Osteoclastic activity (bone resorption) → Ca++ mobilises from bone to blood → digs micropits → and then repair by osteoblastic activity → Ca++ mobilies from blood to bone (bone formation), followed by mineralization (new bone formation)

Remodelling deficit in old age and in menopausal women (lack of estrogen) are noticed → loss of bone formation (trabecular bone, particularly affecting vertebrae, wrist bones and femoral neck) → **Fracture** occurs with minimum trauma.

Increasing bone resorption in relation to bone formation results in OSTEOPOROSIS (THIN BONE)

OSTEOMALACIA is a adult form of rickets, in which there is abnormal bone formation due to inadequate mineralization.

PAGET'S DISEASE is due to excessive osteoclastic activity followed by excessive osteoblastic activity, → fibrosis of bone →↑ (increase) thickness of bone, particularly cranial bone, enlarged skull → abnormal and weak bone.

Fig.71 Regulation of Plasma Level of Calcium

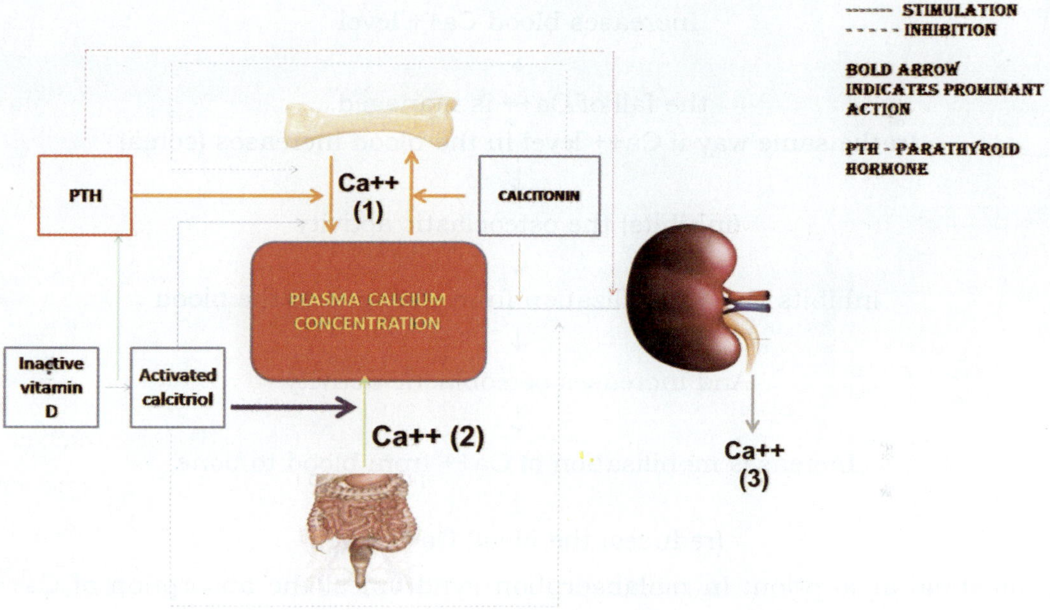

Calcitonin → stimulates bone deposit and inhibit bone resorption. It also increases the excretion of Calcium in the urine. Parathyroid Hormone (PTH) → stimulates bone resorption and inhibits bone deposit and also inhibit Calcium excretion in the urine. It converts inactive vitamin D to active vitamin D

Vitamin D → stimulates absorption of Calcium from intestine and reduces excretion of Calcium in kidney.

Clinical uses of CALCIUM:

1. In tetany (IV Calcium gluconate)

2. In osteoporosis (with Vit.D)

3. In dietary deficiency (in pregnancy and lactation)

Ca++ homeostasis (Fig.71)

Ca++ is in dynamic equilibrium between bone and blood (resorption and bone formation i.e. osteoclastic and osteoblastic activity).

Whenever the blood Ca++ level falls (tetany)

↓

(stimulates) the osteoclastic activity

↓

Stimulates Ca++ mobilization from the bone to the blood

↓

Increases blood Ca++ level

↓

the fall of Ca++ is managed.

In the same way if Ca++ level in the blood increases (coma)

↓

(inhibits) the osteoclastic activity

↓

inhibits Ca++ mobilization from the bone to the blood .

↓

And increases osteoblastic activity

↓

Increases mobilisation of Ca++ from blood to bone

↓

(reduces) the blood Ca++ level.

2. Intestinal absorption: In malabsorption syndromes, the absorption of Ca++ is reduced, may cause osteoporosis.

3. Renal excretion: In chronic renal failure. There is reduced reabsorption of Ca++ and excretion of Ca++ leads to osteoporosis.

PTH deficiency is the common cause of Ca++ deficiency (hypocalcemia)

Metastatic cancer causes (hypercalcemia)

Preparations of Calcium: (oral/ IV)

1. Calcium chloride

2. Calcium gluconate (IV choice)

3. Calcium lactate

4. Calcium dibasic phosphate

Calcium turn over:

Major portion of Calcium is stored in the bone (98%-1.5 G) as crystalline hydroxyl apatite(Calcium Phosphate) deposited in the organic matrix of bone (OSTEOIDS)

CHARACTERISTIC FEATURES OF DRUGS AFFECTING CALCIUM METABOLISM

DRUGS	ACTIONS				Net result Plasma calcium level	R.O.A & DOSAGE	CLINICAL USES	ADVERSE EFFECTS
	Intestinal absorption	Renal excretion	Bone resorption (Osteoclastic activity)	Bone formation (Osteoblastic activity)				
1. CALCITONIN	–	↑	↓	↑↑	↓ Hypocalcemic weak	100 IU S.C/I.M	1.hypocalcemic states(Hypervitaminosis D,Hypercalcemia of malignancy, Supplement Bisphosphonates 2. Post menopausal Osteoporosis(When other drugs fail) 3. Paget's disease (Bisphosphonates is preferred with Calcitonin)	Nausea Flushing
2.PTH (Parathyroid Hormone – secreted from para thyroid gland)	Convert inactive Vit-D3 Cholecalcefe rol to active form Calciferol ↑ (Indirectly)	↓	↑↑	–	Increase plasma Ca++ level ↑ Hypercalcemic ↑ Ca++	S.C.Inj	1.In hypoparathyroidism (Tetany,Convulsion,Laryngospas m, Parasthesia, Cataract. (Vit D is preferred)	Hypercalcemia & Paget's disease are C/I Dizziness, leg cramps

						Route/Dose	Uses	Adverse effects
3.Vitamine D (Vit D2,D3) Synthesized from sunlight exposure->Cholecalciferol (Inactive Vit D3)-> Calcitriol (active)	↑↑	↓	↑	-	↑ Ca++	Oral (Cholecalciferol Vit-D3) 25,000-50,000 IU/Week Calciferol 1µ/oral/day	1. In nutritional Vit D deficiency (Steatorrhoea) 2. In metabolic rickets 3. In renal rickets(Chronic renal diseases) 4. Post menopausal women along with Ca++ 5. Hypoparathyroidism-Calcitriol 6.Psoriasis-Calcipotriol 7. Fanconi's syndrome (↑ P04 level)	Hyper vitaminosis D Hyper calcaemia , weakness, fatigue, vomiting, diarrhea, hypertension, growth retardation in children, Even coma has been reported Rx s.c.Inj. Calcitonin
4.Bisphosphonates (Synthetic) ALENDRONATE Mechanism of action 1.Effective ca++ chelator and gets deposited 2. ↑ Osteoblast, ↓ Osteoclast 3. ↓ Dissolution of bone	Intestinal absorption	-	↓	↑ (BMD)	↓ Ca++	oral	1.Osteoporosis (1st Choice) prevention and treatment 2. Paget's disease 3.Hyper calcemia of malignancy 4. Osteolytic bone metastasis	Gastric irritation, flatulence, headache, body ache(initial fall in ca++ level)

BMD= Bone Mineral Density

↑ = stimulate

↓ = inhibit

DRUGS USED IN OSTEOPOROSIS

Osteoporosis means 'thin bone'. There is reduction in bone mass and reduction in all components of bone Ca++ and others → the bones become fragile. It increases risk of fracture (vertebrae, neck of the femur are common sites).

Osteoporosis is common in post menopausal women due to estrogen deficiency → ↓ (reduction) in bone mass. It increases bone loss.

It is also common in vit. D and calcium deficiency.

I. **BISPHOSPHONATE**: (ALENDRONATE, RISEDRONATE, ETIDRONATE)

Mechanism of action

- They inhibit bone resorption through inhibition of osteoclastic activity and increase bone mass at the hip and spines → reduce the incidence of fracture.

Clinical uses :

1. In osteoporosis (with vit.D and Ca++)

2. In Paget's disease (excessive osteoclastic activity followed by excessive osteoblastic activity → disordered bone remodelling (honey comb structure bone).

3. Hypercalcemia of malignancy

4. Osteolytic bone metastasis-(reduce bone pain, arrest osteolytic lesions).

Dose: Alendronate- 35-70mg/weekly/orally

II. RALOXIFENE (SERM –Selective Estrogen Receptor Modulator)

Mechanism of action Activates oestrogen receptors in bone (while has no stimulatory effect on endometrium or breast to reduce the incidence of cancer) and only reduce bone mineral density loss at spines and hip

III. Recombinant human parathyroid peptides (only in severe cases)

IV. Estrogen: (HRT-Hormone Replacement Therapy)- long term use will lead to endometrial, breast carcinoma and cardiovascular disease risk.

V. Anabolic steroids in men

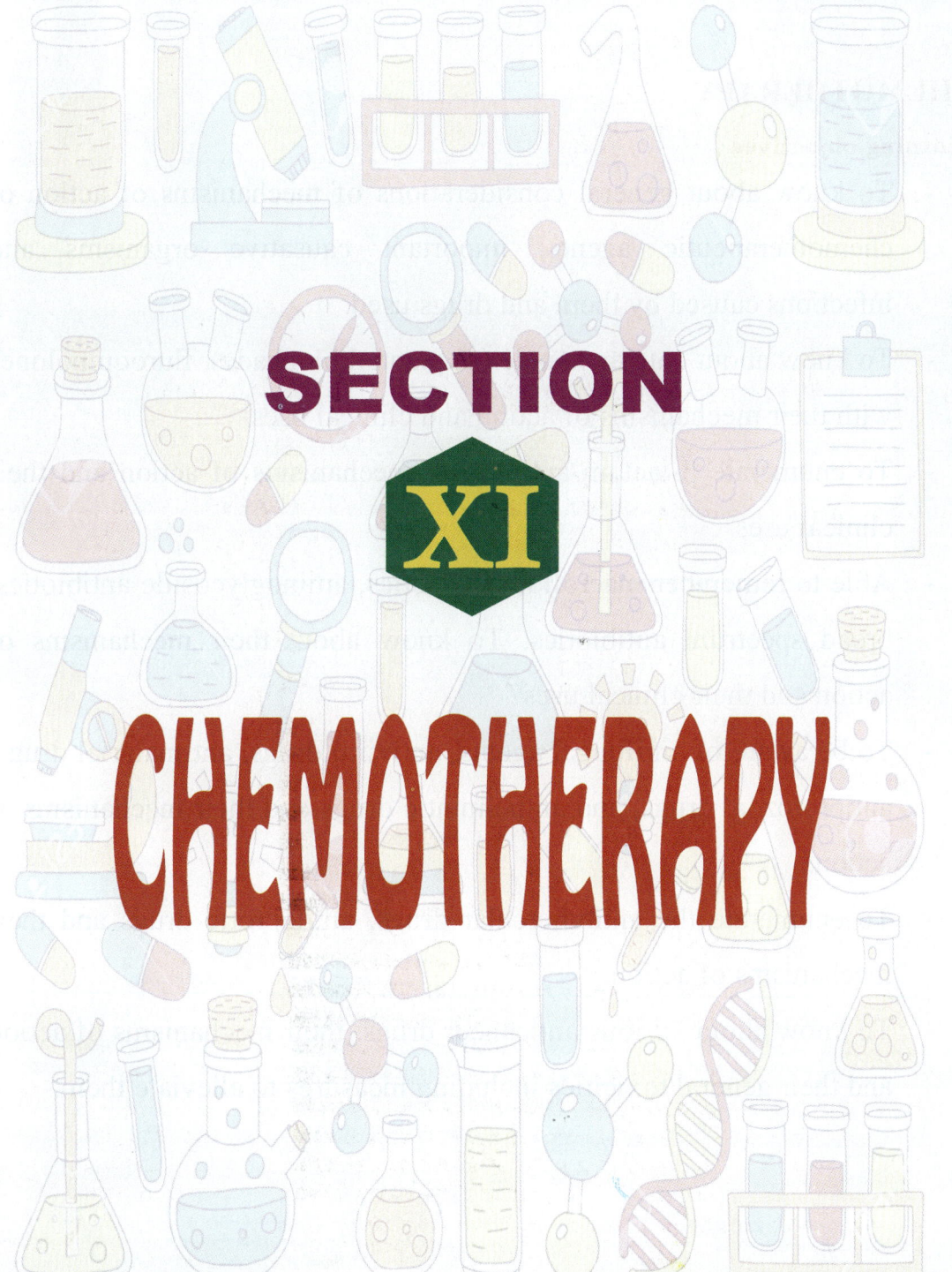

SECTION

XI

CHEMOTHERAPY

CHEMOTHERAPY

Learning objectives

- To know about general considerations of mechanisms of action of chemotherapeutic agents, important causative organisms and infections caused by them and drugs used.

- To know about cotrimoxazole (sequential blockade), fluroquinolones with their mechanisms of action and clinical uses

- To enumerate β-lactam antibiotics, mechanisms of action and their clinical uses

- Able to remember macrolide antibiotics, aminoglycoside antibiotics, broad spectrum antibiotics. To know about their mechanisms of action and their clinical uses

- To be aware of antifungal agents, antiviral drugs, antimalarial drugs, antiprotozoal drugs, and anthelmintic drugs and their mechanisms of action.

- To enumerate the antitubercular drugs, antileprotic drugs and their mechanisms of action.

- To know about various anticancer drugs, their mechanisms of action and their general toxicities including measures to alleviate them.

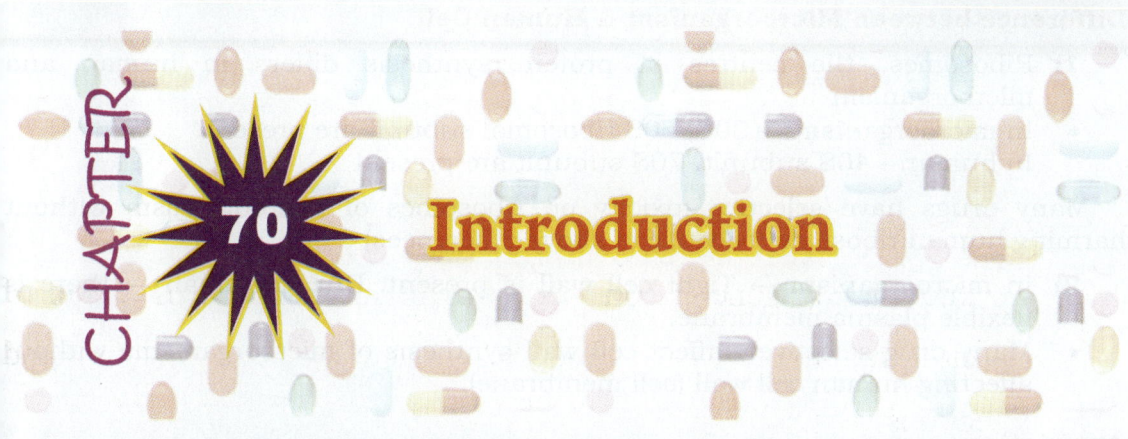

CHAPTER
70

Introduction

Chemotherapy deals with the treatment of infectious diseases by drugs that have selective lethal action on invading pathogens without harming the human cells .

Infectious diseases means, diseases caused by microbes (bacteria, fungus , virus, protozoa and helminths)

- Paul ehrlich (1913) – father of chermotherapy had coined the term Chemotherapy
- Anti microbial agents – (agents acting against microorganism)

Antibiotics	Non antibiotics (synthetic)
From the microorganisms and Kill other microorganisms prevent the growth .	- fluoroquinolones (Norfloxacin, Ciprofloxaction) or
	- sulphonamides (cotrimoxazole)
Penicillins	- antitubercular drugs
Erythromycin	- antimalarial drugs
Tetrayclines	-

Action Of Drugs (Chemotherapeutic Agents)

STATIC – inhibit the growth of microorganism

Fungistatic, bacteriostatic

CIDAL - KILL THE MICROORGANISM

- Fungicidal, bactericidal

STATIC DRUGS - May not be effective in neutropenic/ immunocompromised patients. Cidal drugs are preferred in those conditions.

Difference between Microorganism & Human Cell

1) Ribosomes, the centres of protein synthesis differs in human and microorganism
- In microorganisms – 30S, 50S ribosomal subunit are present.
  In human - 40S subunit, 70S subunit are present

Many drugs have selective toxicity on ribosomes of microorganism without harming human ribosome (because of above differences)

2) In microorganism → Tight cell wall is present. But in human → there is flexible plasma membrane.
- Many drug selectively affect cell wall synthesis of microorganisms without affecting human cell wall (cell membrane).

Antibiotics:

Depending upon the spectrum of activity, they are called as follows:

- narrow spectrum → penicillin G. Erythromycin, Gentamicin. They are either effective against G^{+ve} or G^{-ve} only.
- extended spectrum →Ampicillin, Amoxicillin, (effective aganist G^{+ve} and few G^{-ve} bacteria)
- broad spectrum →effective against G^{+ve}, G^{-ve} ,Chlamydia, Ricketisiae etc., → Tetracyclines , Chloramphenical

Synthetic Antimicrobial Agents

- Cotrimoxazole (Bacrtrim, Septran)
- Ciprofloxacin
- Synthetic antimalarial : Chloroquine
- Synthetic antiamoebic: Metronidazole, Tinidazole
- Synthetic anthelmintic: Albendazole, Diethyl carbamazine citrate (DEC)
- Synthetic antitubercular: INH, Pyrazinamide, Ethambutol

Sites and Mechanism of action of ANTIBIOTICS

- They act mainly by 3 different mechanisms
1) Inhibition of cell wall synthesis (bactericidal)
2) Alteration of cell membrane integrity(bactericidal) inhibition of ribosomal protein synthesis(bacteriostatic)
3) Suppression of DNA synthesis
1) Inhibition of cell wall synthesis.

β- lactam antibiotics
(Penicillins, Cephasporins)
↓
(inhibit) transpeptidase
↓
(inhibit) cross linkage
↓
cell wall becomes weak
↓
Bacteria are burst
↓
leakage of nutrients
↓
bacteria die (bactericidal)

Problems facing the treatment of infectious diseases:

1. Drug resistance
2. Hypersensitivity reactions- Allergy is common, because of antibiotics are derived from microorganisms
3. Immune status : static drugs are not effective in immune-compromised individuals
4. Supra/super infection: New infection is produced

I. BACTERIAL RESISTANCE:

Certain microbes become resistant (unresponsiveness) to the antimicrobial agents due to repeated use.

Resistance is of two types: 1.Natural (clinically not important) 2. Acquired

Natural resistance: Due to synthesis of drug destroying enzymes by bacteria.

Acquired:

1. By mutation
2. By plasmid transfer
3. By methods of transfer of 'r'gene from one bacterium to another through
   i)   Conjucation
   ii)   Transduction
   iii) Transformation
   iv)   By transposons
   v)   Drug permeable: There may be some specific channel 'porins', through which the resistance material will pass
   vi)   Cross resistance → if the organism is resistant to one drug, it is also resistant to other drugs in the same group.

Prevention of drug resistance:

1. There should not be indiscriminate, inadequate use of AMAs (Antimicrobial agents).

The combination of drugs used to prevent the development of resistance as far as possible (antitubercular drugs, anti H. pylori drugs and antiretroviral).

2. Intensive treatment

Super/supra infection: (There is a bacterial flora in the GIT which is protective to our body by killing the invading pathogens). If the bacterial flora is killed by broad spectrum antibiotics, the invading pathogens are not killed and grow fast. The invading pathogens cause infection and that is called super infection.

Appearance of new infection as a result of antimicrobial therapy (particularly by broad spectrum antibiotics) is called as Super/supra infection.

Broad spectrum antibiotics will produce fungal /Cl.difficle (pseudomemberanous enterocolitis) → super infection.

(Glucocorticoids aggravate super infection)

3. Hypersensitivity reactions to AMAs are common
4. Drug allergy: If anybody is allergic to one drug, then he will be allergic to all the drugs in that group.
5. Impaired host defence system (Bacteriostatic drugs are not effective.)
6. Genetic factor

Mechanism of action : of chemotherapeutic agents (in general) (Fig.72)

1. Interference with cell wall synthesis (Penicillins, cephalosporins)

2. Damage to the cytoplasmic membrane: Polymyxin

3. Inhibit the synthesis of protein and impairment of function of the ribosomes (50S, 30S) But in human, there is only 70S, 40S ribosomes

4. Interfere with gyration → INHIBIT GYRASE → ↓(INHIBIT) THE DNA SYNTHESIS: Ciprofloxacin, Rifampicin, Antiviral drugs.

5. Anti metabolite action: Anticancer antimetabolites (Methotrexate) → produce useless metabolites → not at all useful for their growth → Inhibit DNA synthesis → inhibit protein synthesis → Inhibit the multiplication of bacteria.

Fig.72 Sites of Action of Antimicrobial drugs

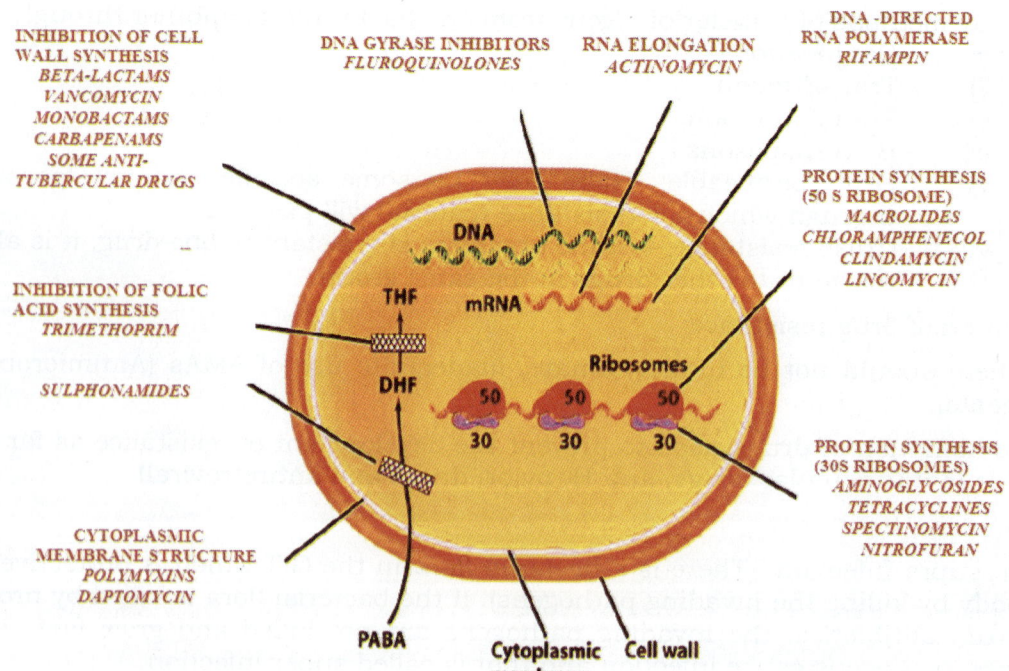

COMBINED USE OF AMAs:

1. To achieve synergestic action.
   (Ampicillin+ Beta lactamase inhibitor, Clavulanic acid)
2. To prevent emergence of resistance microorganisms → INH +Rifampicin+Ethambutol in Tuberculosis
3. To reduce the severity or incidence of adverse effects (AMP-B + Flucytosine in fungal infection)

FAILURE OF CHEMOTHERAPY:

1. Improper selection of drugs.
2. Treatment began too late
3. Poor host defence
4. Infecting organisms present behind barriers (SABE, BBB)

Before going to individual AMA (anti microbial agents) it is better to know about the micro-organisms (mainly bacteria) and the diseases caused by them and the drugs preferred in those conditions

If they ask any short note in any antibiotic, it should be under the following headings

1. Introduction
2. Mechanism of action
3. **Clinical uses** (in the bracket antibacterial spectrum – causative organisms)
4. Adverse effects
5. Dose

ANTIBACTERIAL SPECTRUM	DISEASES	DRUGS PREFERRED
Gram +ve cocci i)streptococci pyogenes, viridans, peptostrepto-cocci	Septicaemia, RTI, Rh.fever, pneumonia, dental abscess (while tooth extraction)	Ampicillin/ Amoxicillin with clavulanic acid
ii)staphylococci	Abscess, Skin and soft tissue infections, osteomyelitis, Endocarditis	Ampicillin/ Amoxicillin with clavulanic acid
Gram –ve cocci i)N.gonorrhoea(gonococci)	Gonorrhoea (urethritis, cervicitis)	Ampicillin/ Amoxicillin/ Cephalosporins/
ii)N.meningitidis (meningococci)	Meningitis	Norfloxacin
Gram +ve bacilli i)clostridium teteni ii)clostridium perfringens	-tetanus -gas gangrene	Penicillin G/ alternate azithromycin

iii) corynebacterium diptheriae iv) clostridium difficile	-diphtheria -psedomemberanous enterocolitis	Metronidazole / tinidazole
Gram –ve bacilli 1)E.coli 2)Proteus 3)klebsiella	U.T.I and hospital acquired pneumonia	Fluroquinolones (Norfloxacin)
4)salmonella typhi	Typhoid fever	Cephalosporins/Norfloxacin
5)shigella	Dysentery	Norfloxacin
6)Helicobacter pylori	peptic ulcer	Tinidazole+ clarithromycin+amoxicillin
7)H.influenza	RTI (Pharyngitis, bronchitis, sinusitis, otitis media)	Ampicillin/amoxicillin with clavulanic acid and cephalosporins/ azithromycin
8)Pseudomonas	Burns infected, hospital acquired pneumonia	Gentamicin
9)Yersinia pestis	Plague	Streptomycin/ doxycycline
10)Vibrio cholera	Cholera	Doxycycline
11)Campylobacter jejuni	Gastroenteritis	Azithromycin
12)G-ve anaerobic i) fusobacterium sp ii) bacteroides fragilis	Cause oral, pharyngeal, lung,brain abscesses during abdominal/ gynaecological surgery,dental abscess during tooth extraction and toothache	Metronidazole /tinidazole / clindamycin
13) bordetella pertussis	Whooping cough	Azithromycin
14) **Acid fast bacilli** Mycobacterium Tuberculosis and	Tuberculosis,	Isoniazid, Rifampicin, Pyrizinamide, Ethambutol, Streptomycin
leprae	Leprosy	Rifampicin, Dapsone.

Sulphonamides and cotrimoxazole

CHAPTER 71

- They are synthetic drugs and are not antibiotics.
- Sulphonamides alone are no longer used except in topical administration .For burns → (Silver Sulfadiazine Ointment) & for ulcerative colitis →(Sulfasalazine (Oral)). Used in bacterial conjunctivitis →Sulfacetamide (Locula)

COTRIMOXAZOLE

It is the combination of sulfamethaxazole (A Sulphonamide) + Trimethoprime (Bactrim, Septran)

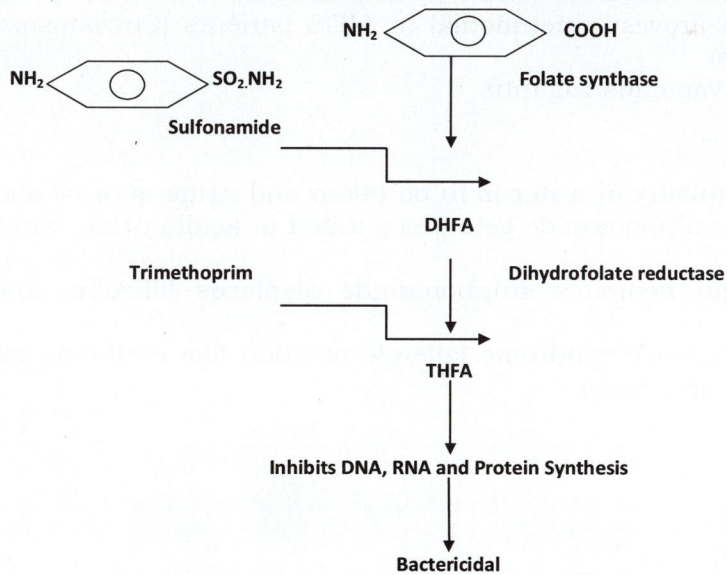

MECHANISM OF ACTION OF COTRIMOXAZOLE

Sequential block of Cotrimoxazole in bacterial folate metabolism

PABA – Para Amino Benzoic Acid

DHFA –Di Hydro Folic Acid

THFA – Tetra Hydro Folic Acid

Mechanism of Action

- Cotrimoxazole is bactericidal (either drug alone is only bacteriostatic).
- Spectrum of antimicrobial activity is extended.
- Synergestic combination
- Sulphonamide, being structural analogue of PABA, enter the synthetic sequence in place of PABA, by competing for the enzyme, folate synthetase and thus form a non-functional analogue of Folic acid which is of no use for the bacterial growth. → bacteriostatic action.
- Trimethoprim - ↓ (inhibits) the enzyme DHFR →↓ (inhibits) the conversion of DHFA to THFA → ↓ (inhibits) DNA synthesis in microorganism → ↓ (Inhibit) completely the protein synthesis → bactericidal.

Clinical uses :

Dose : Trimethoprim 80 mg + sulfamethoxazole – 400 mg 2 tab / twice / daily.

Antimicrobial spectrum: It is effective against G+& G-Bacilli (H.influenzae, N.gonorrhoea N.meningitidis, Salmonella, Shigella, Pneumocysti carini etc.,)

1) In Urinary Tract Infection (E.coli)
2) In Respiratory Tract Infection (H. Influenza)
3) In Typhoid fever (Salmonella)
4) In Gonorrhoea (N. Gonorrhoea)
5) In Bacillary dysentery (Shigella)
6) Bacterial prostatitis (enter effectively into the prostate)
7) Pneumocystis jirovesi (pneumonia) in AIDS patients (Cotrimoxazole is the drug of choice)
8) Trichomonas vaginalis vaginitis

Adverse effects:

1) Crystalluria (plenty of water is to be taken and urine is to be alkalinised). Metabolite of Sulphonamide gets precipitated in acidic urine, which causes crystalluria.
2) Kernicterus (in neonates sulphonamide displaces bilirubin and causes kernicterus).
3) Stevens – Johnson's syndrome (allergic reaction like erythema multiforma and sometime it is fatal)

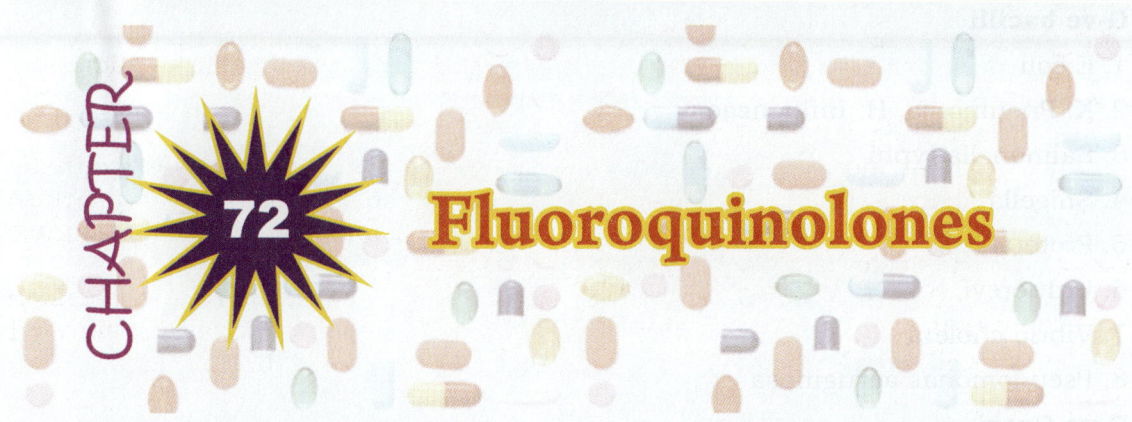

These are quinolone antimicrobials having one or more fluorine substitutions. They are all equal to extended spectrum antimicrobial agents.

1st Generation (1980)

2nd Generation (1990)

1st Generation

1. Ciprofloxacin – Prototype, but replaced by other drugs.

2. Norfloxacin

3. Ofloxacin

4. pefloxacin

2nd Generation

1. Lomefloxacin

2. Levofloxacin

3. Sparfloxacin

4. Gatifloxacin

5. Moxifloxacin

Mechanism of action

Bacterial DNA GYRASE is essential for replication and multiplication

FQs→↓(inhibit) the enzyme DNA gyrase →↓(inhibit) replication and multiplication → bactericidal

- Also in g+ve organisms, FQ → inhibits Topoisomerase II →↓(inhibits) replication and multiplication → bactericidal.

Antibacterial Spectrum:

Highly Susceptible

G-ve bacilli

1. E.coli

2. K. Pneumonia, H. Influenzae

3. Salmonella typhi

4. Shigella

5. Proteus

6. H.ducreyi

7. Vibrio cholera

8. Pseudomonas aeruginosa

G-ve Cocci

1. Neisseria gonorrhoeae

2. N.meningitidis

G+ve cocci

1. Staph. aureus

Other

1. M.tuberculosis

2. MAC (Mycobacterium avium complex)

Active against many beta lactam, Aminoglycosides antibiotics resistant bacteria

Pharmacokinetics

- **High tissue penetrability**
- **High concentration is achieved in muscle, bone, prostate, urine etc.,**

Excretion:

They are excreted as such by Glomerular filtration and tubular secretion, they attain higher urinary concentration than in plasma (useful in UTI) → caution in renal failure.

Clinical uses :

1. In urinary Tract Infection (E.coli, Klebsiella, Proteus) – they bring high cure rates. Effective in complicated cases and those with indewelling catheters / protatitis

2. In gonorrhoea – Single dose -100% cure rate (N.gonorrhoeae)

3. In chancroid – excellent alternate to ceftriaxone (H.ducreyi)

4. In bacterial dysentery & gastroenteritis (Shigella)

5. In typhiod fever (Salmonella typhi) – They are first line drug. They prevent carrier state, since they are bactericidal.

6. In bone, soft tissue, Gynaecological and wound infection (Better penetration into tissues and bones)

7. In RTI (H. influenzae & some streptoccal infections). Useful in pharyngitis, sinusitis, otitis media etc.,

8. In multi drug resistant tuberculosis

9. In G-ve septicaemias

10. In meningitis (N.Menigitidis - meningococci)

11. In conjunctivitis (drop) – G-ve bacteria

Dose : Norfloxacin (norflox) – 400 mg / daily

Pefloxacin, ofloxacin – 400 mg / daily

CAUTIONS : Fluoroquinolones

Recently it has been found out that Fluoroquinolones produce fatal hypoglycemic coma. Blood glucose level should be monitored. If the patients experience any symptoms of hypoglycaemia, they should stop the drugs immediately. They are contraindicated with Sulfonylureas or with any antidiabetic drug which release Insulin.

Fluoroquinolones also cause severe psychiatric disorders. They are contraindicated in any psychiatric disorders.

Adverse effects :

- Nausea,vomiting
- TENDONITIS and TENDON RUPTURE C/I in pregnancy.

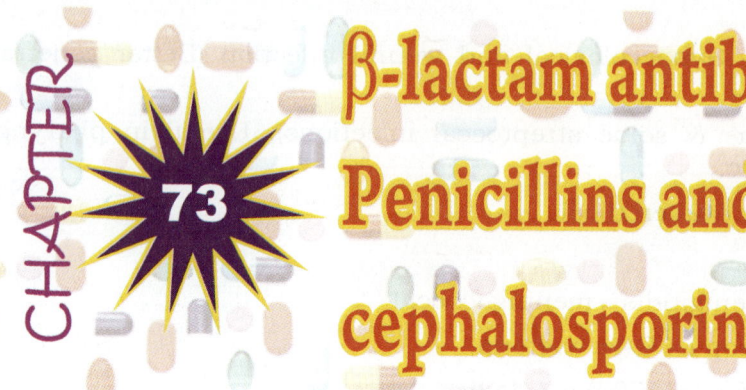

CHAPTER 73

β-lactam antibiotics- Penicillins and cephalosporins

BETA LACTAM ANTIBIOTICS

The structure of these antibiotics are having β lactam ring.

The two groups of drugs are under the β lactam antibiotics (narrow spectrum)

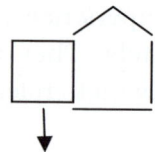

β lactam ring

I. PENICILLINS

Antibacterial spectrum G+ cocci, G+ bacilli, Spirochetes etc., and few Gram –ve bacteria (Ampicillin, Amoxicillin)

CLASSIFICATION OF PENICILLIN
1. Penicillin G (inj) (Benzathine Penicillin G, PAM)
2. oral Penicillin – Penicillin –V
3. extended spectrum Penicillins (oral) – **Ampicillin, Amoxicillin**
4. Penicillinase resistant Penicillins
   - cloxacillin
   - nafcillin
   - methicillin

5. Anti pseudomonal Penicillins – Ticarcillin, Piperacillin, carbenecillin

II. CEPHALOSPORINS
i. Generation (G+ ve cocci)(destroyed by β Lactamase)
   1) Cephalexin (Oral)
   2) Cephadroxil (Oral)
   3) Cephalothin(Oral)
ii. Generation (G-ve cocci+ G – anaerobes)
   Penicillinase resistant
   1) Cefuroxime (oral) only used

iii. **Generation very effective on (G-ve of II Generation + some more) β lactamase resistant.**
  1) Cefotoxime proxetil (oral)
  2) Ceftrioxone (I V)
  3) Cefotaxime (I V)

iv. **Generation– very effective against G-ve cocci – resistant to β–Lactmase**
  1. Cefpirome
  2. cefepime

PENICILLINS

- Narrow Spectrum Antibiotic (G+ Cocci, G+ Bacilli, Spirochetes etc.,
- Extended Spectrum Penicillins (Ampicillin,Amoxicillin are effective against G+ cocci,+ G- cocci and few G- bacill. **Pharmacokinetic: – Pencillin G- is not effective orally. All other Penicillins are effective orally. Actively secreted in the proximal tubule.**

Mechanism of action :

Penicillins bind with PBP (Penicillin Bound Protein)
↓
(Inhibit) the enzyme transpeptidase
↓
(inhibit) cross linking of peptido-glycon strands
↓
(inhibit) the cell wall synthesis
↓
the cell wall becomes weak
↓
the rupture of cell wall
↓
the nutrients of bacteria will leak out
↓
the organisms are killed
↓
bactericidal.

- In G-, they enter through porin in the cell membrane and then inhibit cell wall synthesis.

PENICILLIN – G

Antibacterial spectrum:

- Narrow spectrum antibiotics.
- Effective against g+ cocci & g+ve bacilli and few g-ve organism.

Clinical uses

Penicillin G is the drug of choice for infection caused by organism susceptible to it, unless the patient is allergic to it.

1. Syphilis (Treponema pallidum) has not shown any resistance so far. It is the drug of choice in this condition.
2. Diphtheria – Antitoxin is the first choice. Penicillin G is used with that. It is useful to prevent carrier states.
3. Tetanus and gas gangrene – Antitoxin is more important. Penicillin G is given as adjuvant to kill the causative organism.
4. Penicillin G is the drug of choice for rare infection like anthrax, rat bite fever.
5. For trench mouth or ulcerative gingivitis due to mixed infection by spirochaetes and g^{-ve} anaerobes, penicillin V is combined with Tinidazole.
6. In sub acute bacterial endocarditis (Streptococcus viridans), penicillin-G is given along with Gentamicin.
7. In lobar pneumonia – Penicillin G is the drug of choice, if the organism is sensitive.
8. Prophylactic use:
   i. In Rheumatic fever
   ii. In syphilis
   iii. In bacterial endocarditis (In tooth extraction, endoscopies, catheterization can cause bacteremia, which in patients with valvular defects can cause endocarditis).

Preparation:

1. Procaine penicillin G injection

   0.5 – 1 MU/1M/12 hrly

2. Benzathine penicillin G (Penidure – LA)

   0.6 – 2.4 MU/1M/weakly/for 3 to 4 weeks

Adverse effects:

1. Hypersensitive reaction is common → Anaphylactic shock → death. Adrenaline (1ml of 1:1000 dilution/IM) is life saving drug. Penicillin sensitivity test (intradermal) should be done, before giving Penicillin. Penicillin G combines with body protein and forms haptens, which act as antigen. It produces antibodies. Antigen and antibody reaction takes place on mast cells → release of mediators like Histamine, slow reacting substance-A etc,.) → mild form of hypersensitive reations are like urticaria, pruritus, wheezing and rhinitis. In severe form there is Hypotension and

bronchoconstriction, angioneurotic oedema, loss of consciousness →
Anaphylactic shock → fatal.
2. Pain at the site of IM injection

AMPICILLIN (Roscillin, Ampillin)

- It is an extended spectrum penicillin
- It is effective orally
- It is a gastric irritant
- Food interferes with absorption of Ampicillin

Mechanism of action (As that of Penicillin)
Antibacterial Spectrum:

Effective against g^{+ve}, g^{-ve} cocci, few g^{-ve} bacilli and H.pylori.

Clinical uses:

1) In respiratory tract infection (Pharyngitis, sinusitis, otitis media, lobar pneumonia)
2) In urinary tract infection (E.coli, klebsiella, proteus)- pyelonephritis)
3) In gonorrhoea (N.gonorrhoeae) – urethritis, cervicitis.
4) In meningitis (Meningococci)
5) In H.pylori infection (Peptic ulcer)
6) In cholecystitis (E.coli, klebsiella)
7) In sub acute bacterial endocarditis (streptococcus viridans)

Adverse effects:

It irritates lower intestine due to unabsorbed drug and causes diarrhea (If it is troublesome one antimotility drug like Loperamide). It also inhibits intestinal bacterial flora. Skin rashes is common.

Drug Interaction:

- With oral contraceptive there is failure of contraception (Ref: enterohepatic circulation in general pharmacology)

AMOXICILLIN (NOVAMOX)

- Extended spectrum penicillin
- Completely absorbed from the upper intestine (No gastric irritant and less/no diarrhoea)
- Food does not interfere with Amoxicillin (It can be given at anytime)

Mechanism of action (As that of penicillins)

Antibacterial spectrum: As that of Ampicillin

Clinical uses:

As that of Ampicillin. Now Amoxicillin is preferred over Ampicillin, because of less side effects.

Adverse effects:

- Skin rashes
- No drug interaction with Oral Contraceptive pills
- **Dose:** Ampicillin/Amoxicillin-250mg thrice daily/orally. 250mg/1M/inj.
- Ampicillin is given 2 hrs after food.

β- LACTAMASE INHIBITORS
(CLAVULANIC ACID, SULBACTAM, TAZOBACTAM)

- Many strains of bacteria (Staphylococci, E.coli, H. influenzae, N. Gonorrhoeae) produce enzyme Penicillinase (β-lactamase) which destroy Penicillins, Cephalosporins and make them inactive.
- β- Lactamase Inhibitors→ ↓ (inhibit) the enzyme β- Lactamase produced by the bacteria and protect Penicillins from destruction
- They are combined with Ampicillin /Amoxicillin
- They are not antibacterial – But potentiate the action of β- Lactam antibiotics.
  Clavulanic acid = 500mg (0.5g). 250mg,125mg.

Clinical uses:

With Ampicillin / Amoxicillin against penicillinase producing bacterial infection. Amoxicillin 250 mg + clavulanic acid 125 mg (Augmentin)

1) In PPNG (Penicillinase Producing Niesseria Gonorrhoea - urethritis, cervicitis) infection
2) Mixed aerobic – anaerobic infections
3) Intra abdominal, gynaecological, skin / soft tissue infection – acquired in the hospital

CEPHALOSPORINS

- Narrow spectrum antibiotics
- Mainly effective against G+&G- Cocci

CLASSIFICATION: According To chronological development of drugs.

Mechanism of action – Similar to that of Penicillins.

First Generation:

- Mainly effective against G+Cocci
- Destroyed By β Lactamase enzyme
- Not used clinically (against G+ Cocci- Ampicillin/Amoxicillin / Azithromycin are better)

Second Generation

- Mainly effective against G-cocci & G-bacilli +G- anaerobes
- Resistant to β Lactamase enzyme.
- Only Cefuroxime& Cefaclor (Oral) are used.

Clinical uses :

1) RTI (Against β Lactamase producing H.influenzae)= pneumonia, pharyngitis, otitis media, sinusitis etc., in hospital acquired pneumonia (By H.influenzae, Klebsiella)as well as Penicillin resistant Pneumococci,

Third Generation (commonly asked short note, since they are commonly used) – Extended Spectrum Antibiotic.

DRUGS:

1) Cefotaxime(I.V)
2) Cefotaxime Proxetil(Oral)
3) Cefdinir(oral)
4) Ceftriaxone(IV)
5) Cefpodoxime Proxetil(Oral)
6) Cefixime (oral)

- They are not destroyed by β – lactamase
- Many of them cross CSF and useful in meningitis
- Ceftriaxone → **excreted via bile** (no adjustment of dose is needed in renal failure)
- All other drugs excreted by tubular secretion.

Clinical uses :

Antibacterial spectrum → very effective against g+ & g- cocci g- anaerobes (some drugs) & g- bacilli(few) → R.T.I (Pneumonia) & UTI

1) In meningitis (caused by N.meningitidis, H.influenzae and Pneumococci) since they attain higher concentration in CSF
2) Sepsis in immunocompromised individuals
3) In febrile neutropenia along with gentamicm in immunocompromised individuals
4) In gonorrhoea caused by N.gonorrhoeae (PPNG – Penicillase Producing N. gonorrhoeae) (Urethritis, cervicitis) with Probenecid.
5) In Typhoid fever (caused by S.typhi) particularly in multi drug resistant
6) In complicated UTI (caused by E. Coli, Proteus, Klebsiella).

7) Biliary infection
8) In abdominal sepsis & colorectal surgery (infection caused by g-anaerobes)
9) In RTI- pharyngitis, bronchitis, sinusitis (caused by H. Influenzae, penicillase producing staphylococci infection)
10) Skin & soft tissue infection (caused by staphylococci particularly & g-organisms)
11) In mixed aerobic & anaerobic infection in cancer patients

Adverse effects:

1) Disulfiram like action (some) – alcohol intolerance – Alcohol is to be avaoided
2) Less severe hypersensitive reaction
3) Diarrhoea (oral drugs)
4) Pain at the site of injection
5) Hypoprothrombinemia (bleeding) and with warfarin there is severe bleeding

Fourth Generation Cephalosporins

Drugs:

1. Cefepime(I.M) 2. Cefpirome(I.M)

Antibacterial spectrum: They are more potent against g^{+ve} than the III generation g+ve and the III generation g^{-cocci}

Highly resistant to β-lactamase

Clinical uses:

1. In severe hospital acquired infections (Pneumonia)

2. In Lower respiratory tract infection

Dose of cephalosporins:

- Cefuroxime axetil – 250mg/daily/oral
- Cefixime 100 to 200mg/daily/oral
- Cefpodoxime proxetil 100 to 200mg/daily/oral
- Ceftriaxone 50mg/I.M

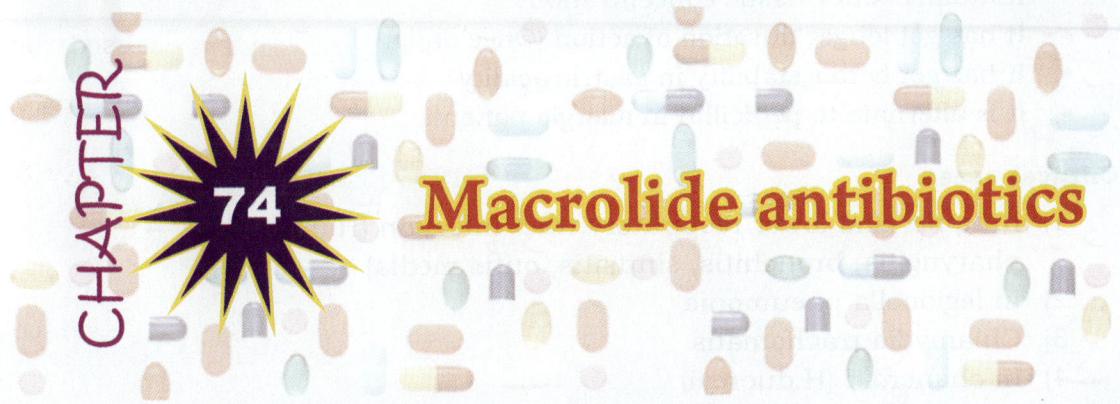

CHAPTER 74

Macrolide antibiotics

- They are having big molecular structure, hence the name.
- They are narrow spectrum antibiotics.

Drugs :

1. Erythromycin
2. Azithromycin
3. Clarithromycin
4. Roxithromycin

Antibacterial spectrum:

Mainly effective against g+ cocci & g+ bacilli, few g- bacilli (Bordetella pertussis, H.pylori, mycobacterium avium complex, M. tuberculosis), legionnaire, Chlamydia, H.influenzae. **They are not effective against g-cocci.**

Mechanism of action: (Fig.73)

They enter into bacteria
↓
bind and inhibit **50 S** ribosome subunit of bacteria (human cells do not have 50 S)
↓
inhibit protein synthesis
↓
inhibit multiplication of bacteria
↓
bacteriostatic.

AZITHROMYCIN (Azithral)

- It is commomly used in this group

- It attains better tissue concentration
- It has got longer duration of action (Once daily)
- It has got better stability in gastric acidity
- It is alternate to penicillin in allergic patients

Clinical uses:

1) In upper and lower respiratory tract infection (H.influenzae → pharyngitis, bronchitis, sinusitis, otitis media)
2) In legionella pneumonia
3) Chlamydia trachomatis
4) In chancroid (H.ducreyi)
5) In whooping cough (Bordetella pertussis)
6) In multi drug resistant tuberculosis

Dose : 250 mg daily

Adverse effects:

Mild gastric upset, abdominal pain, headache and dizziness.

ERYTHROMYCIN

- It is one of the macrolide antibiotics
- It is a narrow spectrum antibiotic
- Antibiotic spectrum: (Ref: before)
- Mechanism of action: (Ref: before)
- **Clinical uses** of Erythromycin (as that of Azithromycin)
- Adverse effects: Safe drug, mild gastric irritant, reversible hearing impairment, hypersensitivity reactions like skin rashes, fever, hepatitis with cholestatic jaundice.

Dose: 250-500 mg/4 times daily.

CLARITHROMYCIN & ROXITHROMYCIN

- They are macrolide antibiotics
- They are narrow spectrum antibiotics

Antibacterial Spectrum:

Similar to azithromycin and H.pylori, mycobacterium avium complex and M.leprae.

Mechanism of action:

Similar to that of macrolide antibiotics.

Clinical uses:

All the uses of Azithromycin and

1) In H.pylori (peptic ulcer) infection – clarithromycin is one of the drugs in anti H.pylori regimen.
2) In mycobacterium avium complex infection
3) In leprosy
4) In multidrug resistant tuberculosis

Dose : 250 mg twice daily

Adverse effects:

Nausea, vomiting and abdominal pain.

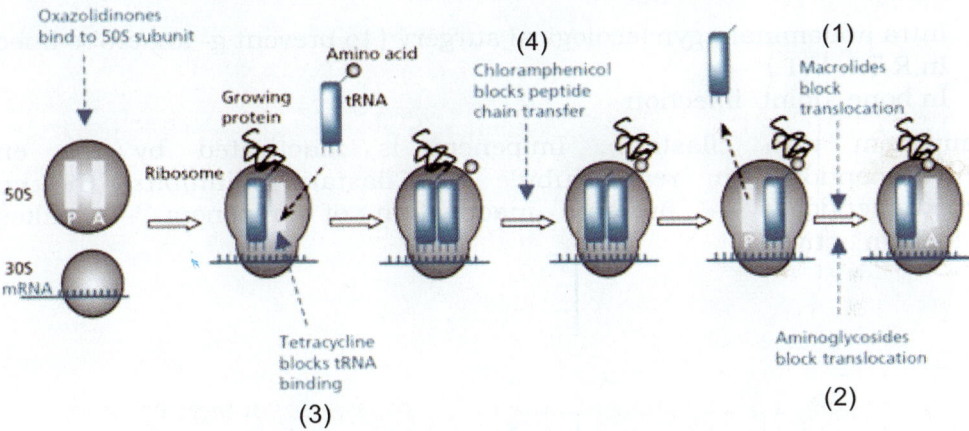

Fig. 73 Mechanism of action of some important antibiotics

1. Macrolides → bind to 50S subunit and block → inhibit the translocation of the growing peptide → not available for binding of next aminoacid → protein systesis stops → Bacteriostatic

2. Aminoglycosides → bind 30S subunit and block → inhibit DNA synthesis → inhibit protein synthesis → Bacteriostatic

3. Tetracyclines → bind and block 30S subunit → inhibit binding of tRNA → inhibit protein synthesis → Bacteriostatic

4. Chloramphenicol → binds and blocks 50S subunit → inhibits the protein synthesis → Bacteriostatic.

AZTREONAM (I V)

- Narrow spectrum antibiotic (mainly effective against g-bacilli)

Mechanism of action :

Similar to penicillin: ↓(inhibits) cell wall synthesis

- Useful in case of penicillin allergy
  1) In R T I (Respiratory Tract Infection)
  2) In Gonorrhoea

IMIPENEM(I V)

- Narrow spectrum antibiotic (effective against g- bacilli + g- anaerobes

Mechanism of action :

Similar to penicillin (↓ cell wall synthesis)

Clinical uses :

1) Intra abdominal , gynaecological surgery (to prevent g- anaerobe infection)
2) In R T I, U T I
3) In bone, Joint infection

Imipenem with cilastatin. Imipenem is inactivated by the enzyme dehydropeptidase in renal tubule → Cilastatin↓ (inhibits) the enzyme dehydropeptidase → prevents inactivation of imipenem → makes the imipenem active

Glycosides and aminoglycosides antibiotics

CHAPTER 75

GLYCOSIDE ANTIBIOTIC

VANCOMYCIN

Narrow spectrum antibiotic (mainly effective against g+ cocci & g+ bacilli (Cl. difficle & few g- cocci)

Mechanism of action :

↓ (inhibits) cell wall synthesis → binds with freshly formed peptidoglycans → inhibits the lengthening of cell wall→ cell wall synthesis is not possible → cell wall become weak → nutrients leak out →bactercidal action

Clinical uses :

1) In M. R. S. A (Methicillin Resistant Staphylococcus aureus) infection
2) In pseudomemberanous enterocolitis (costly, orally not effective. So, cheaper & orally effective Metronidazole is preferred)
3) In meningitis (crosses Blood Brain Barrier effectively)
4) In bacterial endocarditis (with gentamicin)

Adverse effects:

- Fever, chill
- Rarely ototoxic

AMINOGLYCOSIDES

- They contain amino group with glycoside.

Drugs:

1) Gentamicin
2) Streptomycin
3) Kanamycin
4) Neomycin
5) Amikacin
6) Tobramycin

- **Orally not effective, parenterally given, excreted as such in active form in the urine by glomerular filtration.**

Mechanism of action : (Fig.73)

Drugs enter into bacteria via porin channels in the cell membrane by active transport (Oxygen dependent)

↓

Aminoglycosides are not effective against g-ve anaerobes

↓

bind with bacterial **30S** ribosome subunit

↓

(inhibit) irreversible protein synthesis of bacteria (it will not affect human cells, which do not have 30S ribosome)

↓

bactericidal because of irreversible (inhibition) of protein synthesis.

GENTAMICIN

Antibacterial spectrum

G^{-ve} bacilli (Pseudomonas, Proteus, E.coli, Klebsiella), few g^{+ve} cocci

Clinical Uses

1. In Sub Acute Bacterial Endocarditis with β-lactam antibiotic
2. In UTI
3. In burn to prevent Pseudomonas infection
4. In lung abscess, osteomyelitis
5. In meningitis (g^{-ve} bacilli)
6. In pneumonia including community acquired (g^{+} cocci)

Adverse effects:

1. Nephrotoxicity (tubular damage, low G.F.R, loss of urinary concentrating power) → reversible, if the drug is withdrawn immediately → caution in renal failure.
2. Ototoxicity (reversible) except deafness
   Aminoglycosides ear drops can cause ototoxicity
- cochlear damage → hearing loss and deafness (permanent), tinnitus (disappears after stopping the drug)
- vestibular damage → headache, nausea, vomiting, dizziness (disappears after stopping the drug).

3. Neuromuscular blockade → contraindicated when non-depolarizing neuromuscular blocker is used in surgery. It is contraindicated in myasthenia gravis.

   Dose: 1mg/kg/IM. (dose to be adjusted in renal failure according to renal clearance)

- Streptomycin → first line drug in Tuberculosis (100mg/IM/daily). Also used in Plague.

- Kanamycin, Amikacin → useful in multidrug resistant tuberculosis.

Caution in renal failure: Since gentamicin is excreted as such by glomerular filtration, the dose to be adjusted according to renal clearance. So, in renal failure . the dose adjustment is needed according to renal clearance. In old, the dose is to be reduced. (Refer excretion of drugs).

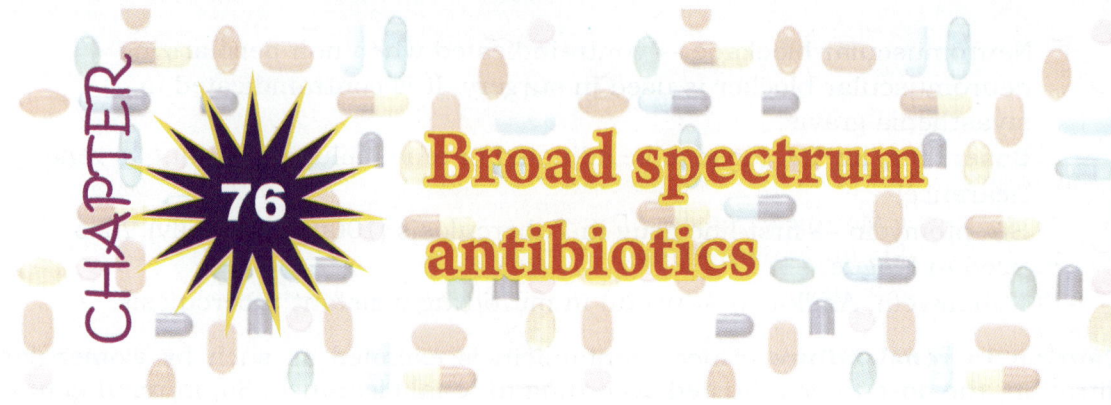

CHAPTER **76**

Broad spectrum antibiotics

The drugs which are effective against wide range of microorganisms (g+,g-, aerobes/anaerobes, spirochetes,rickettsial,chlamydial infections). They are called as broad spectrum antibiotics.

Drugs:

1) Tetracyclines
2) Chleramphenicol

Tetracyclines

They are called, because there are four cyclic rings in their structure

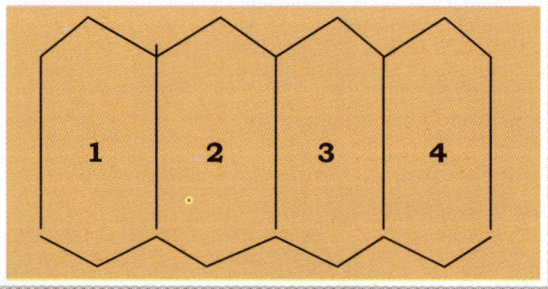

Drugs:

1) Doxycycline
2) Minocycline
3) Tetracycline

Mechanism of action : (Fig.73)

They enter into bacteria by passive diffusion and active transport → bind and inhibit 30S ribosomal sub units → ↓ (inhibit) protein synthesis →↓ (inhibit) multiplication of microorganisms → Bacteriostatic

• Orally effective

- All tetracyclines excreted actively **except doxycycline,** which is metabolized and excreted

Clinical uses of Doxycycline

Advantage of Doxycycline → even in renal failure it is preferred

1) In Rocky Mountain Spotted Fever
2) In Syphilis (in patient allergic to Penicillin –G)
3) In Leptospirosis
4) In Cholera (Vibrio cholerae)
5) In Malaria (Chloroquine resistant falciparum malaria) – As Prophylaxis mainly
6) In Acne vulgaris (Oral)
7) It is effective against MRSA infection
   Dose : 100 mg / daily

Adverse effects:

1) Chelation with Ca^{++} of bone and teeth, particularly in children →deformity of bone and tooth of children
2) Super infection (Ref before) - Fungal candidiasis → Antifungal agent like Nystatin is used
3) Nausea, Vomiting, Diarrhoea
4) Dizziness, Vertigo
5) Photosensitivity reaction particularly in fair complexioned persons.

Drug interaction : with oral contraceptive, it leads to failure of contraception

CHLORAMPHENICOL

- Broad Spectrum Antibiotic
- Not used now a days because of its toxic effect. Restricted only in topical administration on eye for bacterial conjunctivitis.

Mechanism of action :

Combines with 50S subunit of bacterial ribosomes and inhibits protein synthesis → Bacteriostatic

Adverse effects:

1) Gray Baby Syndrome – There is a deficiency of enzyme glucuronyl transferase in foetus and infants → Chloramphenical is not metabolized in them → its concentration in plasma is increased → cyanosis→ the baby looks like Gray Ashen colour (Hence the name), abdominal distention, hypothermia, shock and collapse
2) Bone marrow depression → aplastic anaemia
3) Super Fungal infection.

CHAPTER **77**

Drugs used in urinary tract infection

- Urinary tract infection will be either lower UT infection (urinary hesitancy, irritation, pain) or upper UT infection (pyelonephritis)
- Organisms causing UT infection are – E.coli (very common), Proteus, Klebsiella, Pseudomonas
- Drugs used in UTI should attain higher concentration in the urine
- The drugs should reach in active form through glomerular filtration or tubular secretion to act on bacteria present in urinary tubule.

DRUGS USED:

Normally 3 to 5 days treatment is sufficient

First choice is

1. Quinolones → highly effective against most of the organisms causing UTI & they are cheap
   - Normally drugs should be given after the bacteriological sensitivity test. Before starting AMA (Anti Microbial Agent), urine sample is collected for sensitivity test, After that, any one of the following drugs can be employed empirically
2. Cotrimoxazole, because it is effective against most of the pathogens causing UTI
3. Amoxicillin +Clavulanic acid → for initial treatment in acute infection without bacteriological data
4. Cephalosporins
5. Gentamicin – very effective against most of the pathogens. But narrow margin of safety and should be given by I.M injection → kept as reserve drug & C/I in renal impairment

PROPHYLAXIS FOR UTI

Prophylaxis is needed in the following conditions, where UTI is common

1. Catheterization or instrumentation causing damage to the lining of UT which are susceptible to UTI
2. When indwelling catheters are placed
3. When uncorrectable abnormalities of the UT is present
4. In prostate enlargement or any other chronic obstruction causes urinary stasis

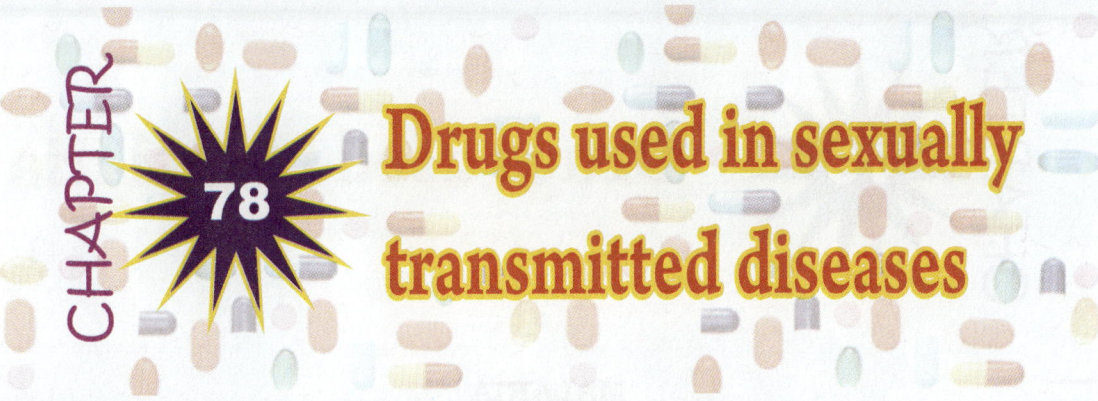

Drugs used in sexually transmitted diseases

TREATMENT OF SEXUALLY TRANSMITTED DISEASES

I.   Gonorrhoea → caused by N.gonorrhoea → urethritis
1. Amoxicillin + Probenecid +Clavulanic acid (first choice)
2. Ceftrioxone
3. Cefuroxime
4. Azithromycin

II.   Syphilis → caused by Treponema pallidum → lesions and itching of genitals → first choice is Penicillin G → Benzathine Penicillin G/IM/ weekly once/ for 4 weeks
   •   In Penicillin G allergic → Doxycycline, Azithromycin

III.   Chlamydia trachomatis → non-specific urethritis, lymphogranuloma venereum
1. Azithromycin (first choice)
2. Doxycycline

IV.   Chancroid caused by H.ducreyi → lesions in the genitals
1. Ceftrioxone (first choice)
2. Azithromycin

V.   Genital hereps simplex (ref antiviral)
1. Acyclovir (first choice)

VI.   Trichomonas vaginalis → vaginitis, itching, lesions in the vagina
1. Tinidazole (first choice)
2. Next Cotrimoxazole

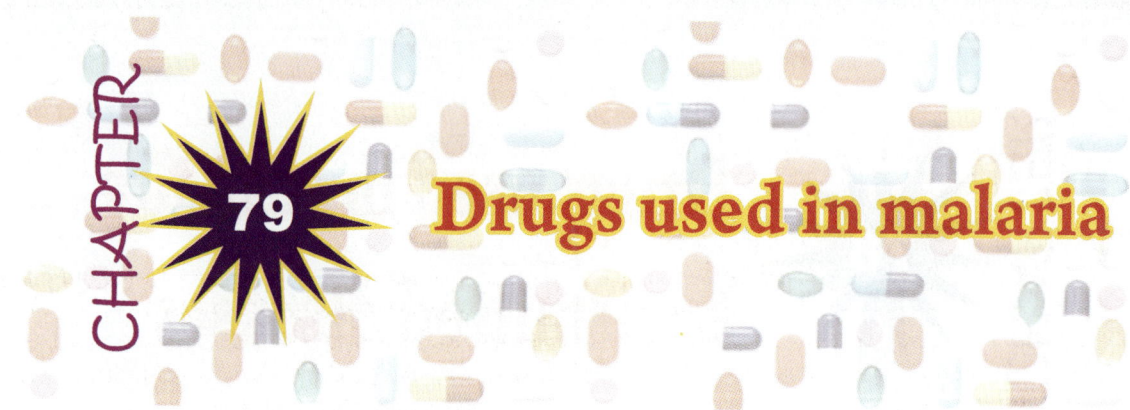

CHAPTER **79** **Drugs used in malaria**

MALARIA

- Malaria is caused by the protozoa Plasmodium. It is transmitted by the female Anapheles mosquitoes from the infected human. The main symptoms of malaria are FEVER, RIGOR, CHILL.
- The clinical symptoms of malarial fever is due to the rupture of R.B.C → release of trophozoites → release toxin → fever, rigor, chill, anaemia, splenomegaly etc.,
- Cerebral malaria is due to P.falciparum causes unconsciousness, coma, sometimes convulsion

DRUGS USED IN MALARIA:

The causative organisms of Malaria are:

1. Plasmodium falciparum
2. Plasmodium vivax
3. Plasmodium malariae

- The most common and dangerous parasite causing malaria is P.falciparum (no relapse)
- P.vivax → which causes relapse
- Earlier chloroquine was highly effective and drug of choice against P.falciparum
- Now most of P.falciparum developed resistance to chloroquine in most parts of the world including India
- Once diagnosed as malarial fever by P.falciparum → chloroquine is started → if fever does not subside within 3 days → then P.falciparum may be Chloroquine resistant. Other suitable antimalarial drugs are started
- Now, the clinicians assuming that all cases are chloroquine resistant falciparum malaria, straightaway, Chloroquine resistant antimalarial drugs, preferrably ARTEMISININ derivatives are prescribed.

CLASSIFICATION OF ANTIMALARIAL DRUGS ACCORDING TO THEIR Clinical uses

I. SUPPRESSIVE PROPHYLAXIS (Chemoprophylaxis)

- Long term treatment → hence, less toxic drugs are to be selected. They are given weekly once. (Chemoprophylaxis is needed to those who are going to travel to endemic area)
  1. Chloroquine 300 mg base / weekly → is 1st choice (if chloroquine sensitive P. falciparum. In resistant malaria, any one of the following drugs is preferred)
  2. Doxycycline 100mg/daily – 1st choice
  3. Mefloquine ⎤
  4. Atovaquone ⎬ /weekly once
  5. Fansidar ⎦

II. GAMETOCIDES: kill gametes and prevent spread → rarely used

1. Chloroquine
2. Artemisinin derivatives
3. Doxycycline
4. Primaquine
5. Proguanil

III. BLOOD SCHIZONTICIDES – CLINICAL CURATIVE (ACUTE ATTACK)

1. Chloroquine. If P. falciparam is sensitive to chloroquine, otherwise any one of the following drugs is used.
2. Artemisinin derivatives
   - Artemether
   - Artesunate
   - Arteether
3. Halofantrine, Lumefantrine combined with Artemisinin (Lumerax)
4. Mefloquine
5. Cinchona alkaloid – Quinine
6. Sulfodoxine + Pyrimethamine (Fansidar)
7. Atovaquone
8. Amodiaquine

IV. RADICAL CURATIVE : (tissue Schizonticide)

Primaquine + any one of the clinical curative drugs are given in case of vivax malaria (to prevent relapse)

Radical curative is complete eradication of malarial parasite (including persistant liver stage)

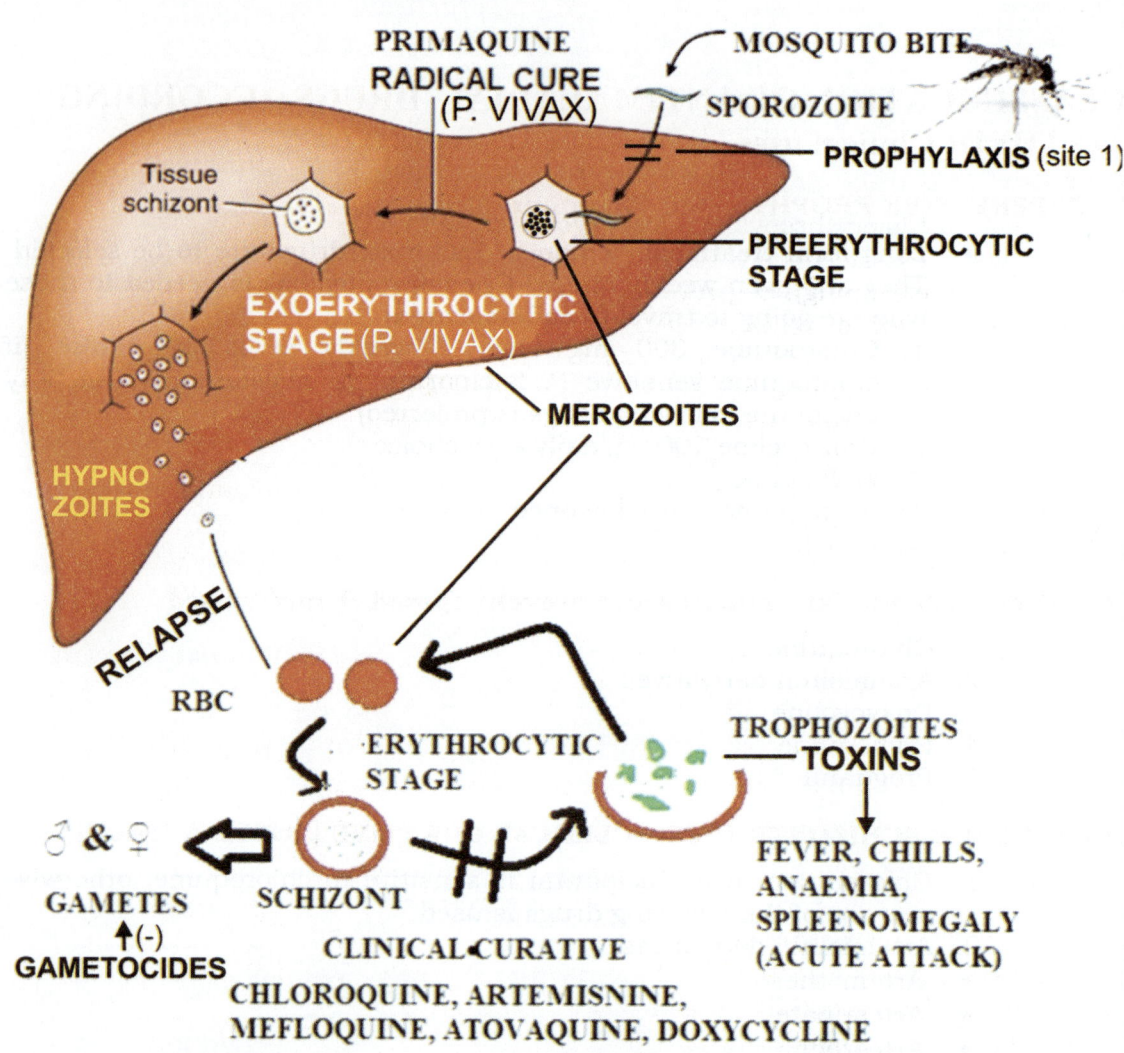

Fig. 74 Life Cycle of Malarial Parasite & Site of action of Antimalarial drugs

Female Anaphele's mosquito → sucks blood from the infected person, while biting. Sporozoites → pre-erythrocytic stage → schizonts → merozoites → enter into RBC → erythrocytic cycle → Schizont → after full development → rupture of RBC → release of toxins (TNF-α, pyrogens etc) → Fever, rigor, chill, anaemia, spleenomegaly (clinical symptoms). Drugs which reverse/prevent clinical symptoms are 'clinical curative' ('erythrocytic schizonticides). Few schizonts (in case of P. Vivex) stays in the liver for long time (6 months) (exo-erythrocytic stage) and then released and produce clinical symptoms (relaps malaria), the drugs acting here as tissue schizonticidal are called radical curative.

Chemoprophylaxis drugs act at the site (1) – prevent pre-erythrocytic schizonts.

Gametocides are drugs, which kill gametes and prevent the spread of infection.

CHLOROQUINE

- It is an antimalarial drug
- It is concentrated in R.B.C, liver and kidney

Mechanism of action: (Fig.74)

- It is erythrocyte schizonticide
- It is selectively taken up and concentrated by RBC → degrades Hb (clumping) → preventing the parasites to be able to utilize it → death of schizonts (schizonticidal) in RBC
- It inhibits conversion of Toxic haem to nontoxic haem → accumulation of toxic haem leads to death of erythrocytic schizonts
  1. Antimalarial action
     - It is fast acting
     - It is highly effective against all species of malarial parasites
     - Fever usually subsides within 3 days of acute attack of malaria (if fever does not subside within 3 days after chloroquine), it is assumed that chloroquine resistant malaria
- It is used as suppressive prophylaxis (if resistant, other drugs to be given)
  2. In Giardiasis
  3. Its Anti-inflammatory action is useful in Rheumatoid arthritis, lepra reaction

Clinical uses of CHLOROQUINE

1. In chloroquine sensitive falciparum malaria
2. Used as prophylactic (1 tab / weekly) & clinical curative (in acute attack) → It is started with 4 tablets (600mg base) in milk/fruit juice and 2 tablets (300mg) base at 6 hours followed by 300mg (base) (2 tab) on 2nd & 3rd day. Total 1.5gm (base) 10 tablets of 250 mg size.
3. In giardiasis (Tinidazole is better)
4. In hepatic amoebiasis (Tinidazole is better)
5. In Rheumatoid arthritis: (ref – DMARDS – Disease Modifying Anti Rheumatic Drug) Hydroxychloroquine → commonly used and less toxic
6. In Lepra reaction (better drugs are available)

Adverse effects:

- Nausea, vomiting (troublesome) → antiemetic is needed and taken after meal
- Myopathy
- Ocular complications like blurring of vision, diplopia, temporary loss of accommodation on long term use (reversible). In children, it is contraindicated, since they are unable to report the defect in time.
- Contraindicated in retinal damage

QUININE

- It is a cinchona alkaloid.

Clinical uses:

1. In cerebral malaria
2. As sclerosing agent in varicose vein.

Adverse effects: cinchonism → tinnitus (ringing of ear)

PRIMAQUINE

- It is an antimalarial drug
- Antimalarial action: It is useful only to prevent relapse of P.vivax
- It is not useful in acute attack (as clinical curative)
- It acts on liver schizonts only.

Mechanism of action: (Fig.74)

Primaquine → liver → releases intermediate substance → oxidants → lethal to tissue schizonts (exo-erythrocytic stage) → ONLY TISSUE SCHIZONTICIDE-USEFUL IN RELAPSE MALARIA DUE TO P. VIVAX (not erythrocytic schizonticide, and hence it is not effective in acute attack of malaria)

Clinical uses:

- For radical curative → in vivax malaria → one drug for clinical curative + Primaquine (15 days) for radical curative (complete cure)

Adverse effects:

- Haemolysis, particularly in the individuals in whom there is G6PDH (Glucose 6 Phosphate Dehydrogenase) deficiency
- It is avoided in pregnancy

ARTEMISININ DERIVATIVES

Artesunate (I /V), arteether (IM), artemether (O/IM)

- They are preferred in chloroquine resistant malaria

Mechanism of action: (Fig.74)

- They damage the cellular membranes of Malarial Parasite due to free radical generation and they are blood schizonticides

ANTIMALARIAL ACTION:

- They are fast acting
- They are highly potent
- They are useful in acute attack → not suitable for prophylactic (more toxic for long term use)

Clinical uses:

- They are useful in chloroquine resistant malaria with other drugs in Multi Drug Resistant malaria & in complicated cerebral malaria

WHO has recommended the following combination of Artemisinin derivatives for chloroquine resistant malaria.

1. Artesunate + Sulfadoxine + Pyrimethamine
2. Artesunate + mefloquine
3. Artesunate + amodiaquine
4. Artesunate + Halofantrine

Dose : Artemether – 40 mg cap, Artesunate – 50 mg tab, Arteether 150 mg/IM inj.

Advantages :

1. Rapid clinical cure
2. The malarial parasites do not develop resistance
3. They show good tolerability.

Adverse effects:

Anorexia, abdominal pain, ↓HR, long term → AV block C/I in pregnancy

Prophylactic	Acute Attack
1. Chloroquine → 300mg/weekly Chloroquine resistant cases: Doxycycline 100mg/ daily Fansidar / weekly Mefloquine/ weekly	In Chloroquine resistant Malaria: 1. Artemisinin derivative 2. Sulphadoxin + Pyrimethamine (Fansidar) 3. Mefloquine 4. Atovaquone 5. Amodiaquine

Endemic area visit

The drug is started 1-2 weeks before, continued as long as in endemic area and 4 weeks after leaving endemic area.

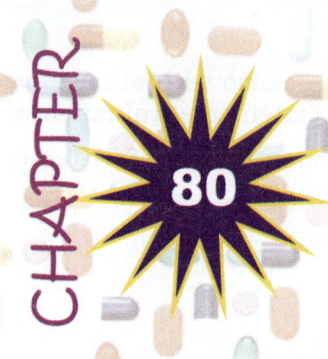

Drugs used in amoebiasis and other protozoal infections

CHAPTER 80

DRUGS USED IN AMOEBIASIS:

Antiamoebic drugs are useful in infection (amoebiasis) caused by the protozoa "Entamoeba histolytica".

CAUSES OF AMOEBIASIS:

1. Poor environmental status – poor hygiene
2. Low socio economic status – poor hygiene

Are responsible for spread of the infection. (contaminated food and drinking water by faecal matter→Amoebic cyst → intestine → trophozoites → either colonic commensal → cyst → passed in the faeces. The trophozoites causes ulcer (dysentery) or pass into liver (liver abscess)The cysts passed in the faeces are contaminated by food and water and helps in the spread of infection by insect to those who consume the contaminated food and drinking water.Trophozoites commonly cause acute dysentery (with blood and mucous in stool) or chronic amoebiasis (with occasional diarrhoea and vague abdominal symptoms) → this is referred as "intestinal amoebiasis"

Occasionally trophozoites pass through blood stream to reach the liver and cause "amoebic liver abscess". This is called as "extra intestinal amoebiasis"

Entamoeba live in symbiotic relationship with bacteria in the colon. The broad spectrum antibiotics (Tetracylines) which inhibit colonic bacteria will kill entamoeba histolytica, indirectly by depriving nutrients from colonic bacteria.

METRONIDAZOLE/TINIDAZOLE:

Now Tinidazole is preferred to Metronidazole, since it produces less nausea and long action.

CLASSIFICATION OF AMOEBICIDAL DRUGS:

I.   Tissue Amoebicidal

        Metronidazole group – Tinidazole, Secnidazole

II.   Luminal amoebicidal

        Diloxanide group – Diloxanide , Nitrazoxamide

III. Antibiotic – Tetracyclines
(other drugs are not used → either not effective or too toxic)

METRONIDAZOLE/TINIDAZOLE:

- It is an antiamoebic drug, commonly used
- Metronidazole is replaced by other drugs in the same group

Mechanism of action

- It is selectively toxic to E.histolytica
  Tinidazole → enters into trophozoites (E.histolytica cells) by diffusion → releases nitro group which contains highly reactive nitro radical, (only in anaerobic condition) which is cytotoxic to the trophozoites. That is the reason Tinidazole group is effective against anaerobic bacteria also → metabolism of anaerobic bacteria is also affected
- It is not directly effective against cyst.
- Metronidazole & its group have been found to inhibit CMI (Cell Mediated Immunity). It induces radiosensitization

Clinical uses :

Metronidazole (Flagyl) dose 400mg|3| daily

It is the only drug, which is effective against BACTERIA, PROTOZOA, HELMINTH & CLOSTRIDIUM (and in infections caused by them).

I. **ANTIBACTERIAL USES (First choice)**
1. In g^-ve anaerobic infection (which is common in abdominal , gynaecological surgery). So this drug is given as prophylactic & also for treatment in g-ve anaerobic infection (brain abscess, endocarditis caused by anaerobic organisms), toothache (gingivitis)
2. In H.pylori infection: (which causes peptic ulcer) It is one of the drugs in anti H.pylori regimen.
3. In clostradial infection – pseudomembranous enterocolitis caused by Cl. difficle associated with the use of extended spectrum and broad spectrum antimicrobial agents.

II. **AS ANTIPROTOZOAL (First choice)**
4. In amoebiasis (both intestinal and extra intestinal amoebiasis)→ It is effective against invasive amoebic dysentery, diarrhoea.
5. In trichomonas vaginalis vaginitis – first drug used in this infection. Till now it is the choice for this infection. Both partners should be treated to prevent cross infections.
6. In giardiasis.

III. **AS ANTHELMINTIC**
7. In Guinea worm infestation

IV. OTHER USES

8. It sensitizes the cancer cells to the action of radiotherapy and anticancer drugs. Anticancer drugs are concentrated in cancer cells.

Adverse effects:

- The most commonest adverse effects are **nausea, vomiting, metallic taste, anorexia and abdominal cramp**
- Prolonged treatment – causes glossitis, peripheral neuropathy

Contraindicated – in neurological diseases

- In pregnancy
- In chronic alcoholism because of its **disulfiram like** action (ref:Alcohol) → and alcohol intolerance and alcohol is to be avoided

TINIDAZOLE (Tiniba)

- All are similar to Metronidazole except
  1. It is better tolerated
  2. Less incidence of side effects like metallic taste and nausea and it is long acting

Dose: 2 g| once daily| as long as required depending upon the infection

DILOXANIDE FUROATE

- It is luminal amoebicidal drug, used in intestinal amoebiasis only
- It directly kills trophozoites which is responsible for the production of cysts
- It has no systemic amoebicidal action
- It is less effective against invasive amoebic dysentery

Clinical uses:

In mild intestinal amoebiasis and in asymptomatic cyst passers. It prevents the spread

Dose: 500mg|3| orally, usually combined with tinidazole for better effect (to eradicate cyst completely)

Adverse effects:

- flatulence, occasional nausea

TETRACYCLINES

- It is indirectly acting amoebicidal drug

Mechanism of action

- E. histolytica has symbiotic action with intestinal flora

- Tetracycline (Doxycycline) by inhibiting the intestinal flora deprive nutrients to E.histolytica and inhibit proliferation of entamoeba

USE

As adjuvant in chronic and difficult to treat cases

Adverse effects:

(refer: Tetracyclines)

DRUGS USED IN OTHER PROTOZOAL INFECTIONS

1. Trichomonas vaginalis vaginitis (Trichomoniasis)
2. Giardiasis
3. Trypanasomiasis
4. Leishmaniasis
I. Trichomonas vaginalis vaginitis (Trichomoniasis)
   Trichomonas vaginalis is a protozoa which cause the infection "Trichomoniasis", characterised by vulvo vaginitis (inflammation, itching, lesions)

   1. DRUGS USED ORALLY
      i. Tinidazole 600mg| daily| 7 days or 2g| single dose
      - It is the drug of choice. The cure rate is > 90%
      - In refractory cases, an additional intravaginal treatment is required
      - Both partners should be treated concurrently to prevent cross infection of each other

   Mechanism of action and Adverse effects: (ref: Tinidazole)

   2. DRUGS USED INTRAVAGINALLY
      i. Diiodoquin
      ii. Quiniodoquin
      iii. Clotrimazole
      iv. Povidone – Iodine
II. DRUGS USED IN GIARDIASIS
   1. Tinidazole
   2. Choloquine

III. DRUGS USED IN LEISHMANIASIS
   - Visceral leishmaniasis (kala-azar) is caused by Leishmania donovani
   - The first choice drug was Sodium stibogluconate (SSG). Many organisms developed resistant to that drugs
   - Mucocutaneous and dermal leishmaniasis are caused by other species are treated by sodium stibogluconate
   - It is transmitted by sandfly

DRUGS

1. Pentamidine
2. Amphotercin-B
3. Paramomycin – locally applied in dermal leishmaniasis
4. Allopurinol

Mechanism of action :

Sodium stibogluconate acts by inhibiting the SH - gp (sulphhydryl) containing enzyme and inhibit energy production in the parasites.

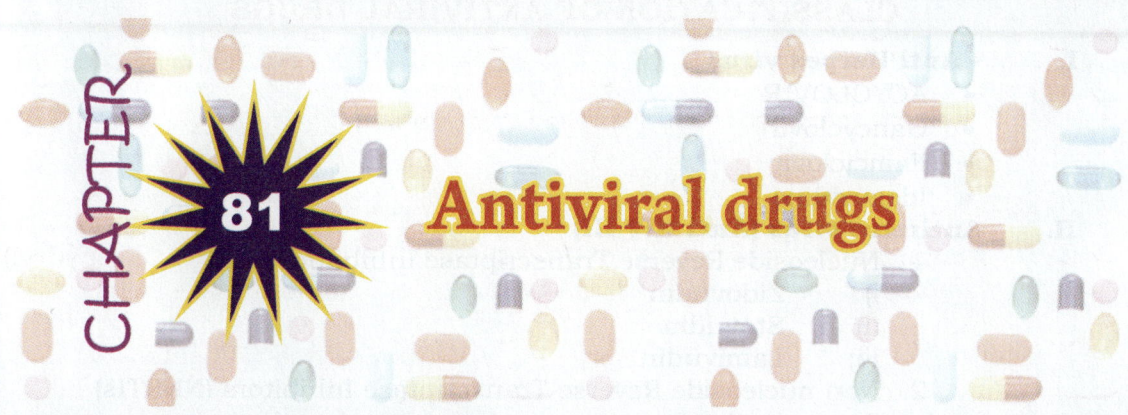

Antiviral drugs

CHAPTER 81

Antiviral drugs act against VIRUSES

- Viruses are essentially nucleic acid
- Viruses are either DNA virus or RNA virus
- Viruses are intracellurly growing microorganisms
- VIRUSES are obligate intracellular parasites
- Virus cannot prepare its own food
- Commands host (human) cell to synthesize viral proteins and thus replicates (host cells may or may not die)
- VIRUSES are active only when it is within living cell of human or plant (Outside the host cells). The virus is inert material.

I. The drugs that are effective against DNA viruses :
- Herpes simplex – Type I & II (HSV)
- Varicella – Zoster virus (VZV) HHV   →   Herpes virus
- Epstein – Barr Virus (EBV) HHV$_4$
- Cytomegalo virus (CMV) HHV$_5$
    Hepatitis viruses (A,B,C)

II. RNA VIRUSES against which the drugs are effective:
- HTLV = Human T- Lymphotropic virus
- HTLV III = also called HIV – Human AIDS virus
- HTLV II = Human T – Lymphotropic virus (Hairy cell leukemia)
- H_1N_1 = Influenza virus

III. VIRAL VACCINES
Polio, rabies, mumps, measles, varicella, hepatitis – B, influenza, HIV vaccines (on the way) etc.,
    The antiviral drugs should enter into host cell and selectively affect virus without affecting the host cells
        Only few drugs are effective
        Main targets of drugs are nucleic acid synthesis of virus, entry of virus and release
        Another problem is RESISTANCE
- Resistance is common among Retrovirus (HIV).
- Hence 2 or 3 drugs combinations are given.

CLASSIFICATION OF ANTIVIRAL DRUGS

I.   **– Anti Herpes virus**
- ACYCLOVIR
- Gancyclovir
- Famciclovir
- Idoxuridine

II.   **Antiretro virus (Anti HIV III)**
1. Nucleoside Reverse Transcriptase Inhibitor (NRTI)
   - i) Zidovudin
   - ii) Stavudin
   - iii) Lamivudin
2. Non nucleoside Reverse Transcriptase Inhibitors (NNRTIs)
   - i) Nevirapine
   - ii) Efavirenz
3. Protease Inhibitor (PIs)
   - i) Indinavir
   - ii) Ritonavir
   - iii) Saquinavir

III. **Anti – influenza virus**
- **i)** Amantidine
- **ii)** Rimantidine
- **iii)** Oseltamivir
- **iv)** Zanamivir

IV.   **Non selective antiviral**
- i) Interferon –α
- ii) Ribavirin

ACYCLOVIR

- it is an antiviral drug
- it is effective against Herpes virus

Clinical uses and Antiviral spectrum

Anti viral spectrum: Acyclovir is effective against Herpes simplex Type I and Type II Herpes Zoster, Varicella Zoster, Epstein Barr virus. Herpes infection affects mouth, face, eye, skin, genital, rectum, brain etc.,

Clinical uses

Antiherpes virus reduce duration and severity of illness.

In immunocompromised patients the antiherpes drugs are given by IV route.

In severe cases the duration of treatment is prolonged.

Preparations : Oral / topical / parenteral

1. In genital Herpes simplex infection (oral, topical)
2. In mucocutaneous H-simplex infection
3. In H.simplex encephalitis & neuralgia
4. In H.simplex keratitis (Topical)

5. In H.zoster infection (CNS)
6. In chicken pox (varicella zoster)- Acyclovir is the drug of choice

400 – 800 mg|3| daily| as long as required

Mechanism of action:

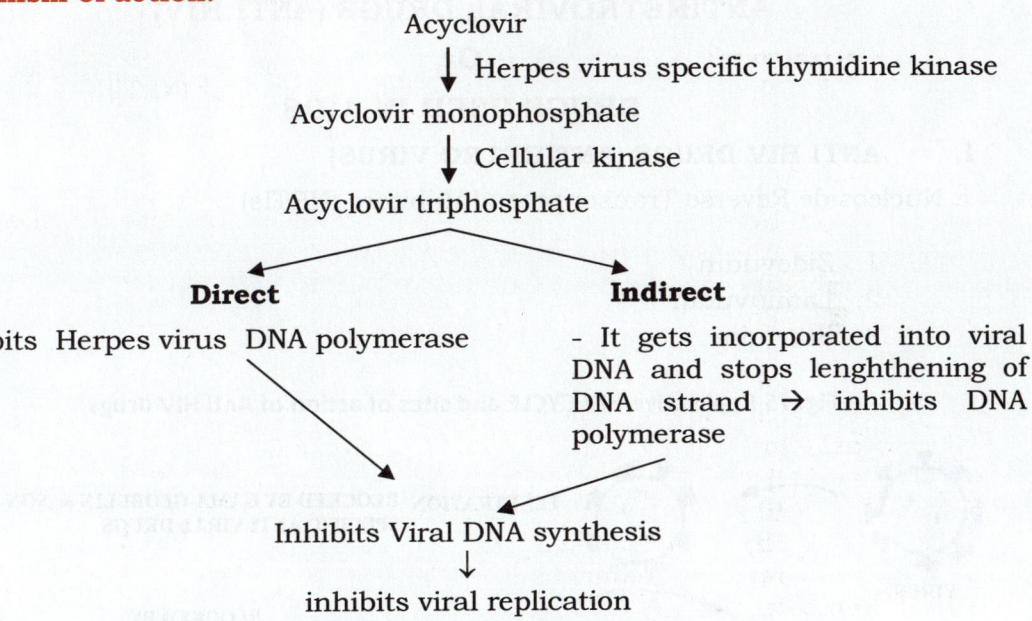

Acyclovir

↓ Herpes virus specific thymidine kinase

Acyclovir monophosphate

↓ Cellular kinase

Acyclovir triphosphate

Direct   **Indirect**

It inhibits Herpes virus DNA polymerase   - It gets incorporated into viral DNA and stops lenghthening of DNA strand → inhibits DNA polymerase

Inhibits Viral DNA synthesis

↓

inhibits viral replication

- crosses cornea, BBB, excreted **UNCHANGED** in urine
- caution in renal failure

Adverse effects: headache, neurological manifestations (tremor, hallucination etc)

IDOXURIDINE

- First antiherpetic drug, (antiviral drug)
- It is effective only against DNA virus
- It is thymidine analogue (Pyrimidine antimetabolite)

Mechanism of action:

Idoxuridine

↓

Competes with thymidine

↓

Gets incorporated into viral DNA

↓

Faulty DNA is formed

↓

It directs synthesis of wrong protein

↓

Non-infective viral particles are released

Antiviral spectrum – It is effective against H.simplex only → topical administration in Kerato conjunctivitis

Adverse effects: Ocular irritation, photophobia, oedema of eye lids

ANTIRETROVIRAL DRUGS (ANTI HIV)

Or

DRUGS USED IN AIDS

I.   ANTI HIV DRUGS (ANTIRETRO VIRUS)

i. Nucleoside Reverse Transcriptase Inhibitors (NRTIs)

    1. Zidovudin

    2. Lamiuvudin

    3. Stavudin

Fig. 75 Replicative HIV CYCLE and sites of action of Anti HIV drugs

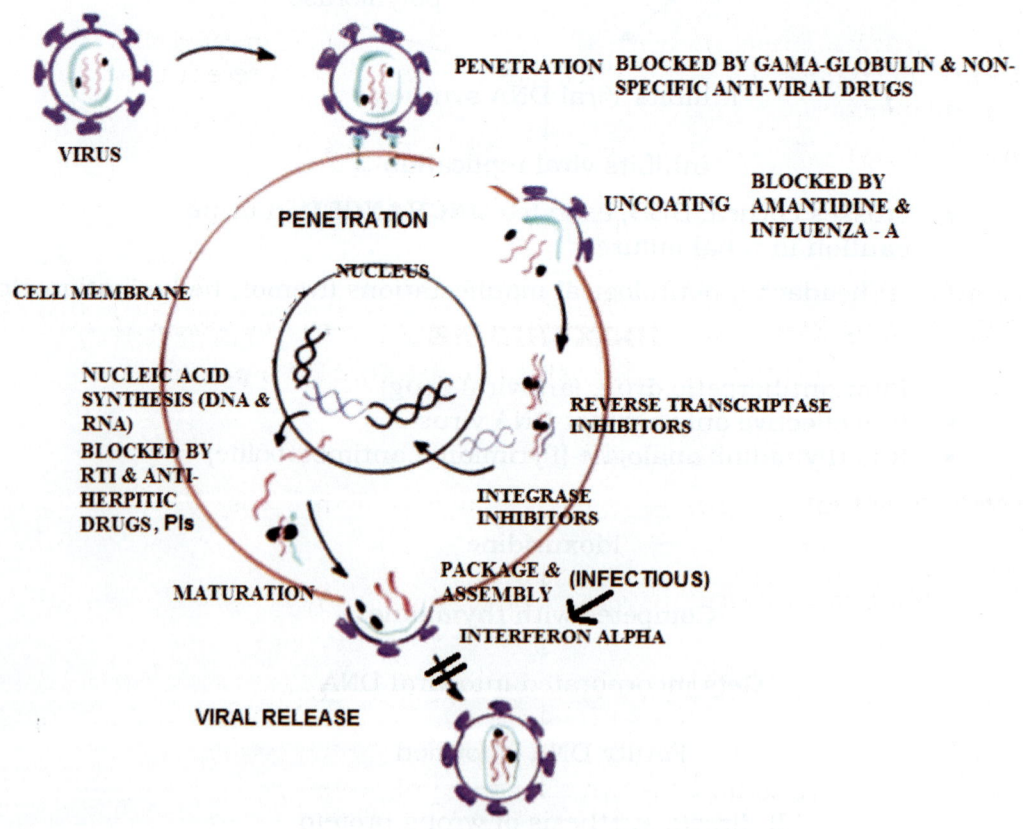

ii. Nonnucleoside Reverse Transcriptase Inhibitors (NNRTIs)

   1. Nevirapine

   2. Efavirenz

iii. Protease Inhibitors

   1. Ritonavir

   2. Saquinavir

   3. Indinavir

  II. Entry Inhibitor: Enfuvirtide

 III. Integrase Inhibitor:Raltegravir

NUCLEOSIDE REVERSE TRANSCRIPTASE INHIBITOR (NRTI)

ZIDOVUDIN

- It is an antiretroviral drug

Mechanism of action: (Fig.75)

All the Antiretroviral drugs increase the CD4 count, which in turn increase the body defence mechanism by stimulating B & T lymphocytes, prevent the attack by opportunistic infections.

It inhibits the enzyme Reverse Transcriptase (virus directed)

- It has got high affinity for the enzyme
  Single stranded viral DNA

Inhibited by Zidovudin → virus directed **Reverse Transcriptase**
(RNA Dependent DNA polymerase)

Inhibits↓ Double stranded viral DNA

Inhibits ↓ This DNA translocates to the nucleus

Inhibits ↓ Integration with chromosomal DNA of host cell

Inhibits ↓ Viral genomic RNA & m- RNA

Inhibits ↓ m-RNA directed viral proteins

Inhibits ↓ Finally viral particles, assembly and maturation

Adverse effects of ZIDOVUDIN:

- Mainly due to partial inhibition of cellular DNA polymerase → anaemia, neutropenia (corrected by the transfusion of Erythropoietin/ Granulocyte colony stimulating factor (G CSF)
- Anorexia, abdominal pain, headache
- Myopathy (less common)

D/I – paracetamol, antifungal agents increase the toxicity of Zidovudin

Dose: 500mg/4/ daily in divided doses

Clinical uses : It is not used alone due to development of resistance

- In HIV infection
- As prophylactic (somewhat effective)
- Common combination regimen (according to HAART – Highly Active Anti Retroviral Therapy (HAART)
  1. INRTI + 1 PI
  2. NRTI + 1 NNRTI
  3. Two NRTIs

LAMIVUDIN

- Anti HIV, also Antihepatitis – B
- All other actions and uses are same as that of Zidovudin

NON-NUCLEOSIDE REVERSE TRANSCRIPTASE INHIBITORS (NNRTIs)

- Nevirapine and Efavirenz
- They are anti HIV drug

Mechanism of action: (Fig.75)

NNRTIs do not require any activation through phosphorylation(Unlike NRTIs). They inhibit the reverse transcriptase enzyme. They block the conversion of RNA to DNA and further inhibit the maturation and multiplication of virus → improved CD4 count → control immune deficiency syndromes.

-If used alone, resistance develops rapidly. So, usually they are combined with other anti HIV drugs

Adverse effects of NNRTs: skin rashes, Steven-Johnson syndrome. Some are enzyme inducers (usually combined with Protease Inhibitors, which are enzyme inhibitors)

Caution with enzyme inducer like Rifampicin, which reduce the efficacy of Nevirapine

Clinical use : only in HIV infection (in AIDS)

Dose : 200-400mg| daily

They are anti HIV drug

PROTEASE INHIBITORS

Example: Indinavir, Ritonavir, Saquinavir

- They are anti HIV drugs

Mechanism of action: (Fig.75)

- Inhibit Protease enzyme.→ Proteas enzyme is needed for the late stage protein synthesis → maturation and infectivity of HIV
- The enzyme is also responsible for the production of 'Reverse Transcriptase Enzyme'
- Indinavir →↓(inhibits) protease enzyme →↓(prevents) the development of the mature AIDS virus and its infectivity →↓ (prevents) further round of infection
- Resistance develops, if it is used alone. Always given with other groups of anti HIV drugs

Clinical use : only in AIDS

Dose: 750 mg|3|daily

Adverse effects:

1. 'Altered' distribution of fat (Buffallo hump) , truncal obesity (like GC)
2. 'Altered Metabolism' →↑(increase) concentration of lipid, → aggravate atherosclerosis, and aggravate DM
3. 'Altered' coagulability: Increase bleeding tendency in haemophilia

Common drug interactions:

- They are enzyme inhibitors of drugs metabolized by CYP3A4. Protease inhibitors increase the toxicity of the following drugs (due to increased plasma level)
- Cisapride(arrhythmia)
- Statins(rhabdomyolysis)
- Midazolam (respiratory depression)
- Enzyme inducer like rifampicin decrease the level of Protease Inhibitors.
- St.John's wart antagonizes the antiviral action of PIs

TREATMENT OF AIDS (HIV)

Retrovirus is a Human immunodeficiency virus, the most notorious organism in developing resistance for a single drug treatment. So, for the treatment of AIDS, it is better to give 2 or 3 drug combination in order to overcome the development of resistance.

The antiretroviral drugs are only symptomatic and not curative. They only prolong the survival time and improve the quality of life.

AIDS is characterized by immune deficiency state. The retrovirus suppress the cell mediated immunity by destroying T-lymphocytes and CD4, which are very important for the body defense mechanism.

But the AIDS in pregnancy can be managed by giving Zidovudine in pregnant woman. It will cure the baby and free from AIDS.

The most important symptoms of AIDS are due to immune deficiency and superinfection (Fungus, Tuberculosis, Virus) which is treated by proper antimicrobial drugs. It becomes very difficult to treat in severe cases.

The commonly used treatment regimen is HAART (Highly Active AntiRetroviral Therapy) with combination of 3 or more drugs whenever indicated.

Since none of the currently available regimens can eradicate HIV from the body of the patients. The aim of the treatment should be to control maximally. The immune-deficiency syndrome is controlled by stimulating the immune system, thereby increasing the CD4 count to counter the superinfection.

The Preferred regimens are:

I. 2NRTI+NNRTI (PI-Sparing) – Zidovudine+Lamivudine+Efavirenz

II. 2NRTI+PI - Zidovudine+Lamivudine+Indinavir

III. 3NRTI - Zidovudine+Lamivudine+Abacavir (only when a NNRTI or PI cannot be used in patients receiving rifampicin, which is an enzyme inducer)

INTERFERONS (IFNs)

- Orally it is not effective → given parenterally

Mechanism of action:

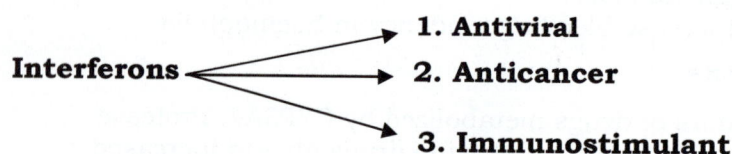

- In response to viral infection → release of Interferons and production of endogenous glycoproteins, cytokines (by host cells) → act against virus (non specific) → inhibit viral replication at multiple steps (i.e., viral penetration, synthesis of viral m-RNA, assembly of viral particles and their release)
- Interferons inhibit many DNA, RNA viruses
- They are host specific i.e., human Interferons (α,β,γ)
- They are produced by DNA recombinant technology
- They activate T-lymphocytes which produce anticancer and Immunostimulant actions. They increase host diffense mechanism. (Fig.80)

Clinical uses :

1. In chronic Hepatitis B & C
2. In AIDS related Kaposi's syndrome
3. In hairy cell leukaemia
4. In AIDS patients (as adjuvant with antiretroviral drugs)
5. In chronic myelogenous leukaemia & multiple myeloma
6. In non-Hodgkin's lymphoma

Adverse effects of INTERFERONS:

- 'Flu' like syndromes
- Neurotoxicity → numbness, tremor etc
- Myelosuppression → Neutropenia, thrombocytopenia
- Thyroid dysfunction

AMANTADINE

- It is an anti-influenza 'A' virus

Mechanism of action:

- It inhibits at early step, i.e., uncoating as well as late step (viral assembly)
- viral particles release is inhibited

Clinical uses :

1. As Prophylaxis of Influenza – A (during an epidemic or seasonal)
2. In the treatment of Influenza – A
3. In Parkinsonism (Dopamine agonist) Promoting synthesis and release of DA at the basal ganglia

Adverse effects:

- Insomnia, anorexia, dizziness, hallucination, postural hypotension

OSELTAMIVIR, ZANAMIVIR

- Useful in H_1N_1 Influenza virus (Swine Flu)

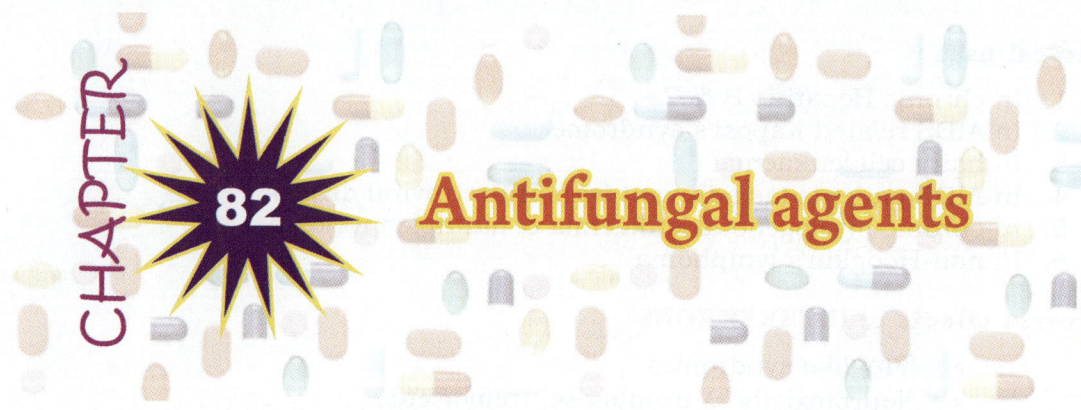

CHAPTER 82 — Antifungal agents

Antifungal agents prevent/cure fungal infections.

- Fungal infections are termed as "Mycoses" (singular: Mycosis)
- Clinically fungal infection are classified as follows:
  1. Superficial fungal infection affects skin and mucous membrane (itching, dermatitis and secondary infection). They are called as superficial mycoses.
  2. Systemic (deep) fungal infections → deep mycoses cause pneumonia, meningitis, etc.,
- Some fungal infections cause hypersensitivity reactions (asthma, dermatitis)

A. SUPERFICIAL FUNGAL INFECTIONS

- These are very common
- Dermatophytes → Tinea (Ringworm) fungal infection. It is termed as follows according to site of infection
  Skin & its appendages
  I. Tinea/Ring worm
      - Tinea corporis (body)
      - Tinea capitis (scalp)
      - Tinea cruris (genital)
      - Tinea pedis (clefts in between fingers, toes→ athletes foot)
      - Tinea versicolor (skin)
      - Tinea barbae – beard portion

  II. Candidiasis (candida albicans)
      Affects mucous membrane
      1. Oral- thrush
      2. Intestinal candidiasis – diarrhoea
      3. Vaginal candidiasis (lesions in vulva, vagina & itching)
      4. Ocular candidiasis – keratitis
      5. Occasionally in moist area of skin (under mammary gland)
      6. Pityrosporum ovale (fungus – yeast) causes dandruff (seborrheic dermatitis)

B. SYSTEMIC MYCOSES: (very rare, but common in AIDS patients)

1. Systemic candidiasis are U.T.I, meningitis, endocarditis and allergic (eczema, asthma, gastritis)
2. Blastomycosis causes meningitis
3. Histoplasmosis causes pulmonary infection
4. Cryptococcosis causes endocarditis
5. Aspergillosis causes pneumonia

Predisposing factors

- Deficient of host defence due to any cause
- Wide spread use of oral broad spectrum antibiotics (Tetracyclines) cause fungal superinfection (ref: Introduction to Chemotherapy), Orophanyngeal candidiasis (when Beclomethasone is used in bronchial asthma)
- Anticancer drugs depress Bone Marrow cause neutropenia → Body defence mechanism is decreased → fungal infection becomes common.
- In AIDS patients and by the use of immunosuppressant drugs → fungal infections are very common → both superficial and deep (systemic) mycoses. It is called as opportunistic infections.
- The indwelling catheter and dentures are prone to fungal infection.

CLASSIFICATION OF ANTIFUNGAL AGENTS

I. Antifungal antibiotics
1. Amphotericin- B (AMB)
2. Nystatin
3. Griseofulvin

II. Antimetabolites
1. Flucytosine (5 FC)

III. Azoles
1. Topical
   i. Clotrimazole (candid, candiderm)
   ii. Miconazole
   iii. Biconazole
2. Systemic
   i. Ketoconazole (in systemic, it is toxic). It is used only in dandruff (topical application in the form of shampoo – Nizral).
   ii. Fluconazole
   iii. Itraconazole (zocon, fluc-AF-150)

IV. Others
1. Terbinafine (Zimig, Sebifin – 250)
2. Whitfield's ointment – cheapest for Tinea infection (Benzoic acid + Salicyclic acid)

AMPHOTERICIN – B (AMB)

- It is an antifungal agent
- It is obtained from Streptomyces nodosus

Mechanism of Action :

- AMB has got high affinity for ergosterol present in fungal cell membrane → combines with it and forms 'MICROSPORE' → through which ions, amino acids leak out of fungal cell → Death of fungus → Fungicide
- It also attaches cholesterol in human cells and produces toxic effect to human cells to some extent.

Antifungal spectrum (broad spectrum antifungal agent):

- It is effective against Candida albicans, Histoplasma, Crytococcus, aspergillus etc., (systemic/ deep mycoses)
- It is not much effective in dermatophytes
- It is not effective against bacteria, since there is no ergosterol in bacterial cell membrane
- **It is not effective orally** (not absorbed) and it is given by I.V inj.
- It does not cross BBB → in meningitis, it is given by intrathecal injection.

Clinical uses :

1. Topical → in oral, vaginal, cutaneous candidiasis, otomycosis.
2. It is slightly immunostimulant and useful against deep mycoses in AIDS patients.
3. In deep mycoses target delivery preparation is available. Azoles are preferred.
4. In leishmaniasis (kala azar). Better drugs are available.

Dose : Liposomal Amphotericin (Ref: Dosage forms of drugs - Page No.19) – 10-50 mg/IV

Adverse effects:

Highly toxic → chill, fever, headache, pain, fever, dyspnea
- Long term toxicity → nephrotoxic, anaemia due to B.M. depression

Mechanism of action of AMB & Nystatin

Amphotercin – B and Nystatin

↓

Bind to ergosterol present in fungal cell membrane

↓

Form pores & channels in the membrane

↓

Permeability of the membrane increases

↓

Leakage of intracellular (ions, aminoacids) contents of fungi

↓

Death of fungi (fungicidal)

NYSTATIN

- It is an antifungal antibiotic
- Systemic, it is more toxic than AMB
- Use is restricted only topically, **it is not absorbed orally** and there is no systemic toxicity

Mechanism of action: similar to AMB

Clinical uses & ANTIFUNGAL SPECTRUM :

It is effective mainly in **superficial candidiasis**
It is not effective in dermatophytes
1. It is used in intestinal candidiasis → 5 lakh unit tablet (oral). Azoles are preferred.
2. In Monilial vaginitis (vaginal tab) → azoles are preferred
3. Oral candidiasis (thrush) → tablet is sucked or crushed & mixed with honey and applied on the affected area.
4. In oropharyngeal candidiasis as lozenges

GRISEOFULVIN

- It is an antifungal antibiotic from Penicillium griseofulvum
- Orally effective (topically not effective)
- Antifungal spectrum: It is only effective against Dermatophytes (orally given). Azoles are preferred. Griseofulvin is a narrow spectrum antifungal drug.

Mechanism of action: It interferes with mitosis → stunted hyphae → loss of infectivity by fungi.

Adverse effects:

Peripheral neuritis, alcohol intolerance because of its disulfiram like reaction (Ref: Alcohol) → alcohol is to be avoided

AZOLE DERIVATIVES

Topical

- Clotrimazole
- Miconazole
- Ketoconazole (only in dandruff)

Systemic

- Fluconazole
- Itraconazole

Antifungal spectrum

- They are broad spectrum antifungal agents
- They are effective against superficial and deep mycoses

     i.   Candida albicans
     ii.   Dermatophytes
     iii. Histoplasma
     iv. Aspergillus
     v.   Pityrosporum ovale (dandruff) → local application of ketoconazole

- Also effective against g⁺ anaerobic bacteria
- Also effective against leishmaniasis

Mechanism of action of Azoles:

They↓ (inhibit) fungal CYP-450 called 'Lanosterol 14 α demethylase →↓(inhibit) synthesis of ergosterol, which is necessary for fungal cell membrane →↓(inhibit) fungal cell membrane synthesis → nutrients will leak out → fungi die → fungicidal action

Mechanism of action of TERBINAFINE & AZOLES

Toxic ← Increase the Plasma Level, ↑ Squalene

(fungicidal) ⥮ Terbinafine inhibits Squalene 2-3 epoxidase

Inhibits Lanosterol synthesis

⥮ Azoles inhibit CYP-450 dependent 14α -demethylase

Inhibit Ergosterol synthesis

(Inhibit cell membrane synthesis)

Contents leak out

Fungi die (Fungicidal)

Clinical uses of AZOLES:

1. In superficial fungal infections (clotrimazole)
    i.   Athlete's foot
    ii.   Oral, cutaneous, vaginal candidiasis
    iii.   Otomycosis
    iv.   Oropharyngeal candidiasis is common after inhalational GC, beclomethasone.
    v.   All Tinea (ring worm) infections → all dermatophytes infections
2. In systemic (deep) mycoses (Fluconazole, Itraconazole)
    i.   Dermatophytes (nail infection) 150mg/weekly/4 weeks (oral)
    ii.   Systemic and mucosal candidiasis
    iii.   Fungal keratitis (topical)
    iv.   Cryptococcal, Aspergillus meningitis

3. **Other USES** : In dandruff (topical ketoconazole)
4. In leishmaniasis
5. In cushing's syndrome: ketoconazole inhibits GC synthesis

Adverse effects of Azoles:

Nausea, vomiting, abdominal pain, headache

Adverse effects of KETOCONAZOLE

- Drug interation – it is an enzyme inhibitor → increases toxicity of many drugs
- Inhibits Androgen synthesis, GC synthesis
- Loss of libido, menstrual irregularities
- Hepatotoxic

Dose of Azoles : Clotrimozole (candid) cream – 1%, 100 mg/vaginal tablet

Fluconazole (Zocon) – 100-200 mg/oral as long as required, 200 mg/IV, 0.3% eye drops.

Itraconazole – 200 mg/OD/orally/as long as required, depending upon the infection.

TERBINAFINE

- It is a new antifungal agent
- It is mainly effective against superficial fungal infection (dermatophytes, candida)

Mechanism of action: (refer before)

> It inhibits Squalene epoxidase and increases concentration of squalene, which is toxic to fungi → fungicidal
- Also inhibits synthesis of ergosterol

Clinical uses :

1. In Tinea/ ringworm infections
2. In cutaneous/mucosal candidiasis (next to azole)

Adverse effects:

- Gastric upset, taste disturbances, haematological disorders

CHOICE OF DRUGS IN FUNGAL INFECTION

I. For Deep mycoses:
   1. Cutaneous, disseminated candidiasis----AMB, Nystatin,Itraconazole
   2. Aspergillosis,Cryptococcosis, Histoplasmosis, Blastomycosis---AMB, Itraconazole,Fluconazole

II. For superficial fungal infection:

Dermatophytosis	Clotrimazole	Itraconazole
Superficial candidiasis	Nystatin	Clotrimazole
Dandruff	Topical shampoo Ketoconazole (Nizral) shampoo	

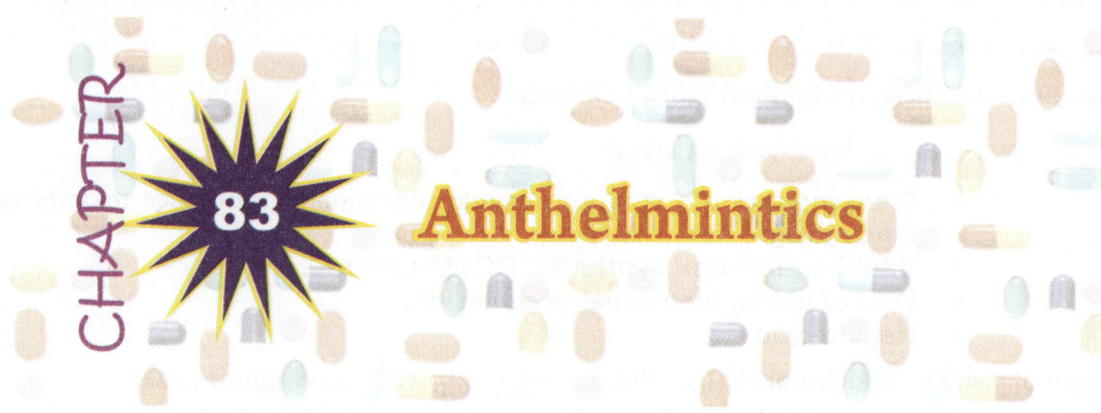

CHAPTER **83** **Anthelmintics**

- Anthelmintics are drugs either kill (vermicide) or expel (vermifuge) the infesting helminths

I.   Drugs used mainly in Nematodes (Round, Hook, Pin, Whip and Thread worms)
  1. ALBENDAZOLE
  2. Mebendazole
  3. Pyrantel pamoate
  4. Levamisole (also immunostimulant)

II. Drugs mainly used in Cestodes (Tape worm)
  1. PRAZIQUANTEL
  2. Niclosamide

III. Drugs mainly used in Filariasis
  1. Diethyl Carbamazine Citrate (DEC)
  2. Ivermectin
  3. Albendazole (high dose)

ALBENDAZOLE

- It is the broad spectrum anthelmintic
- It is effective against most of the Nematodes (round, hook, whip, thread, pin worms)
- Tapeworm (only in neurocysticercosis) – It is infestation of CNS by larva characterized by seizure and neurological dysfunctions
- It is also effective against filariasis
- It is effective in thread worm causing 'cutaneous larvae migrans' (erythema)

Clinical uses

- It is a broad spectrum Antihelmintic drug
  1. It is effective against all Nematodes (Round worm, Hook worm, Pin worm, Thread worms & Whip worms) single dose → 400mg to all (< 2 years → 200mg)
  2. In visceral larvae migrans (400 mg/OD / for 3 consecutive days.)

3. In tapeworms (400 mg/OD for 3 days treatment)
4. In neurocysticercosis → (400 mg/OD/for one month).
5. In Hydatid cyst → (400 mg/OD/for one month).
6. In Filariasis: A single dose with Diethyl Carbamazine (DEC) citrate are used in antifilarial mass programme. They suppress microfilaria and disease transmission.

Mechanism of action:

Albendazole
↓
It binds with β – tubulin of the parasites
↓
attacks the β – tubulin, which is very important for the entry of glucose (nutrient)
↓
(inhibits) glucose entry into parasitic cells
↓
now glucose of the host cannot enter inside the parasitic cell
↓
no ATP synthesis
↓
no energy production
↓
death of the parasites
↓
vermicidal action

- It also produces microfilaricidal action

Adverse effects:

- Well tolerated, mild nausea, diarrhea
- Alopecia, jaundice in long term use

MEBENDAZOLE

- All like that of Albendazole
- But less potent
- Not effective against filariasis, cutaneous larvae migrans & tapeworms

PYRANTEL PAMOATE

- It is effective against few nematodes
- It is useful in combined infestation of Hook worm and Round worm

Mechanism of action:

- It activates Nicotinic cholinergic receptors of parasite →
- Persistent depolarization → spastic paralysis→
- Detached from the intestinal mucosa → expelled in the faeces

- Mammalian Nicotinic receptors are not affected (very low affinity)
- Very useful in intestinal obstruction by Round worm (due to its intestinal relaxant action)

PRAZIQUANTEL

- It is an anthelmintic drug
- It is effective against trematodes, cestodes (Tapewroms)
- It is not effective against Nematodes
- It crosses BBB and useful in neurocysticercosis (by Tape worm)

Mechanism of action:

- It is taken up by worms and causes leakage of intracellular calcium → contracture and paralysis → the tape worms loose their grip from intestinal mucosa → and are expelled in faeces.
- Flukes and schistosomes are also dislodged from veins and tissues

Clinical uses :

1. In Tapeworms → single dose → 500mg| daily
    - It kills tape worm larvae within the cyst → no chance of developing systemic cysticercosis
    - In neurocysticercosis
    - In schistosomiasis and other flukes

Adverse effects: (minimum) nausea, abdominal pain, headache, dizziness

DIETHYL CARBAMAZINE CITRATE (DEC)

- First choice drug in filariasis

Mechanism of action:

DEC is highly selective effect on microfilariae→ clears microfilariae within 7 days → microfilariae present in nodules and transudates are not affected

- Alteration of microfilariae membrane
- Microfilariae are easily phagocytosed and cleared by body defence mechanism

Clinical uses :

1. **In filariasis:** 2mg|kg|TDS are 100mg tab for 3 weeks. Elephantiasis due to chronic lymphatic obstruction and hydrocele are not affected by D.E.C (only surgery)
2. Tropical Eosinophilia
3. It is used in antifilarial mass programme with Albendazole

Adverse effects:

Nausea, anorexia, headache

Febrile reaction → urticaria, bronchospasm due to death of microfilariae and adult worms

Mazotti reaction → within 2 hours produces fever, pruritus, postural hypotension etc., The symptoms disappear after withdrawing the drug.

IVERMECTIN

- It is effective in tapeworm infestation.
- It is an important anthelmintic drug.
- It is semisynthetic macrocyclic compound derived from S. avermetilis

Mechanism of action of Ivermectin:

After Ivermectin, the parasites develop tonic paralysis and they loose grip from the intestinal mucosa. They are excreted in the faeces.

- It also potentiates GABA in the worm, and is useful in expelling the worms.

Clinical uses of Ivermectin:

1. In filariasis: It is effective when given along with DEC
2. It is effective against tape worms
3. It is effective against scabies and lice (oral)
4. It is also effective against thread worm infestation (single dose of 0.1- 0.2 mg/kg)
5. In cutaneous larva migrans (next to Albendazole)

Adverse effects: pruritus, giddiness, nausea, abdominal pain, constipation

Dose: 0.1-0.2 mg/kg/oral as long as required

Choices of Anthelmintic drugs:

WORMS	FIRST CHOICE	ALTERNATE DRUG
1.Round worm	Albendazole	Piperazine
2.Hook worm	Albendazole	Levamizole
3.Whip worm	Albendazole	Levamizole
4.Trichirosis	Albendazole	Mebendazole
5.Pin worm	Mebendazole	Albendazole
6.Thread worm	Ivermectin	Albendazole
7.Filariasis	DEC	Ivermectin
8.Orchocerciasis	Ivermectin	DEC
9.Guinea worm	Metronidazole	Albendazole
10.Cutaneous larva migrans	Ivermectin, albendazole	Thiabendazole
11.Flukes:1)Schisto somiasis	Praziquantel	
12.Blood flukes	Praziquantel	Albendazole
13.Liver flukes	Praziquantel	Albendazole
14.Neurocysticercosis	Albendazole	Praziquantel
15.Hydatid diseases	Albendazole	Praziquantel

Cysticercosis - infection with larval form of Taenia solium

Cutaneous larva migrans - creeping eruption, pruritus appeared to migrate caused by burrowing of larva of round worm

Hydatid cyst - A larval form of tape worm enclosed in a bladder like cyst

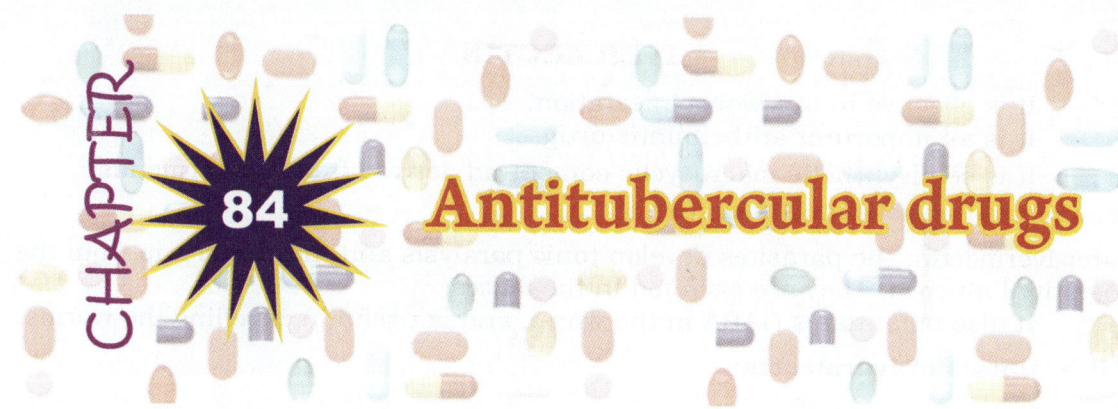

CHAPTER 84 **Antitubercular drugs**

Causative organism for tuberculosis is Mycobacterium tuberculosis

Tuberculosis (TB) is a chronic granulomatous disease caused by M.tuberculosis bacilli characterized by persistent cough, esophageal bleeding, thick sputum, chest infection. TB is contagious disease. It is highly susceptible in AIDS patients. At later stages it causes lesions in lung, bone, skeletal muscle, brain etc.,

Tubercle bacilli reside in the body in 3 stages

1. Dormant stage
2. Intracellular
3. Extracellular

Some information about TB.

1. M.tuberculosis bacilli is slow growing. So, the treatment is prolonged
2. The bacteria are lodged inside the macrophages. Most of the antibiotics fail to penetrate the lipid membrane of macrophage and bacterial cell membrane to reach the bacteria, hence most of the antibiotics are not effective against tuberculosis.
3. The mycobacteria are notorious for their ability to develop resistance against the drugs. Hence multidrugs regimen is preferred to prevent the development of resistance by mycobacteria.
4. Pools of bacteria
   - i. Intracellular (within macrophage)
   - ii. Caseous pool (in the caseous cavities)
   - iii. Free pool (metabolically active and are most susceptible to antitubercular drugs)
     - Rifampicin is effective against all the 3 pools
5. The aims of treatment
   - i. To prevent emergence of resistance
   - ii. To prevent relapse (to eradicate completely the mycobacteria from the body)
   - iii. To make the patients as quickly as possible non infectious (make the sputum +ve, which spreads infection, into sputum −ve)

Tuberculosis -**Symptoms and Signs: (Fig.76)**

Cough   Afternoon Fever

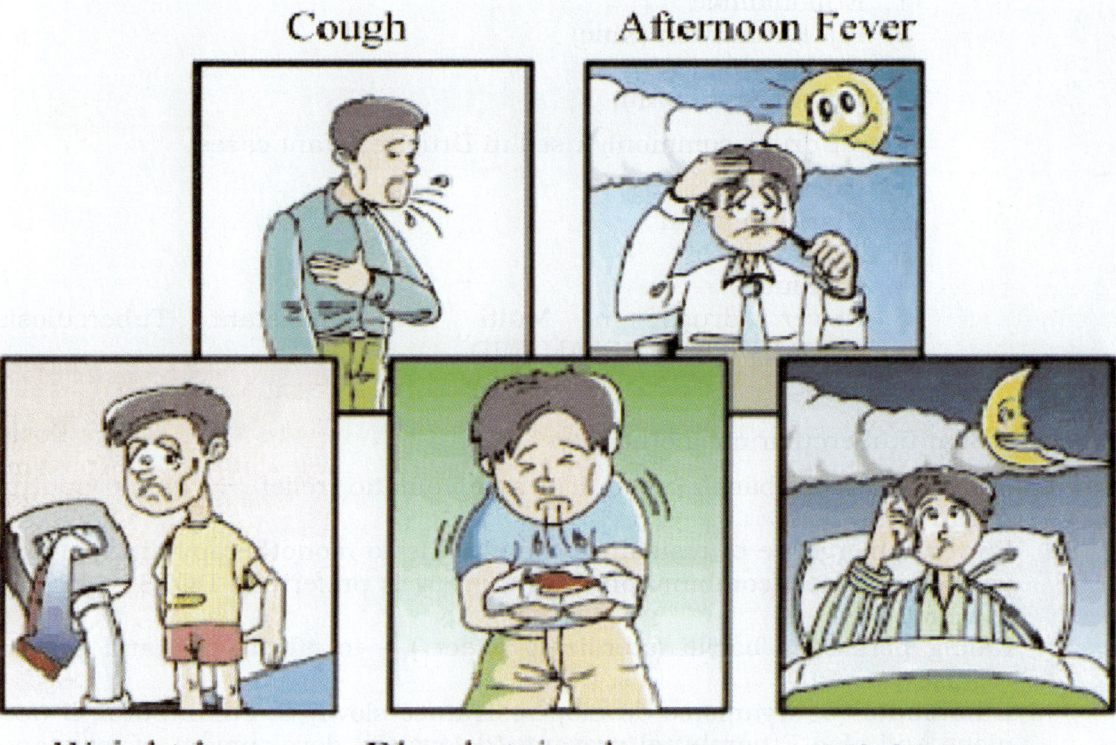

Weight loss   Blood stained sputum   Night sweats

Fig.76 Symptoms of Tuberculosis

DRUGS

I.   First line drugs (high antitubercular activity, low toxicity and acceptable) → routinely used
1. Isoniazid (H) – INH (Isonictonic acid Hydrazide)
2. Rifampicin (R)
3. Pyrazinamide (Z)
4. Ethambutol (E)
5. Streptomycin
       - Reserved
       - parenterally given
       - inconvenient

II.   Second line drugs
       Low efficiency, highly toxic

Useful in multi drug resistant tuberculosis

1. Ethionamide
2. Inj. Kanamycin (Kmc)
3. Cycloserine (Cys)
4. Inj. Amikacin (Am)

Newer drugs commonly used in Drug resistant cases:

1. Ofloxacin
2. Clarithromycin
3. Azithromycin
4. Rifabutin
5. Newer drugs in Multi Drug resistant Tuberculosis: BEDAQUILINE, DELAMANID

The goal of antitubercular chemotherapy

1. Killing dividing bacilli → quick symptomatic relief → quick sputum negativity
2. Prevent emergence of resistance mainly due to monotherapy and patient's poor compliance (combination drug therapy is preferred). DOTS regimen is to be followed.
3. Killing persisting bacilli (sterilizing effect) – to effect cure and prevent relapse
4. Ethambutol → organisms develop resistance slowly to ethambutol, if used alone and also Ethambutol prevents/delays the development of resistance by organisms to the other drugs
5. Drugs to be given to act against all subpopulations of bacilli – H,Z,R,E

ISONIAZID (H)

ISONICOTINIC ACID HYDRAZIDE

- First line antitubercular drug
  I.   Antitubercular action
       i.   It is primarily tuberculocidal
       ii.   It acts on both intracellular and extracellular bacilli
       iii. It is equally effective both in acidic and alkaline medium
       iv.   It is one of the cheapest antitubercular drugs
       v.   However, most atypical mycobacteria are not inhibited

Isoniazide- Inhibits mycolic acid synthesis of cell wall

Drug action: Isoniazid (INH)

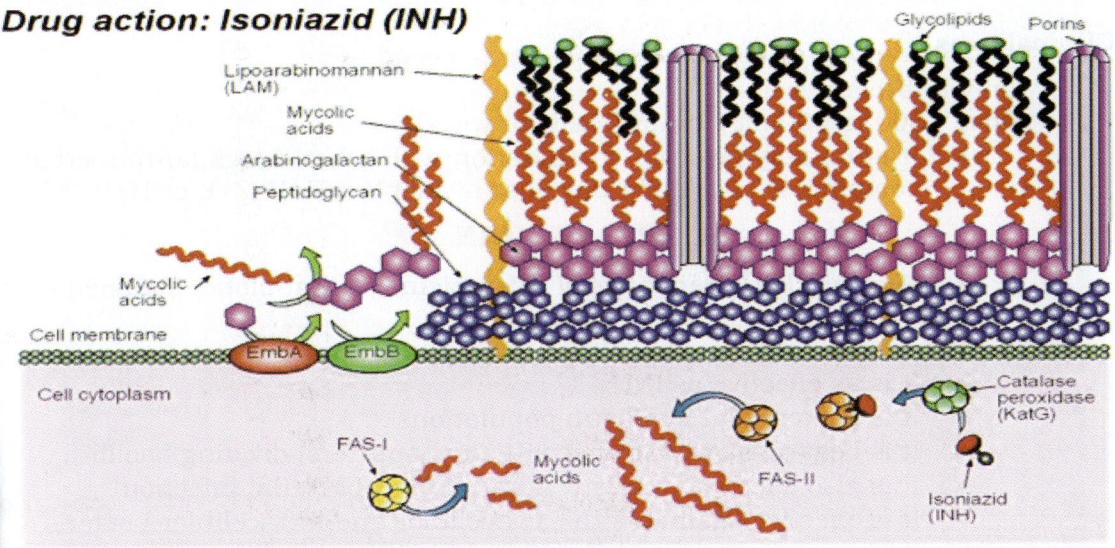

The first-line antibioic drug isoniazid (INH) interferes with cell wall biosynthesis in Mycobacterium tuberculosis. INH is a prodrug and is converted to an active form by catalase peroxidase (KatG). Activated INH inhibits the action of enoyl-acyl carrier protein reductase (InhA). InhA is an important enzyme component of the fatty acid synthetase II (FAS-II) complex. FAS-II is involved in the synthesis of long-chain mycolic acids. Mycolic acids are essential structural components of the mycobacterial cell wall and are attached to the arabinogalactan layer.

Fig.77 Mechanism of action of Isoniazid

Mechanism of action of INH: (Fig.77/78)

- The sensitive mycobacteria concenterate INH and convert it into active metabolite
- It inhibits synthesis of 'mycolic acid', the unique component of bacterial cell wall → contents leak out of bacteria → tuberculocidal action (not effective on any other bacteria, which do not have mycolic acid in the cell wall)
- Resistance develops rapidly, if used alone (always combined with other antitubercular drugs)
- It is orally active

Pharmacokinetic :

- There are two types of acetylators (fast & slow).
- But if INH is used daily, the acetylators status will not affect the metabolism of INH

Adverse effects:

- PERIPHERAL NEURITIS → due to Vit B_6 utilization for the metabolism of INH → so vit B_6 deficiency → paresthesia, numbness, mental disturbances, rarely convulsion
  (to prevent this, Vit B_6 (pyridoxine) is given 10mg/daily)

- HEPATITIS – common in old and alcoholic (reversible)
- Fever, acne, arthralgia

Clinical uses :

1. Only in tuberculosis
   Dose : 300 to 600 mg/ orally/ daily or weekly
     - It is usually given in combination with other drugs (antitubercular combipack – pack of 1 day dose available = H+R+Z+E or H+R+Z)

RIFAMPICIN

- Semisynthetic derivative of Rifampicin – B (Antibiotic) obtained from S.mediterranei

1. Antitubercular activity
   - It is as effective as INH
   - It is bactericidal in all sub populations
   - It is best on slowly or intermittently (spurters) dividing bacilli
   - It is also effective in many 'Atypical mycobacterial infection'
   - It is effective against both extracellular and intracellular bacteria
   - It has good sterilizing effect (kills persisting bacilli)
2. Antibacterial spectrum
   - Apart from M.tuberculosis, it is also effective against M.leprae
   - Staph.aureus (Methicillin Resistant Staph.aeurius)
   - N.meningitides
   - H.influenza
   - E.coli, Proteus and legionella

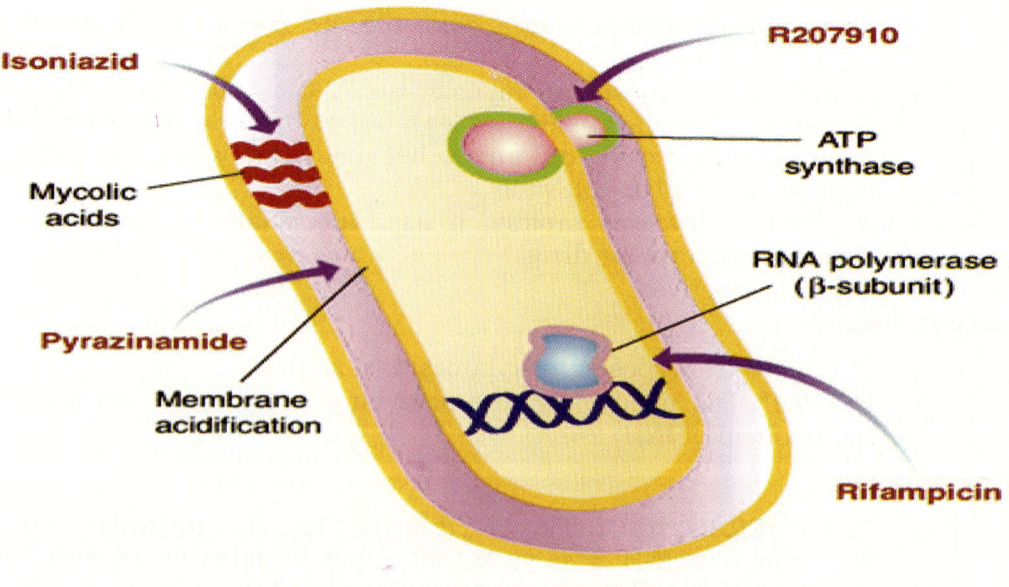

Fig.78 Sites of action of Antitubercular drugs

Mechanism of action: (Fig.78)

Rifampicin
↓
Inhibits DNA dependent RNA polymerase
↓
inhibits RNA synthesis
↓
inhibits nucleic acid synthesis
↓
tuberculocidal action

- It penetrates cavities & caseous masses and kill the organisms there

Adverse effects:

- HEPATITIS → major adverse effect on long term use
- 'Respiratory syndrome' → breathlessness
- 'Cutaneous syndrome' → flushing, pruritus, watering of eye
- 'Flu syndrome' → chill, fever, headache, bone pain
- 'Abdominal syndrome' → nausea, vomiting, abdominal cramp
- Orange red colour urine → harmless

DRUG INTERACTION:

- It is a potent 'enzyme inducer' → increases metabolism of warfarin and reduces efficacy of warfarin and increases the metabolism of oral contraceptive (failure of contraception)

Clinical uses :

1. In Tuberculosis with other antitubercular drugs
2. In Leprosy with other antileprotic drug
3. As prophylaxis of meningococcal infection
4. It is second choice drug in MRSA infection and legionella infection
5. In brucellosis with Doxycycline
   - First line therapy in Brucellosis
     Dose : 10mg/kg/daily or 600 mg/ weekly

PYRAZINAMIDE (Z)

- It is one of the first line antitubercular drugs, commonly used in TB Antitubercular activity:
- It has got only antitubercular action
- It is weak tuberculocidal drug
- It is highly lethal to intracellularly located bacilli (inside macro phages) and at sites showing inflammatory response (pH is acidic)
- It has good sterilizing capacity

- It is highly effective during first 2 months of therapy, when inflammatory changes are present
- It is effective only in acidic medium
- It is not effective against extracellular bacilli (where pH is > 7.5)

Mechanism of action: (Fig.78)

Like that of INH, it inhibits the synthesis of mycolic acid by affecting different fatty acid synthesis → tuberculocidal

- Mycobacteria develope resistance rapidly, when it is used alone
- It shows good penetration into CSF

Adverse effects:

- Hepatotoxicity (reversible) → Contraindicated in liver diseases
- Hyperuricemia → decrease Uric acid secretion → aggravate Gout
- Fever, arthralgia

Dose: 1500mg / daily

ETHAMBUTOL (E)

- It is first line drug used in Tuberculosis
  Antiturbucular activity
- The fast multiplying bacilli are more sensitive
- It is effective against many atypical mycobacteria
- It hastens the rate of sputum conversion

Mechanism of action:

- Arabinogalactan is an important component of mycolic acid
- It inhibits synthesis of Arabinogalactan → interferes with mycolic acid incorporation into mycobacterial cell wall → tuberculostatic
- Resistance develops slowly to it and also it prevents the development of resistance to other antitubercular drugs
- **It is secreted in urine and excreted as such**
- Caution in renal failure

Adverse effects:

- Patient's acceptability is good
  1. Loss of visual acuity, colour vision, field defects due to optic neuritis
- Young children (below 6 years) could not report the defects in time and then condition becomes worse in them (if the defect is found out earlier → withdrawal of drug is sufficient to reverse the defect). Hence it is contraindicated in young children.
  2. Hyperuricemia – if needed uricosuric agent is to be prescribed
     Dose: 1000mg/daily/orally

STREPTOMYCIN

- It is kept as reserve first line drug because it has to be given daily by I.M inj. (inconvenient to the patients)
- However, in MDR (Multi Drug Resistant) cases, it is given with second line drugs
- It is less effective than INH, Rifampicin
- It has got poor penetration into cells and CSF (Cerebro Spinal Fluid)
- It has got poor action in acidic medium (only effective extracellular bacilli)
- Resistance – develops rapidly, if it is given alone
- It is not commonly used due to I.M inj and toxicities

Adverse effects and Mechanism of action: (Ref: Gentamicin)
DOTS (Direct Observation Treatment Short course) according to WHO
Advantages:

1. Since it is supplied by health workers at door delivery, for free of cost, there is no question of financial implication/ omitting the tablet from taking daily (good patient's compliance)
2. Resistance will be prevented
3. Relapse – rare
4. Complete cure

CATEGORYWISE TREATMENT REGIMENS FOR TUBERCULOSIS (1997)

TB Category	Initial phase	Continuous phase	Total duration (momths)
I	2 (HRZE (S))$_3$	4 HR/4 H$_2$ R$_2$ Or 6 HE	6
II	2 (HRZE S)$_3$ + 1 (HRZE)$_3$	5 HRE or (5 H$_2$ R$_2$ E$_2$)	8 8
III	2 (HRZ)$_3$	4 Hr/4 (H$_2$ R$_2$)$_2$ 6 HE	6 8
IV (multidrug resistant cases)	For H resistance - RZE for 12 months For H+R resistance – ZE + S + Kmc+Am/Cr+ Cipro/ofl. for 12 months		

The numerical in subscript = no. of doses / week (for ex: $H_2 R_2$ means twice daily/week). If there is no subscript numeral then the drug is given daily.

The numeral in the beginning indicates no. of weeks. Example : 2 HRZE (for 2 weeks)

Doses:

INH :

- Daily dose → 300 mg
- Weekly dose → 600 mg

Rifampicin:

- 600mg/ daily
- 3 doses per week (600 mg)

Pyrazinamide:

1500 mg/ daily
- 1600 mg/ 3 doses per week

Ethambutol:

- 1000mg/ daily
- 1000 mg/ 3 doses per week

ROLE OF GLUCOCORTICOIDS:

In tuberculous meningitis, inflammation in the meninges is common. That inflammation prevents the entry of antitubercular drugs effectively into meninges. So, GC is given along with antitubercular drugs to remove inflammation, so that the antitubercular drugs effectively reach the meninges to act.

TUBERCULOSIS IN AIDS PATIENTS

- Drugs are same as in non- HIV cases, but prolonged treatment

Initial 2 $(HRZE)_3$
Continuous phase 7 $(HR)_3$ $\quad\Big|\quad \rightarrow \quad$ total of 9 months

Treatment categories and sputum examination schedule in DOTS (Direct Observation Treatment Short Course) Chemoptherapy in India

Category	Initial Phase	Continuous	Total duration (in months)
I	2 $(HREZ)_3$	4 $(HR)_3$	6 months
II	2$(HREZ\ S)_3$ 1 $(HREZ)_3$	5 $(HRE)_3$	8 months
III	2 $(HRZ)_3$	4 $(HR)_3$	6 months

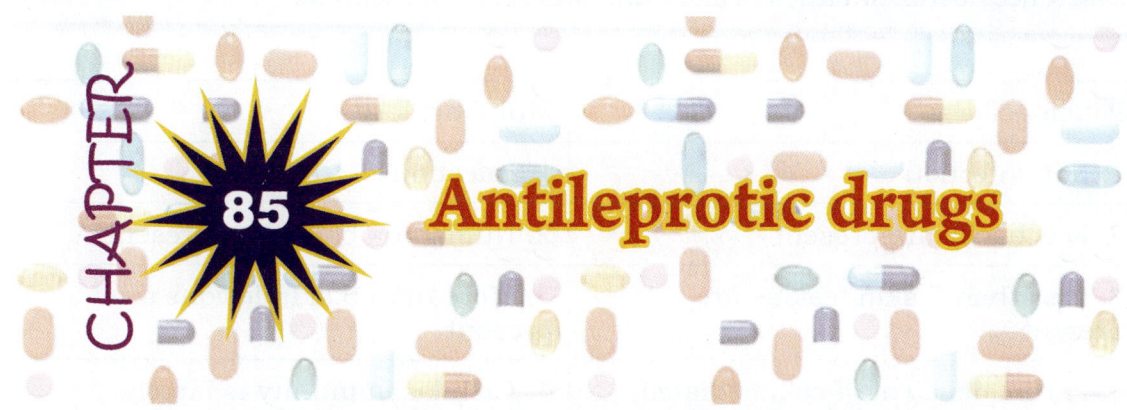

CHAPTER 85   **Antileprotic drugs**

Leprosy is a chronic granulomatous infection caused by acid-fast bacilli Mycobacterium leprae, which is related to Mycobacterium tuberculosis.

Mycobacterium leprae cannot be grown on culture media, so sensitivity testing in vitro is not possible. The M. leprae lie within the macrophages and remain dormant but alive. As long as it is in dormant stage, there will not be any clinical manifestation. Only the susceptible individuals, in whom the cell mediated immunity is deficient, suffer clinically.

Infection is spread from person to person when bacilli are shed in nasal secretion and skin lesions. It affects the peripheral nervous system, the skin and various tissues.

Types of Leprosy

1. Paucibacillary (tuberculoid leprosy) - TL
2. Multibacillary (lepromatous leprosy) – LL

ANTILEPROTIC DRUGS

  I.   Dapsone
 II.   Clofazimine
III.   Rifampicin
IV.   Other drugs
         1.   Fluoroquinolones: Ofloxacin, Pefloxacin.
         2.   Macrolide antibiotics: Clarithromycin, Azithromycin
         3.   Minocycline

Differences between Paucibacillary and Multibacillary leprosy

Paucibacillary	Multibacillary
1. Non infectious	1. Infectious
2. Few bacilli are present	2. Numerous bacilli are present
3. Less than 5 skin lesions are present	3. More than 5 skin lesions are present
4. Partial deficient of cell mediated immunity	4. Cellular immunity is largely deficient
5. Mainly nervous system is affected	5. Skin and mucous membrane are affected
6. Lepromin test is positive	6. Lepromin test is negative

DAPSONE

It is an important antileprotic drug.

Mechanism of action :-

PABA (Para Amino Benzoic Acid) is taken up by the bacteria with the help of folate synthetase. PABA is converted into folic acid and then into tetra hydro folic acid (which is essential for the synthesis of DNA and Protein). The bacteria will multiply.

Dapsone structurally resembles PABA. It competes with that and is taken up by the bacteria instead of PABA and converted into non functional metabolite. The DNA and protein synthesis and multiplication of bacteria are inhibited. It is a bacteriostatic.

Clinical use : In leprosy of all types

Adverse effects :

- methaemoglobinemia is common in person with deficiency of G6PDH (Glucose 6 – Phosphate Dehydrogenase) enzyme. Dapsone should be avoided if Hb is less than 7 g%.
- loss of appetite, nausea, pruritus, drug fever etc.,

Dose :

For multibacillary

- Dapsone 100 mg/daily + clofazimine 50 mg/daily for one month followed by 300 mg/once a month for 24 months+ Rifampicin 600 mg/once a month for 24 months

For Paucibacillary

- Dapsone 100 mg/daily + Rifampicin 600 mg once a month for 6 months

Lepra reaction: After drug treatment
- It occurs in LL type (Type II), if the bacterial load is high
- There is Jarish Herxheimer type of reaction → due to release of antigen from killed bacilli → 'sulfone syndrome' → fever, malaise, lymph node enlargement, jaundice, anaemia, existing lesions enlarge, swollen, painful, several new lesions may appear
- It may be mild, moderate or severe (Erythema nodosum leprosum (Type II)

Treatment:
- Temporary discontinuation of Dapsone → Reversal reaction in TT is seen. It is a Delayed type of hypersensitivity reation to M.leprae
- Clofazimine 200mg/daily (anti-inflammatory & antileprotic action)
- Other drugs used → Analgesic, antipyretic, antibiotic, chloroquine, thalidomide, GC (Glucocorticoid) are used "in severe cases".

RIFAMPICIN

- Antitubercular as well as anti-leprotic drug
- It renders rapidly the leprosy patients to become non contagious
- Upto 99.9% of M.leprae are killed in 3 to 7 days

Mechanism of action: Ref: Antitubercular drugs

USES:

(ref: Antitubercular drugs)
1. In Leprosy
2. In Tuberculosis
3. In other bacterial infection

Adverse effects: not much, since it is given once a month. However it is to be avoided in Liver damage

CLOFAZIMINE

- Antileprotic and anti-inflammatory

Mechanism of action:

- It is bacteriostatic
- It accumulates within phagocytes
- It combines with DNA of M.leprae →↓(inhibits) RNA formation, which is necessary for protein synthesis or DNA duplication, which is necessary for bacterial duplication
- It interferes with template function of DNA

Clinical uses :

- In leprosy (Dapsone +Clofazimine) → prevent emergence of resistance
  Dose: Multibacillary → 300mg/once a month + 50mg/daily for 24 months
- In lepra reaction → both anti-inflammatory and anti-leprotic actions are useful

Adverse effects:

- Reddish-black discolouration of skin
- Conjunctival pigmentation → cosmetic problem
- Dryness of skin (Atropine to be avoided), itching
- Gastroenteritis → loose stool, abdominal pain, anorexia and weight loss

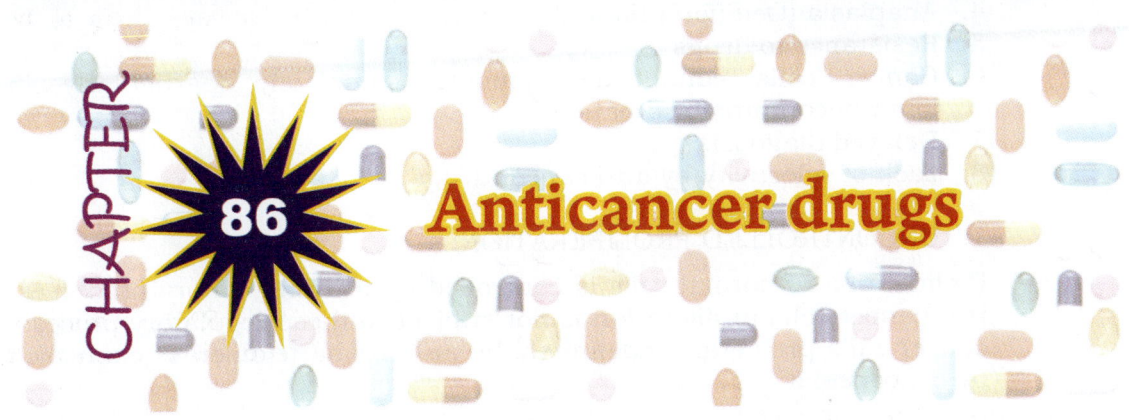

CHAPTER 86 — **Anticancer drugs**

Anticancer drugs either kill cancer cells or modify the growth.

"Cancer" can be defined very broadly as a disease in which there is uncontrollable multiplication and spread (within the body) of abnormal forms of the body's own cells.

Causes of Cancer:

- Virus such as – HPV (Human papilloma virus), Epstein-Barr virus (EBV)
- Environmental and occupational hazards such as exposure to chemical carcinogens like tobacco, alcohol, azodyes, asbestos, benzene etc.
- Genetic factor such as damaged $Cp5_3$ gene which converts pro oncogen to oncogen

Main approaches (Goal of Treatment)

1. Surgery
2. Radiotherapy
3. Immunotherapy
4. Chemotherapy (10-15%)

$\rightarrow$ 50% cure can be achieved

- role of each depends on the type of tumour and the stages of development
- anticancer drugs are used with surgery, radiotherapy and immunotherapy
- anticancer drugs are used either to cure or prolong remission/palliation (alleviation of symptoms) and used as adjuvant chemotherapy after surgery or radiotherapy.

I. Some basic informations about cancer cells and the difficulties in treating cancer by drugs:
   1. Uncontrolled proliferation
   2. Invasiveness
   3. Capacity to metastasize

4. Anaplasia (Dedifferentiation)
5. Resistance to drugs
6. Cancer cells cannot be removed completely (particularly in immunocompromised patients)
7. Delayed diagnosis
8. Lack of selectivity by anti cancer drugs

1. UNCONTROLLED PROLIFERATION:

Proliferation of normal cells is controlled by body regulatory processes. But cancer cells proliferation is not subject to these regulatory process, cancer calls proliferate indefinitely by an enzyme telomerase expressed by cancer cells.

Example : liver cells grow even after removal of 2/3rd of cancer cells

2. INVASIVENESS:

- Normal cells → no invading capacity → but cancer cells → invade neighbour tissues. Cancer of mucous memberane of rectum invades the neighbour rectal tissues

- 3. Capacity to Metastasize (secondary tumour). The tumour cells are released from the primary tumour → through blood vessels, lymphatic system →reach different sites → various tissues are affected → it is advanced stage of cancer → bad sign

- 4. Anaplasia : Cancer cells grow remorselessly but do not differentiate properly. Example : cancer cells in pancreas → do not behave as normal/pancreatic cells.

- 5. Another problem in treating cancer is , the cancer cells cannot be removed completely by body defence mechanism Example : In case of bacterial infection (even 90% killed → remaining 10% is removed by body defence mechanism. But in case of cancer, even 0.09% cancer cell is left out → multiply fast)

- 6. Resistance – Cancer cells are subjected to develop resistance for the available anticancer drugs, if used alone (like tuberculosis, H.pylori, HIV infection), so combination of drugs is given.

- 7. Delayed diagnosis may be due to unawareness.

- 8. Lack of selectivity by anticancer drugs. Anticancers drugs also inhibit the normally fast growing cells in the body (inhibit BM, inhibit GIT, inhibit Gonads, inhibit hair follicles)

Types of cancer

Tumour can be benign or malignant. Benign tumours are resembling normal cells, slow growing and harmless.

Cancer or malignant neoplasm or malignant tumour follow the characteristic of cancer cells and they are harmfull.

Benign tumours usually end with 'oma'. For example : Fibroma (fibrous tissues) Adenoma (glandular epithelium) Melanoma (pigment cells), Papilloma (surface epithelium).

- Malignant cancers are either solid tumour or haematology-cal malignancies. Solid tumours of epithelial tissues (oral cancer, head and neck, lung, breast, prostate, colon etc.,)
- Sarcoma (bone), myeloma, tumour of haemopoietic tissues.
- Haematological malignancies include the following:
- Lymphoma i.e., tumours of lymphatic system include hodgkin's lymphoma (B-cells) and non-hodgkin's lymphoma (extra nodal – blood vessel, bone marrow etc.,
- T-cell lymphoma
- Leukaemia (it is a type of blood cancer due to abnormal proliferation of leukocytes.)
- Acute leukaemia – bleeding is common due to over production of immature cells which consequently prevent the normal production of RBC and platelets.

Classification of Anticancer drug

Drugs acting directly on cell cycle (cytotoxic)
1. Alkylating agents
   i. Cyclophosphamide
   ii. Mechlorethamine (MOPP regimen in Hodgkin's disease)
      a) Mechlorethamine
      b) Oncovin (vincristine)
      c) Procarbazine
      d) Prednisolone
   iii. Busulphan
2. Antimetabolites
   i. Folic acid antagonist → Methotrexate
   ii. Purine antagonist → Azathioprine, 6- mercapto purine 6MP)
   iii. Pyrimidine antagonists → 5 Fluoro Uracil (5FU)
3. Vinca alkaloids
   i. Vincristine
   ii. Vinblastine
4. Antibiotic
   i. Actinomycin – D
   ii. Bleomycin
   iii. Doxorubicin
5. Enzyme → L – Asparaginase
6. Monoclonal antibodies – Rituximab, Alemtuzumab
7. Interferons
8. Ribavarin
9. Others → Cisplatin, Paclitaxel, Etoposide
10. Drugs altering hormonal "status" Hormones and antogonists

- GC, Androgens, Estrogen, antioestrogens (Tamoxifen), 5α – reductase Inhibitor (Finasteride) alter living mucosal epithelium

Common toxicities of cytotoxic (Anticancer) drugs (except L-Asparaginase)

- Anticancer drugs kill rapidly multiplying cancer cells as well as rapidly multiplying normal cells (BM, GI mucosa, hair cells, gonads, etc)
1. Depress Bone marrow → aplastic anaemia, agranulocytosis, leukopenia ↓ inhibits body defence mechanism → spread of infection, thrombocytopenia (bleeding) are the most serious adverse effects (to prevent this toxicity → inject platelets, colony stimulating factor)
2. Inhibit Lymphocyte function → suppression of cell mediated as well as humoral mediated immunity → susceptibility to all INFECTIONS (fungal, viral infections) → delayed wound healing
3. Inhibit G.I.mucosa → stomatitis, diarrhoea, haemorrhage, nausea, vomiting (anticancer drugs release 5HT in the GIT → stimulate $5HT_3$ receptor in vagal afferent → and also stimulate CTZ → nausea and vomiting. To control vomiting, a $5HT_3$ antagonist, ondansetron (highly specific antiemetic) is to be given.
4. Skin → Alopecia (very common)
5. They ↓ inhibit Gonads → impotence (male), inhibit ovulation which will lead to amenorrhoea and sterility (female)
6. Hyperuricemia → due to massive destruction of cells → ↑ (increased) purine metabolism → increased production of uric acid → hyperuricemia → aggravate gout
   Allopurinol is a Xanthine oxidase inhibitor decreases the formation of uric acid.
7. Teratogenicity leads to abortion, death of foetus. They are avoided in pregnancy.

Other methods of toxicity amelioration:

1. Toxicity blocking drug → to improve therapeutic index → 'Folinic acid' is given as rescue. The normal cells are rescued more than cancer cells, when Folic acid antogonists are given.
2. Drugs are given in pulses with 2-3 weeks intervals so that the normal cells to recover more quickly than cancer cells
3. Combination of drugs are used to overcome the emergence of resistance by cancer cells and also for synergistic action and less toxic effect

MOPP regimen → Methotrexate/ Mechlorethamine + Oncovin (Vincristine) + Purinethol +Prednisolone VAMP (in Hodgkin's carcinoma) – Vincristine + Amethopterine (Methotrexate) +6 MP + Prednisolone → in acute Leukaemia.

CISPLATIN

It is an anticancer drug.

Mechanism of action: It inhibits ↓DNA synthesis of cancer cells and inhibits the multiplication of cancer cells.

Clinical uses :

1. In solid tumours (Testicular, ovariam, lung, prostate, head and neck cancer)

Adverse effects:

Ref : General Toxicity.

MONOCLONAL ANTIBODIES

Mechanism of action : They bind more cancer cells and inhibit VEGF (Vascular Endothelial Growth Factor) and EGF (Epidermal Growth Factor)

- They are useful in various types of cancer

L – ASPARANGINASE

- It is an enzyme from E.Coli
- It is an anticancer drug
- It differs from other anticancer drugs in Mechanism of action, toxicity and USES

Mechanism of action: Some tumour cells depend on L-asparagine for their multiplication (Lymphoblastic leukaemias, reticulum cell carcinoma)

- **L**-asparaginase → converts L-asparagine to L-asparate → non availability of L- asparagine to malignant cells (Lymphoblastic leukaemia cell) → ↓ (inhibits) multiplication of those malignant cells → other cells are not affected.

Clinical use : In Lymphoblastic leukaemias

Adverse effects: No general toxicity. Only nausea, fever, allergic reactions

ANTIMETABOLITES

- These are the drugs, which resemble structurally the metabolites (purine, pyrimidine, Folic acid), which are necessary for the synthesis of DNA and multiplication of cells.
- When these drugs are administered compete with metabolites and forms useless (non-functional) metabolites and inhibit the synthesis of DNA, in turn inhibit the multiplication of cells (particularly fast

multiplying cells like cancer cells and some other fast multiplying cells.)

- These drugs disrupt the metabolism of cancer cells (more) and normal human cells (less) and harm to host cells to some extent

They are

(1) Folic acid antagonist: Methotrexate

(2) Purine antagonist: 6 MP (Mercaptopurine, Azathioprine)

(3) Pyrimidine antagonist: Cytarabine, 5 FU (Fluora uracil)

Purine antagonist – 6MP, Azathioprine

Mechanism of action :

6 MP (structurally resembles purine metabolite)
↓
Inhibits Conversion of Iodine Monophosphate to Adenonine, guanine
↓
Useless (non functional) metabolites are formed
↓
inhibits Purine synthesis
↓
inhibits DNA and protein synthesis of cancer cells
↓
inhibits Proliferating cancer cells

Clinical Uses: In many malignancies :

1. As anticancer agent → childhood leukaemia, choriocarcinoma & others
2. As immunosuppressant: Azathioprine inhibits B and T-Lymphocytes and useful in autoimmune diseases (myasthenia gravis, rheumatoid arthritis, psoriasis, haemolytic anaemia) and to prevent graft rejection in organ transplantation.

Adverse effects: General toxicity of anticancer drugs (BM depression, GIT toxicity (nausea, vomiting, ulcerative mucositis, alopecia, nephrotoxicity)

FOLIC ACID ANTAGONIST – Methotrexate

- It is one of the most important anticancer drugs
- It is one of the drugs in drug combination regimen used in cancer

Mechanism of action:

Methotrexate structurally resembles Folic acid. Methotrexate → incorporated into metabolites instead of FA → useless metabolite (not useful in DNA synthesis) is formed → no DNA synthesis → inhibits DNA synthesis of cancer cells → inhibits multiplication of cancer cells → inhibits only proliferating cancer cells and B / T-lymphocytes.

Mechanism of action

Methotrexate (resembles FA)
↓ Inhibits DHFA reductase
Blocking the conversion of DHFA to THFA,
which is essential component for DNA synthesis in cancer cells
↓
produces useless (non-functional metabolites)
↓
Inhibits DNA and RNA synthesis
↓
Inhibits Protein synthesis
↓
Inhibits Proliferating cancer cells, B and T-lymphocytes

Clinical uses AS ANTICANCER :

1. In various types of tumour → in choriocarcinoma, acute leukaemia in children, breast, head, neck, cervical, lung carcinomas.
2. As immunosuppressants :
   i)   Useful in autoimmune diseases (myasthenia gravis, rheumatoid, arthritis, psoriasis, haemolytic anaemia)
   ii) To prevent graft rejection in transplantation

Dose : Methotrexate : 2.5-5 mg/daily/oral;

In cancer – 250/1000 mg/IV

Adverse effects: **(refer Gen. toxicity)** and folic acid deficiency (Folinic acid is to be given after FA antagonist treatment, so as to allow normal cells to regain faster than the cancer cells as rescue.)

5FLUORO URACIL (5FU) – PYRIMIDINE ANTAGONIST

Mechanism of action

5FU (resembles natural metabolite Pyrimidine)
↓
5 Fluoro 2 deoxy uridine monophosphate
↓
Inhibits Thymidylate synthetase
↓
Blocks conversion of deoxy uridylic acid to deoxy thymidylic acid
↓
Useless (non-functional) metabolite is formed
↓
Failure of synthesis of Pyrimidine
↓
Inhibits DNA synthesis and inhibits protein synthesis in cancer cells
↓
Inhibits Proliferation of cancer cells

Clinical uses : As anticancer : Carcinoma of lung, breast, ovary, cervix, prostate, head and neck, GIT adenocarcinoma.

Adverse effects: Similar to methotrexate

ALKYLATING AGENTS

Example: - Cyclophosphamide   (Nitrogen mustards)

     - Mechlorethamine

They are anticancer drugs

Mechanism of action: Cytotoxic and radiomimetic

- They act on dividing as well as resting cancer cells
- They transfer 'alkyl group' – hence 'alkylating agent'

Alkylating Agents
↓
Form highly reactive quarternary ammonium derivative
↓
ethylene iminium cation
↓

$$-N- \text{ (reactive group)}$$

↓
transfer alkyl group
↓
alkylate groupings like aminoacid sulphhydryl into cancer cells
↓
amino acids are unavailable for normal metabolic reaction
↓
Inhibits DNA synthesis
↓
Inhibits Multiplication of cancer cells, B and T-lymphocytes

Clinical uses :

1. In various malignancies Hodgkin's lymphoma, actue leukaemia, cancer of lung, prostate, ovary and breast
2. Cyclophosphamide → also used as immune suppressant
   i. In autoimmune diseases (myasthenia gravis, rheumatoid arthritis, psoriasis, haemolytic anaemia)
   ii. To prevent graft rejection in transplantation

Dose : Cyclophosphamide : 2-3 mg/kg/oral

In cancer : 10-15 mg/IV infusion.

Adverse effects: (ref: general toxicity)
Cyclophosphamids should be given along with mesna. Cyclophosphamide is conveted into toxic metabolite, acrolein, which causes cystitis and haemorrhage from urinary bladder. Mesna binds with acrolein, gets excreted and prevents those adverse effects of Cyclophosphamide.

PROCARBAZINE

- In MOPP regimen, it is one of the components
- Effective anticancer drug

Mechanism of action : Depolymerizes DNA and causes chromosomal damage. It inhibits DNA and protein synthesis of cancer cells.

Clinical Uses:

- In Hodgkin's diseases
- In non Hodgkin's lymphoma
- In Carcinoma of lung

Adverse effects:

- All common toxicity of anti cancer drugs and disulfiram like reaction
- Alcohol is to be avoided

HORMONES AND ANTAGONISTS

1. Glucocorticoids is used in acute childhood Leukaemia and in Lymphomas as MOPP regimen
2. Estrogen is used in prostate carcinoma
3. Antiestrogen, tamoxifen are used in breast cancer
4. Anti androgen, flutamide is used in Prostate carcinoma
5. Finasteride is used in Prostate carcinoma (refer finasteride)
6. Androgen is used in endometrial carcinoma
7. progestin is used in endometrial carcinoma
8. GnRH analogue is used in carcinoma of breast/ prostate

   They do not produce adverse effects of anticancer drugs on BM, GI mucosa, gonads, skin, etc.,

RADIOACTIVE ISOTOPES ^{131}I

They emit β rays, which destroy cancer cells of thyroid and is useful in thyroid carcinoma.

- radiophosphorous ^{32}p is used in polycythemia vera
- radio gold ^{98}Au is used in malignant pleural and peritoneal effusion

VINCA ALKALOIDS

- These are mitotic inhibitors
- They bind to microtubular protein, tubulin
- They cause disruption of mitotic spindle
- They interfere with cytoskeletal function
- The chromosomes fail to move apart during mitosis → metaphase arrest occurs

Clinical Use:

In Hodgkin's disease, childhood acute Leukaemia, Wilm's tumour, Ewing's sarcoma, lymphosarcoma etc.,

Adverse effects: common toxicity of anticancer drugs.

ANTICANCER ANTIBIOTICS

Rubidomycin, Doxorubicin, Bleomycin, Mitomycin source: All antibiotics are derived from species Streptomyces

Mechanism of action: All produce same mechanism

They inhibit DNA dependent RNA synthesis → inhibit protein synthesis → inhibit proliferation of cancer cells.

Clinical Uses: In combination with other drugs → useful in acute lymphatic leukaemia, acute myeloblastic leukaemia, epidermo carcinoma of skin, oral cavity and genito urinary tract, Hodgkin's lymphoma etc.,

Adverse effects: as in common toxicity

Bleeding due to suppression of clotting factors, toxic hepatitis.

SECTION

XII

MISCELLANEOUS

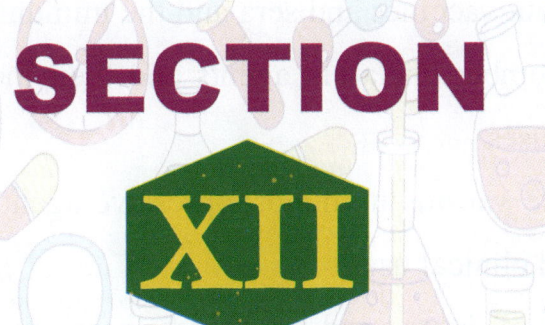

MISCELLANEOUS

Learning objectives

- To know about vaccines and sera and the immunization schedule
- Able to remember chelating agents and their mechanisms of action and clinical uses
- To enumerate various immunosuppressive agents, their mechanisms of action and clinical uses
- To be aware of drugs used in scabies, psoriasis, acne vulgaris, skin and mucous membrane disorders
- To be aware of drugs used in geriatrics, paediatrics
- To know about chronopharmacology, and their clinical significance
- Able to remember the basic principles of drug interactions and their clinical significance.
- To know about pharmacovigilance and its importance.

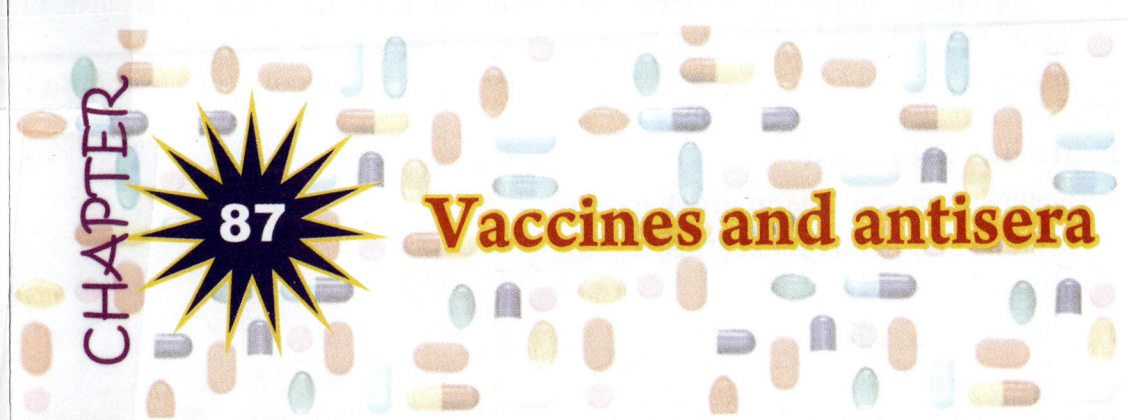

CHAPTER 87

Vaccines and antisera

VACCINES AND ANTISERA:

Vaccines and Antisera are biological products which enhance the immunological defence of the body against foreign bodies (mainly against the microorganisms and toxins)

Vaccines provide two types of immunity

Active immunity: Here the vaccines act as antigens, which induce production of specific antibodies by recipient himself. Act as prophylactic only

Passive immunity : (Immunoglobulin and Antisera). Already prepared antibodies are given to the recipient (the antibodies are produced by another person or animal who have been actively immunized). The antisera and immunoglobulin are also curative

The method of administration of vaccines/sera is called immunization/vaccination

Active immunization is more efficacious and long acting than the passive immunisation

Active immunity is slow acting (1-7 days), but passive immunity gives immediate protection

Hence, the vaccines are mainly used for prophylactic purpose. The antisera is mainly for the treatment as well as prophylactic for short period

The active immunity is very difficult in debilitated patients or immuno-compromised individuals, who may not be able to generate an adequate antibody response and require passive protection

Vaccines are of 3 types

1   Inactivated vaccines consist of microorganisms killed by heat or by chemicals

2   Live attenuated vaccines contain live bacteria or viruses which have been rendered avirulant. The live microorganisms, however grow and multiply, which are sufficient to cause disease in AIDS, immunocompromised, leukemia, GC therapy etc., So, the live vaccines are contraindicated in them.

3   Toxoids: modified bacterial exotoxin, so that the toxicity is lost but antigenicity is retained

Immunization   schedule   will   be   discussed   in   detail   in   Community Medicine/Paediatrics

Bacterial vaccines:

1 Bacillus Calmette Guerin (BCG) for TB

2 Typhoid and Paratyphoid (TAB)

3   Cholera

4   Whooping cough

5   Meningococcal

6   Haemophilus influenza type 'b'

Viral vaccines:

1   Poliomyelitis

2   Rabies

3   Influenza

4   Hepatitis-A

5   Hepatitis-B

6   Mumps (live attenuated)

7   Measles ("   )

8   Varicella ("   )

Toxoids:Tetanus +Diphtheria

Triple antigens (DPT) MMR-Measles, Mumps, Rubella

Actions of vaccines :

The antibodies developed in response to live vaccines inactivate the bacteria/virus when they subsequently enter the body.

Toxoids: The antibodies produced by toxoids neutralize the elaborated exotoxin.

Viral vaccines generally afford more prolonged protection than bacterial vaccines.

ANTISERA and Immunoglobulins (Igs)

Antisera: The sera containing antibodies obtained from an animal (horse) immunized either by injection of antigen or by infection with microorganisms containing antigens.

Anaphylactic shock can be produced by antisera (Adrenaline 1:1000) should be kept ready.

Immunoglobulins (IGs) are human gammaglobulins which carry antibodies,

- They are more efficacious than antisera.
- Hypersensitivity reactions are rare.

Antisera	Immunoglobulins
1) Antitetanus serum (ATS)	1) Tetanus immunoglobulin
2) Antirabies serum (ARS)	2) Rabies immunoglobulin
3) Antisnake venum (ASV) serum	3) Normal human gammaglobulin
4) Antidiphtheria serum (ADS)	4) Anti-D immunoglobulin

1) For Tetanus
   i) Tetanus immunoglobulin – is used as prophylactic in high risk patients and also as therapeutic
   ii) Antitetanic serum (ATS) – is inferior to tetanus immunoglobulin and used only if Tetanus immunoglobulin is not available.
2) For Rabies
   i) Antirabies serum is used in individuals after suspected exposure. It is injected subcutaneously around the bite.
   ii) Rabies immunoglobulin is injected subcutaneously around the wound for immediate protection, since Antirabies serum will produce active immunity only after 1-2 weeks.
3) For Snake bite:
   i) Antisnake venum (ASV) serum contains antibodies to the venoms of cobra, krait and Russel viper, which 1 ml neutralizes, 0.6 mg of standard cobra venum, 0.6 mg of standard Russel viper's venom, 0.45 mg of standard krait venum.
4) Anti-D-immunoglobulin (Anti Rh – Gammaglobulin) to prevent Haemolytic Disease of new born (HDN):

Rh – system of blood is named because it was found in Rheusus monkey. The person's RBC, which carries Rh(O) antigen, is called as Rh+, and lack of that is called as Rh-. Rh+ is very common. But Rh- blood is very rare. Normally plasma does not have anti Rh-antibodies. But if a Rh- person receives Rh+ blood, then the body starts to make anti-Rh+ antibodies which will be circulating in the blood. For the first time, infusion of Rh+ blood into Rh- patient, there will not be any reaction. But the Rh- patients receive Rh+ blood for the second time, then there will be incompatibility with anti Rh+ antibodies and haemolysis may occur.

In Pregnancy : Such type of above incompatibility may occur in pregnancy and cause haemolysis in foetus, called as Haernolytic Disease of the New born (HDN). Normally there is no direct contact between foetal and maternal blood during pregnancy. Suppose maternal blood is Rh- and foetal blood is Rh+, there is a possibility of small amount of foetal blood (Rh+) may leak and mix with maternal blood, during pregnancy / abortion. The mother will start making anti Rh+ antibodies. The new born baby would not be affected for the first time. But in subsequent pregnancy the mother's anti Rh+ antibodies can cross placenta and enter into foetal circulation. If the foetus is Rh-, then there will not be any problem, since there is no incompatibility. But if the foetus is Rh+, then there will be incompatibility with anti Rh+ antibodies and haemolysis may occur in the foetus, which is called as Haemolytic Disease of New born (HDN).

HDN can be prevented by giving Rh- mother an injection of an anti-Rh-gammaglobulin (Rho(D) immunoglobulin) soon after delivery or abortion. These antibodies will bind to foetal Rh- antigen and neutralized it. The mother's own immune system is spared from generating antibodies against these Rh+ antigens. The foetus of next pregnancy is also protected and is not at risk because the mother has no memory B-cell. The usual dose is Rho(D) immunoglobulin 2 ml (300 mg) / IM.

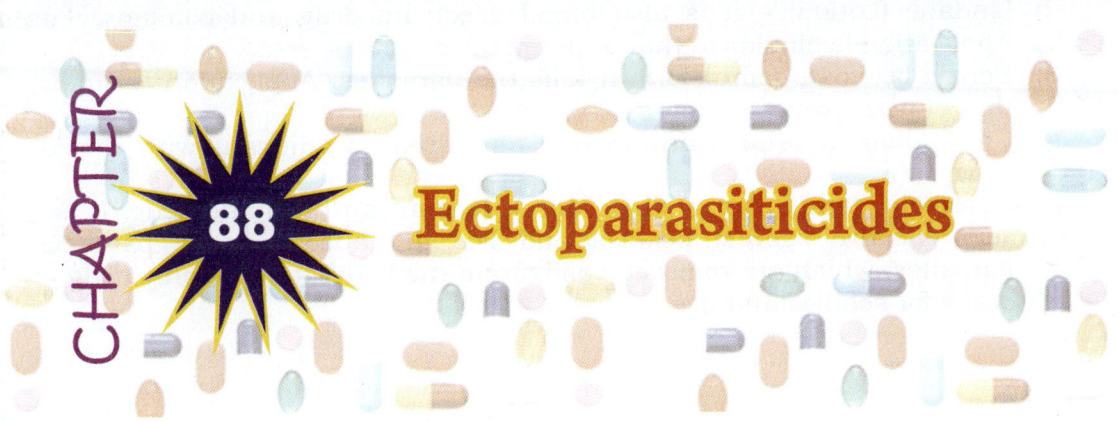

CHAPTER

88

Ectoparasiticides

Scabies and Lice are ectoparasites that live on body.

These are drugs used to kill parasites that live on body call as Ectoparasiticides.

(i)   Scabies – Sarcoptes scabies (itch mite)
(ii)   Lice - Pediculus sp (wingless insect)

The drugs used in scabies and lice are same.

They infect human skin and hair.

Scabies : It is highly contagious caused by the anthropod 'Sarcoptes scabei' (itch mite). The mites burrow through epidermis and lay eggs, which cause itch by forming papules. There may be secondary infection by bacteria, which requires antibiotic therapy. The finger web is the first site to be affected and spread other parts of the boy (forearm, neck, genital and lower legs). The other family members are also treated simultaneously. The clothes used by the patients are kept separately and washed thoroughly in hot water.

Pediculosis : The lice thrive on head. They cause itching. Very common in women. They suck blood and transmit typhus and relapsing fever which is very rare.

DRUGS USED in Scabies and lice:

1   Permethrin (cream, lotion)

2   Lindane (lotion)

3   Benzyl benzoate (oily liquid)

4   Ivermectin (Oral)

1) Permethrin: It is commonly used. It is Broad spectrum scabicide and pediculoside. It kills the parasites by causing neurological paralysis of parasites, which are then removed easily from the body after washing. It is available as cream 10% to be applied all over the body except eye (since it causes irritation) after a scrub bath and then washed after 24 hrs. If it is not cured after single application, repeated after 1-2 weeks.

2) Lindane (Lotion) – it is also broad spectrum drug and commonly used. Application is similar to that of permethrin.

3) Benzyl benzoate (emulsion). It kills the parasites. Application is similar to that of permethrin.

4) Crotamiton: It is also antipruritic and used as adjuvant with the above drugs.

5) Ivermectin (oral – 8 mg/single dose). It is an anthelmintic drug. It is also very effective against scabies and lice. It causes spastic paralysis of parasites, which are removed easily from the body. It is the only drug given orally for scabies and lice.

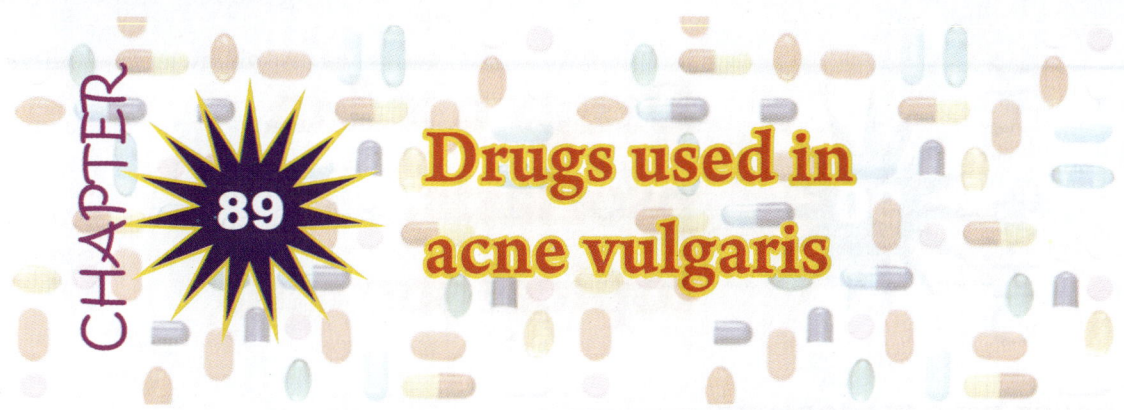

CHAPTER 89

Drugs used in acne vulgaris

Acne vulgaris is a skin infection caused by the organism, 'Propionibacterium acne'.
It is common in adult boys and girls.
There is excess production of Androgen
↓
stimulates sebaceous follicles of face
↓
produce excess sebum
↓
get colonized by bacteria and yeast
↓
during colonization
↓

bacterial lipase produce fatty acids
↓
irritate follicular duct
↓
retention of secretion
Hyperkeratosis
↓
comedones(pimples) are formed
↓
rupture into dermis
↓
inflammation and pustulation.

DRUGS:

I Benzoyl peroxide (gel, cream) It is one of the most effective and widely used drug.

Mechanism of action

- It combines with water and liberate nascent oxygen, which kills P. acne, the itch mite and lice.
- It has got additional comedolytic and keratolytic properties.
- It reduces the production of irritant fatty acids in the sebum.

2 Retinoic acid (Tretinoin): potent comedolytic and highly efficacious in acne. Promote lysis of keratinocytes. Prevent formation of comedone. No antibacterial activity

3 Azelaic acid: It is a natural product from Pityrosporum ovale. Used in acne. Many anaerobes, especially P. acnes present in acne is inhibited.

4 Systemic therapy: Antibiotic –(i) Doxycycline (oral) – prevent colonization of bacteria and hence inhibit the formation of sebum. (ii) Isotretinoin (Oral)- reduces production of sebum. Contraindicated in pregnancy

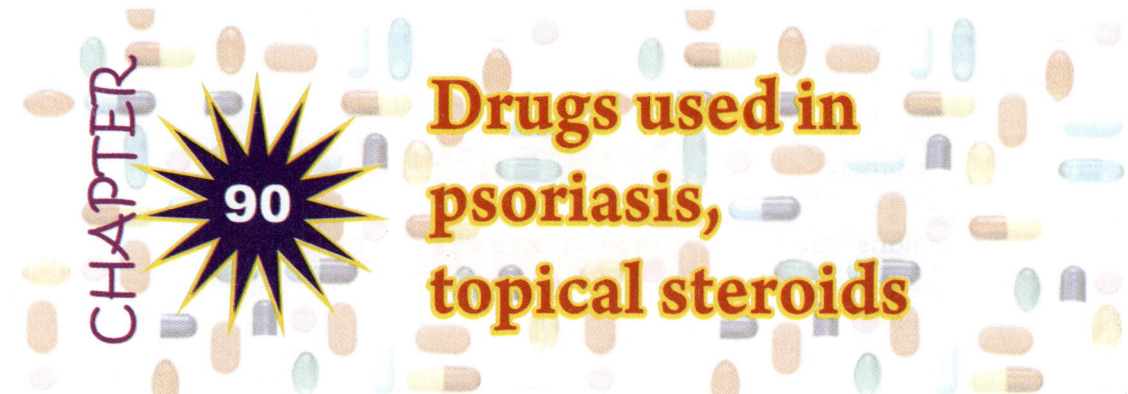

CHAPTER 90

Drugs used in psoriasis, topical steroids

DRUGS USED IN PSORIASIS

Psoriasis is due to an immunological disorder manifested as localized or wide spread erythematous scaling, lesions or plaques

There is excessive epidermal proliferation with dermal inflammation

1   Immunosuppressive agents: METHOTREXATE, GLUCOCORTICOIDS

Mechanism of action : Antiinflammatory and antiproliferative, hence useful in psoriasis.

2   Calcipotriol (ointment): inhibits the proliferation of epidermal cells

3   Phototherapy: PUVA-(Psoralen-Ultra Violet-A): binds with affected cells → inhibits DNA synthesis and proliferation of epithelial cells

4   Coal tar and Acetracin (Mechanism of action of Coal tar) : It is phototoxic like PUVA. It inhibits DNA synthesis and proliferation of epidermal cells. It is combined with GCs in severe cases for its anti inflammatory action. Mechanism of action of Acetracin : It binds with retinoic acid receptors in epidermal cells and inhibiting the proliferation and maturation of epidermal cells.

TOPICAL STEROIDS (GLUCOCORTICOIDS)

They are used for their anti-inflammatory, Immunosuppressive, antiproliferative and antiallergic actions

Useful in various dermatological disorders

DRUGS:

I.   Potent:

   1. Betamethasone benzoate

   2. Clobetasol propionate

   3. Dexamethasone sod.sulphate

   4. Fludrocortisone

   5. Triamcinolone acetonide

II. Moderate and mild potent:

    1. Hydrocortisone acetate

Guidelines for the use of steroids

1. Absorption from skin in infants and children is greater. So, milder agents are to be used.

2. For acute lesions- moderately potent drugs are to be used

3. They are used along with proper antimicrobial drugs in impetigo, secondary infected dermatoses

Clinical uses :

Respond well in

1. Atopic eczema, varicose eczema

2. Allergic contact dermatitis

3. Lichen simplex

4. Psoriasis of face

5. Uses on eye – Topical – in keratitis, iritis, iridocyclitis, allergic conjunctivitis etc.

Respond poorly (Strong /potent steroids are needed) in

1. Cystic acne

2. Alopecia areata

3. Nail disorders

4. Psoriasis of palm, sole, elbow and knee

Adverse effects: thinning of epidermis, striae, easy bruising, delay in wound healing, fungal and bacterial infection

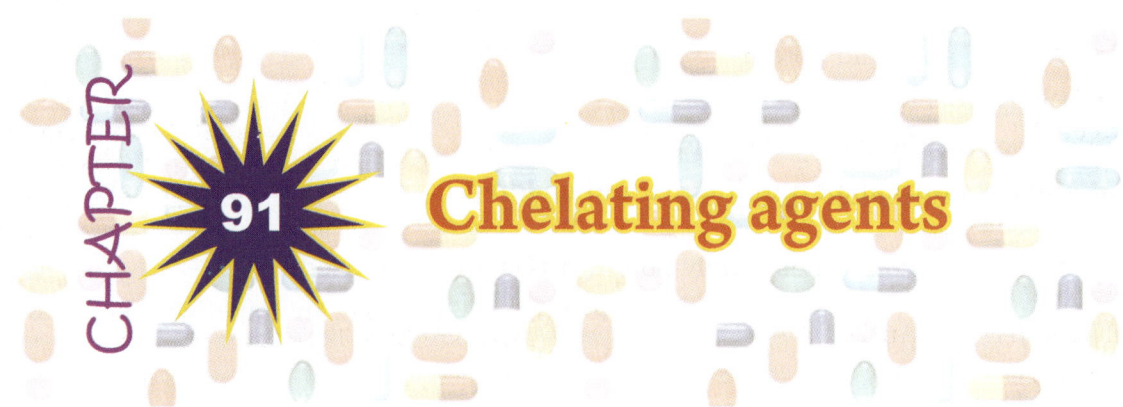

Chelating agents are used in heavy metal poisonings

Heavy metals are Arsenic, Copper, Lead, Mercury, Iron etc

Heavy metal poisoning: Heavy metals have electro positive charge combine SH-groups (Electro negative charge) of vital enzymes and inactivate them and hence the various toxic symptoms

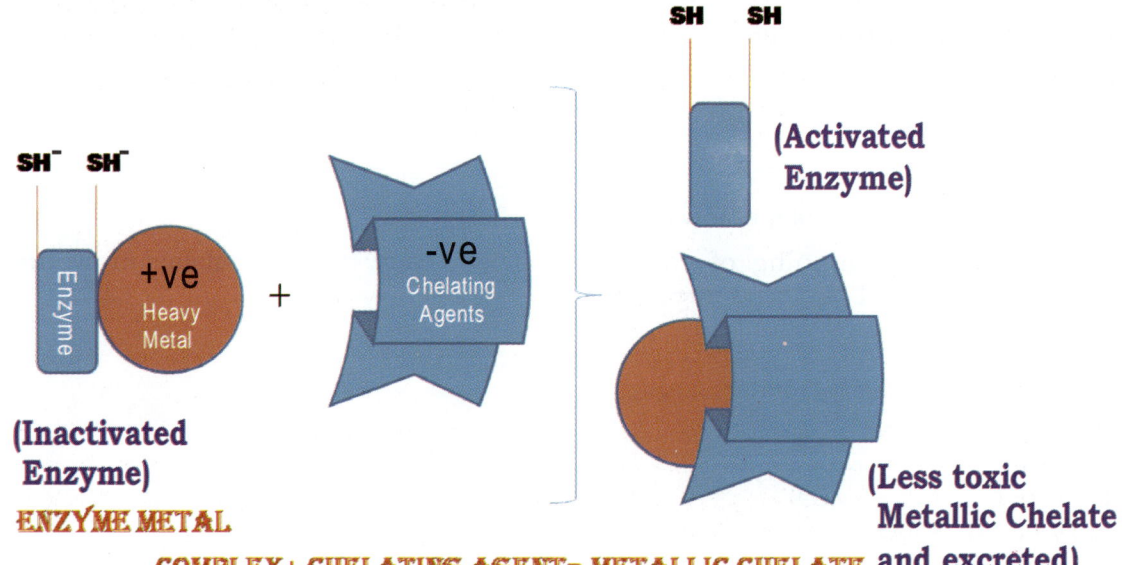

FIG: 79 - GENERAL MECHANISM OF ACTION OF CHELATING AGENTS

HEAVY METALS COMBINES WITH ENDOGENOUS ENZYMES → ENZYME-METAL COMPLEX (ENZYMES BECOME INACTIVE AND ALSO EXERTS TOXIC ADVERSE EFFECTS).

CHELATING AGENTS SHOW AFFINITY TO THE ENZYME-METAL COMPLEX → LIBERATION OF ENZYME AND FORMS METAL-CHELATE COMPLEX (NON-TOXIC, WATER SOLUBLE AND ELIMINATES THROUGH URINE)

Mechanism of action of chelating agents: (Fig.79)

'Chele'=crab's claw (like crab's claws catch their prey and eat, the chelating agents (-vely charged) combine with the heavy metals(+vely charged) → chelating agent-heavy metal complex → Nontoxic and easily excreted →free the enzyme to be active by releasing 'SH' group to the enzyme.

DRUGS:

1 BAL(British Anti Lewisite) DIMERCAPROL:-Universal heavy metal antagonist

2 D-Penicillamine (copper poisoning)

3. Desferrioxamine (Iron poisoning)

4 EDTA (Lead poisoning) (Ethyle Diamine Tetra Acetic Acid – edidate)

Clinical uses :

1. In chronic heavy metal poisoning, which occur among workers in industries using heavy metals.

Chronic heavy metal poisoning is common among workers in industries using heavy metals for manufacturing paints, batteries, Aluminium products, steel and also in persons consuming Arsenic obtained from subsoil(nausea, vomiting)

2. In acute poisoning, who has ingested in large quantity (insecticides, rodenticides(rat killer),containing Arsenic)

D-PENICILLAMINE

- It is a chelating agent
- It is the degraded product of Penicillin, but doesn't have antibacterial activity

Mechanism of action : Ref:before

Clinical uses :

1. Drug of choice in Copper poisoning

2. Drug of choice in the management of Wilson's disease (accumulation of Copper in brain, liver, kidney, cornea etc). Ceruloplasmin helps in the excretion of Copper.In Wilson's disease, due to genetic defect there is a deficiency of the enzyme and there is no excretion of Copper which gets accumulated.

3. In cystine stone (Copper complexes with cystine and gets deposited in the urinary tract)

4. In scleroderma crisis: It increases the solubility of collagen

Adverse effects: Vit B_6 deficiency, aplastic anaemia

DESFERRIOXAMINE

It is an Iron chelating agent.

Mechanism of action : ref: before

Clinical uses :

1. In Iron poisoning (1 g is capable of chelating 85 mg of elemental iron)

2. To prevent overload of Iron, (in transfusion siderosis) when the blood is infused in thalassemia patients

Adverse effects: diarrhoea, hypotension, respiratory distress syndrome etc.,

B.A.L (DIMERCAPROL)

It was first used in II world war to antagonize the Arsenic gas poisoning

ORALLY NOT EFFECTIVE

Mechanism of action : ref before

1. In all heavy metals poisoning (universal heavy metal antagonist)

Adverse effects: Pain at the site of injection, tachycardia, rise in BP, vomiting, etc.,

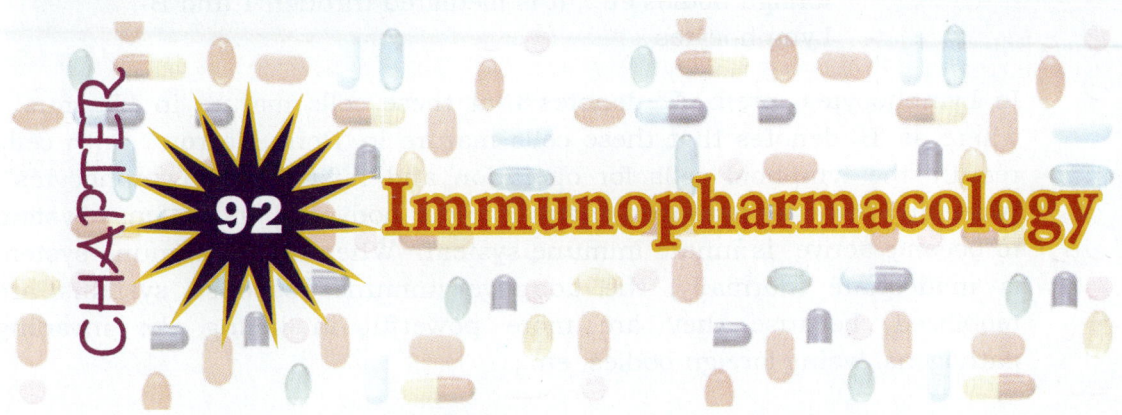

CHAPTER 92 **Immunopharmacology**

➢ It deals with the drugs affecting immune system.

Two groups of drugs are available ⟶ Immunosuppressive

⟶ Vaccines (reinforce immune defence against invading pathogens (Immunomodulator / Immunostimulant)

Immune system in our body plays an important role in protecting the body from the invading pathogens and foreign bodies. Immuno modulation is very important to keep the body free from diseases.

➢ The immune system in the body should be kept in balance. If the immune system is depressed (AIDS, Immuno suppressive drugs treatment) or if it is reactive (auto-immune diseases, graft rejection) will lead to harmful effect to the body.

➢ In immune deficiency syndrome (AIDS), there will be super infection of fungus, virus, tuberculosis, etc., which are responsible to bring down the quality of life and death. There is no effective immunostimulant drugs to treat that condition.

➢ In increased activity of humoral or cell mediated immunity will lead to autoimmune diseases, graft rejection in organ transplantation. (Immunosuppressive drugs are useful in the above two conditions).

IMMUNE SYSTEM

Introduction: Immune system in our body is controlled by two systems

- Innate immune system(since birth it is active/natural/nonspecific) mediated through killer cells
- Adaptive immune system or acquired immune system, which is active only when there is invading of exogenous pathogens,

foreign bodies etc., It is mediated through T and B-Lymphocytes

In Lymphocytes, prefix 'T' denotes that these cells mature in 'Thymus' , where as 'B' denotes that these cells mature in 'Bone Marrow'. Both cells require the lymphoid cells for operation and referred as "Lymphocytes". When any invading pathogen enters into our body, the first defense system to become active is innate immune system. When innate immune system is inadequate (normally) the adaptive immune response systems are mobilized, because they are more powerful in killing the invading pathogens, lysing foreign bodies, etc.,

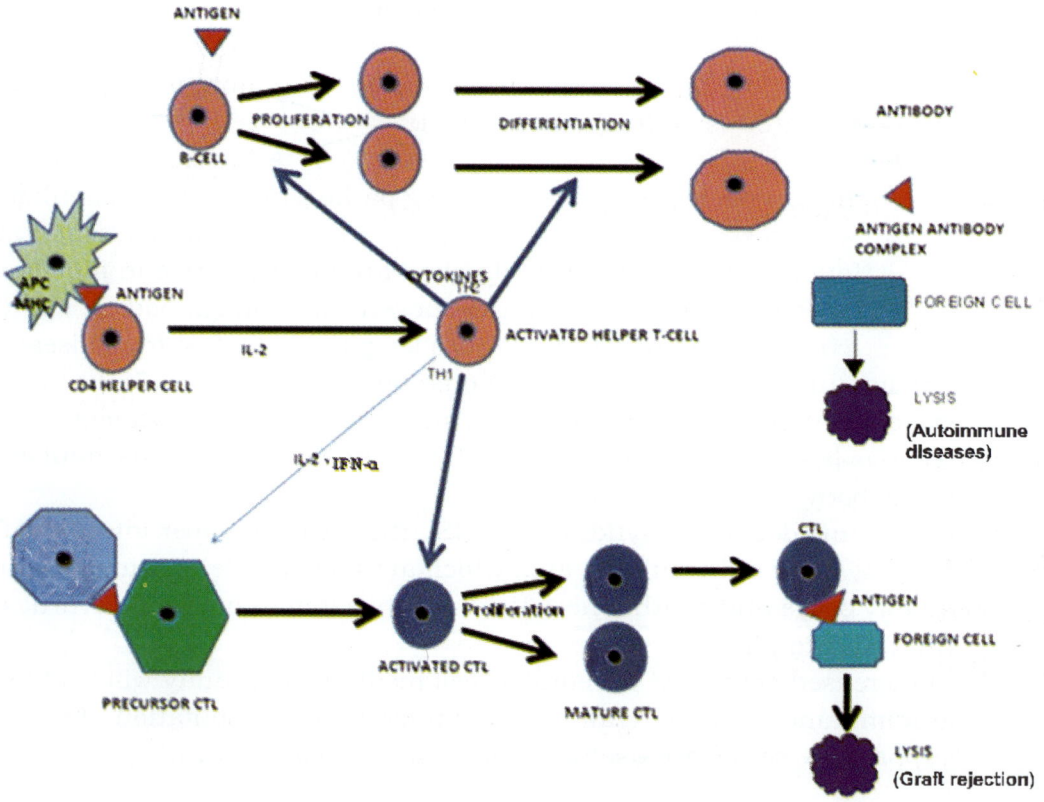

APC – Antigen Presenting cell, MHC – Major Histocompatibility complex, TH1 & TH2 – Helper T-cells 1 and 2, CTL – Cytotoxic T-Lymphocytes (Tc)

Fig. 80 MECHANISM OF HUMORAL MEDIATED IMMUNITY AND CELL MEDIATED IMMUNITY

I. Humoral Immunity (Fig.80)

The antigen (Ag) – (invading pathogen, Foreign body) is processed by macrophages or other antigen presenting cell (APC) coupled with class II major histocompatability complex (MHC) and presented to the CD_4 helper cell, which are activated by IL-1, proliferate and secrete cytokines – in turn promotes proliferation and differentiation of antigen activated B-cells into antibody (Ab) secreting plasma cells. Antibodies finally bind and inactivate the antigen (invading pathogens, foreign bodies).

Antigen   Antigen
↓   ↓

Ag+MHC-I   Ag+MHC-II
↓

APC
↓

Binds and activates T-Lymphocytes IN THYMUS
↓

Precursor CTL with CD8+   AND   Helper T cell with CD4+

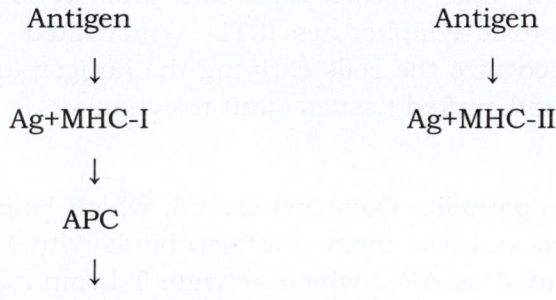

↓   ←IL-1,IFN-α ← TH1 ⟋ ⟍ TH2 → CYTOKINES

Activated CTL with CD8+   ↓
↓   stimulate B- Lymphocytes

Recognise the foreign antigen   (proliferation and differentiation)

(Pathogens, grafted tissues)   ↓

lysis pathogens and grafted tissues   Stimulate plasma cells
↓   ↓

GRAFT REJECTION   increased production of antibodies
↓

React with antigen and kill extracellular pathogens and destroy body's non-self tissues. (Autoimmune diseases)

II.   CMI (Cell Mediated Immunity) (Fig.80)

In cell mediated immunity – endogenous foreign antigen (Intracellular pathogens/ foreign bodies, grafted tissues) is recognized by MHC-class I protein and form complexes with antigen to represent as APC, which activate the T- Lymphocytes processed and presented to CD4+ helper T-cells and cytotoxicT cell precursor with surface marker CD 8+.The CD4+Helper T cell→ which elaborate TH1,which mediate cellular immunity andTH2, which mediate humoral immunity. The TH1→ releases IL-2 and other cytokines, that in turn stimulate proliferation and maturation of precursor cytotoxic lymphocytes (CTL) → activated and then to mature CTL, which recognize the cells carrying the antigen and lyse them → lysis of pathogens and grafted tissues (graft rejection)

MHC (Major Histocompatibility Complex)-class I, which helps cytotoxic T- cell to recognize the non-self and lyse them. Antigen binds with MHC to form Ag-MHC complex to be presented as APC, which activate T-Lymphocytes first to initiates the CMI.

So, CMI is mainly mediated by T-Lymphocytes, through cytotoxic T-Lymphocyte (CTL) bearing a cell surface marker CD8+ (CD8+ T_c-cell).

AUTOIMMUNE DISEASE:

Example: Myasthenia gravis. Due to some reason, the body's self protein becomes non-self (foreign protein-Antigen). It starts producing antibodies. Then antigen/antibody reaction takes place on the non-self tissue, which is then destroyed. In myasthenia gravis, the nicotinic receptors behave as non-self (Antigen) and starts producing nicotinic receptor antibody. Then antigen/antibody reaction takes place on nicotinic receptors, which are then destroyed. The number of nicotinic receptors is reduced and less availability of nicotinic receptors for the action of ACh and progressively the skeletal muscle is relaxed, which will lead to myasthenia gravis.

The immunosuppressive drugs, which inhibit B-Lymphocyte proliferation and inhibit the antibody production will be useful in autoimmune diseases.

CD=Cluster of Differentiation. These are hundreds in number. They are also called as human leukocyte antigen.

Some of the important CD_s and their functions are

CD_3 - On T-cells activation of T-Lymphocyte,

CD_4 - T-cells activation, on TH_1/TH_2 cells,

CD_8 - On Tc Lymphocyte, T-cell activation,

CD_{20}, CD_{40} – B-cell activation

CD_{80} – Activation of both B & T-Lymphocytes.

CD_4, CD_8 are act as markers on lymphoid cells.

CD_4, CD_8 are important. They are synthesized and released from Lymphocytes in response to antigen challenge (invading pathogens, foreign bodies). They are important in stimulating the B- and T- Lymphocytes proliferation to activate humeral mediated immunity (B-Lymphocytes dependent) and cell mediated immunity (T-Lymphocyte dependent) to defend the challenging antigens. If CD_4, CD_8 markers count is decreased, it will lead to immune deficiency syndromes (As in AIDS) prone to super infections.

IMMUNOSUPPRESSIVE AGENTS

The drugs which suppress the both types of immunity (Humoral mediated and cell mediated) are called Immunosuppressive agents.

They are useful in autoimmune diseases and to prevent graft rejection in organ transplantation

IMMUNOSUPPRESSIVE DRUGS:

    I.   Cytotoxic drugs:
    1. Antimetabolites:
        i)   METHOTREXATE
        ii)   Azathioprine
    2. Alkylating agents: Cyclophosphamide
    II.   GLUCOCORTICOIDS
    III.   Calcineurin inhibitors: CYCLOSPORINE, Tacrolimus

IV.   Cytokine inhibitors.
   1. TNF-α inhibitor: Infliximab, Adalimumab
   2. IL-2 inhibitors: Daclizuomab

V   Monoclonal antibody: Muromomab

VI   Misc: Rho (D) Immune Globulin (Ref: Antisera)

   i.   Mechanism of action of cytotoxic drugs: (antimetabolites and alkylating agents)
      -    They inhibit DNA synthesis of B and T- lymphocytes → inhibit T-cell and B-cell proliferation and activation → immunosuppressive action → inhibit the T- cell mediated immunity (treatment of graft rejection) and antibody mediated immunity (useful in autoimmune diseases.)

Clinical uses: 1. As anticancer 2. As immunosuppressive: i) In autoimmune diseases (Rheumatoid arthritis, myasthenia gravis, hemolytic anemia etc.,) ii) To prevent graft rejection in organ transplantation.

Adverse effects: Ref: general toxicity of anticancer drugs.

II.   GLUCOCORTICOIDS : Inhibit both T-cell and B-cell proliferation and hence immunosuppressive
III.   Calcineurin inhibitor

CYCLOSPORINE

- It is obtained from a fungus.
- It is a calcineurin inhibitor.
- It is highly effective to prevent graft rejection in organ transplantation.

Mechanism of action of cyclosporine:

Cyclosporine → inhibits calcineurin enzyme → inhibits helper T-cell activation→ inhibits the release of IL-2, IFN-¥, → inhibits the activation and proliferation of CTL(Tc-CD4+)→ suppress CMI → no lysis of grafted tissues → prevent graft rejection.

   -    Also partly inhibits TH2 → inhibits proliferation of B-cell→ inhibits the production of antibodies → suppresses Antibody mediated immunity→ suppresses autoimmune diseases

Foreign antigen (grafted tissues) → APC +MHC-I (Antigen Presenting Cell + Major Histocompatibility Complex-Class-I), which helps Tc (CTL) to recognize only foreign antigens (grafted tissues) → T-cell activation

↓

↑ Calcineurin enzyme

↕ ← inhibited by Cyclosporine

↓ inhibits TH cell activation (Helper T- cells)

↓

↓ inhibits TH1 activation

↓

↓ inhibits release of IL-2, TNF-α

↓

↓ inhibits activation and proliferation of CTL (Tc-CD4+-Cytotoxic T -Lymphocytes

↓

↓ (suppresses) CMI (Cell mediated immunity)

↓

prevents the lysis of grafted tissues

↓

prevents the graft rejection

Clinical uses:

I.   To prevent graft rejection in organ transplantation. It is effective when it is administered before transplantation (10-15 mg/oral/daily, 12hrs before transplantation and continued as long as required). If rejection occurs, then 3-5 mg/kg/1V infusion is given.

II.   In autoimmune diseases: It is a second line drug. It is given along with GCs, methotrexate in myasthenia gravis, rheumatoid arthritis, psoriasis, nephritic syndrome.

Dose: Cyclosporine 10-15 mg/ orally / daily as long as required.

Adverse effect: Nephrotoxic, neurotoxic, hepatotoxic ↑ B.P, hyperuricaemia, hirsutism, gingival hyperplasia, super infections of fungus, virus (proper anti-microbial agents are given).

V.   CYTOKINES INHIBITORS:
1.   TNF-α- inhibitors and IL- 2 inhibitors:
Mechanism of action: TNF-α , IL-2 →bind to activated lymphocyte (CTL) → initiate the proliferation of T-lymphocytes → initiate cell mediated immunity → lysis (rejection) of grafted tissues.

Cytokine inhibitors inhibit all the above steps → suppress cell mediated immunity → immunosuppressive action → prevent graft rejection. They are also anti-inflammatory by inhibiting cytokines activity.

Clinical uses of cytokines inhibitors:

1. In rheumatoid arthritis (anti-inflammatory and inhibits cell mediated immunity)
2. In Crohn's disease
3. To prevent graft rejection in organ transplantation.

VI.   Monoclonal antibody : (ref: monoclonal antibody for mechanism of action)

VII. Misc: Rho (D) immune Globulin (ref: Vaccines and antisera)

IMMUNOSTIMULANTS

The immunostimulants are not effective in AIDS and they can be used only as adjuvant with anticancer drugs

Drugs:

1. B.C.G. (Bacillus Calmette Guerin): Stimulates T-cells and NK cells. Mainly useful in urinary bladder cancer.
2. Levamisole: Anthelminitic drug. It stimulates both T-cells and B-cells functions. It is used in colorectal cancer (combined with anticancer drugs)
3. Thalidomide: It is an anti-inflammatory and immunomodulatory. It decreases TNF-α level in the blood. It is used in rheumatoid arthritis, lepra reaction and in certain malignancies.
4. Interferon-α- It activates T- Lymphocytes, NK cells and acts as immunostimulant. (ref: Interferon-α.) used in AIDS as adjuvant

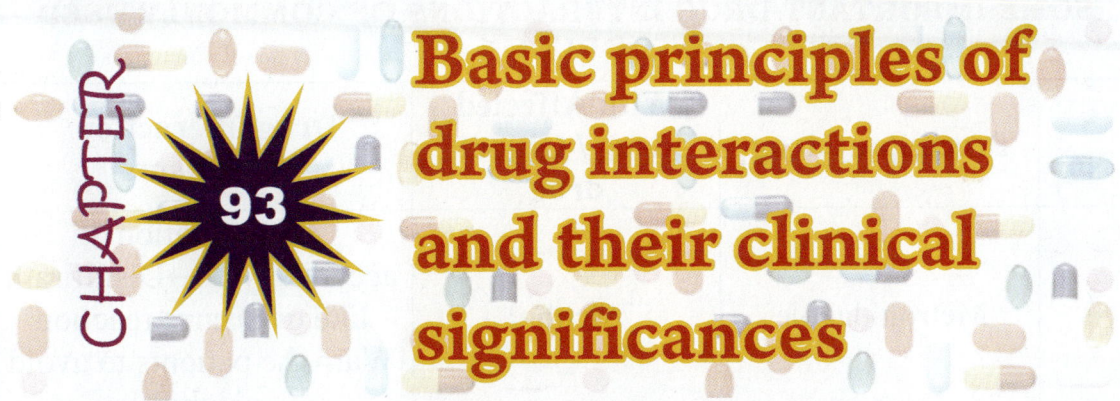

Basic principles of drug interactions and their clinical significances

CHAPTER 93

Toxicity due to drug interaction is different from drug toxicity.

Drug toxicity is due to the over dose of a SINGLE drug. But toxicity is due to drug interaction, in which two or more drugs are involved. One drug increases the toxicity of another drug(in therapeutic dose)

Drug interaction refers to modification of response to one drug by another drug when they are given simultaneously. The response may be increased or decreased for the same therapeutic dose.

The percentage of drug interaction is proportional to number of drugs combined.

The drug interactions are broadly classified into

1. Pharmacokinetic drug interaction: due to their pharmacokinetic properties

2 Pharmacodynamic drug interaction: due to their pharmacodynamic properties

1. Pharmacokinetic drug interactions

i) Due to absorption: Tetracyclines+ calcium containing milk products= Tetracyclines chelate Ca++ and precipitate → absorption of Tetracyclines are reduced

ii) Due to metabolism: (Ref: metabolism, enzyme induction and enzyme inhibition)

iii) Due to distribution (Ref: distribution of drugs-protein bound drugs)

iv) Due to excretion: (Ref: excretion of drugs)

2. Pharmacodynamic drug interaction:

i) Combining two of more drugs, which are having similar pharmacological actions (additive toxic effects) Example : Diazepam and alcohol

3. Pharmaceutical drug interactions (Nurses should be careful)

i) Example : IV infusion – precipitation of two solution, if mixed together. (dextrose + some antibiotic like Gentamicin)

SOME IMPORTANT DRUG INTERACTIONS OF COMMONLY USED DRUGS

S No	Precipitant drug	With Affected drug / Object drug	Drug interaction/ comments
1	Metronidazole	Alcohol	Accumulation of acetaldehyde →Disulfiram like or bizarre reaction Warn the patients to avoid alcohol.
2	Ciprofloxacin, Norfloxacin	Aminophylline, Warfarin	Inhibition of metabolism of object drug → increase the toxicity of object drugs – either change the drug or monitor/reduce the dose of object drugs.
3	Zafirlukast Erythromycin, Clarithromycin, ketoconazole, Itraconazole, Protease inhibitor (enzyme inhibitor of CYP 3A4)	Terfenadine, Astemizole, Cisapride	Inhibition of metabolism of object drug →increase blood levels→increase the toxicity of object drugs (dangerous ventricular arrhythmia – Torsades de pointes). Concurrent use is avoided.
		Cyclosporine, Phenytoin, Warfarin, Sulphonyl urea, Diazepam	Inhibition of metabolism → increase the toxicity of object drug. Avoid concurrent use or monitor/reduce the dose of object drugs.
		Statin	Higher risk of myopathy → avoid concurrent use
4	Tetracycline, Amoxycylline, Ampicillin	Oral Cortraceptive Pills (OCP), or alternate	Failure of contraception (Ref: before) concurrent use is avoided.

		contraceptive method is followed, Oral anti-coagulants	Inhibits bacterial flora →inhibits the synthesis of vitaminK →bleeding – monitor INR of OAC
5	Cephalosporins	Oral anticoagulant	Additive hypoprothrombinemia leads to increased bleeding → reduce dose of anticoagulant by monitoring INR
6	Allopurinol	Ampicillin	Increased incidence of skin rashes
		Warfarin 6MP Azathioprine	Inhibit the metabolism of object drug Increase the toxicity Reduce the dose of object drugs
7	Co-trimoxazole Aspirin	Phenytoin Warfarin Sulphonyl urea	Displacement of Plasma Protein Binding → toxicity of object drug – avoid concurrent use/monitor the dose of object drugs.
		Thiazide diuretics	Thrombocytopaenia – concurrent use is avoided
		Oral contraceptives	Failure of contraception Advise: alternative contraceptive method is to be followed
8	Niacin Fibrates	Statin	Increased risk of myopathy Caution: when concurrent use

9	Iron salts Antacids	Tetracyclines Fluroquinolones	Reduce absorption by forming complexes → failure of antimicrobial effect, 2-3 hrs gap should be there between the administration of two groups
10	Diuretics	Tetracyclines	Increase urea production – Avoid concurrent use
		Lithium	Decrease excretion of Lithium →increases the toxicity of Lithium →reduce the dose of Lithium
		Digoxin	Hypokalaemia produced by diuretics, increase the toxicity of digoxin – Avoid concurrent use
11	NSAIDs	FQ	Increase CNS toxicity and precipitate seizures →avoid concurrent use
		Warfarin	Increase bleeding →avoid concurrent use
		β-adrenergic blockers, ACE inhibitors	Decrease efficacy →avoid concurrent use
		Frusemide	Decrease diuretic action →avoid concurrent use
		Glucocorticoids	Increase gastric bleeding →avoid concurrent use (if needed, paracetamol is preferrable)
12	ENZYME INDUCERS Phenobarbitone	Methotrexate Protease inhibitors Warfarin	Induction of metabolism → reduce efficacy of object drugs. Avoid

	Rifampicin Carbamezapine Phenytoin	Oral contraceptives Sulphonyl ureas Corticosteroids	concurrent use/increase the dose of object drugs
13	<u>Bacteriostatic</u> Tetracyclines Macrolides Chloramphenicol Clindamycin	<u>Bacteriocidal</u> Penicillins Cephalosporins	Both the groups will antagonize each other concurrent use to be avoided
14	Metoclopramide Chlorpromazine Haloperidol	L-Dopa + Carbidopa	Reduce the efficacy of anti-parkinsonism drug. Avoid concurrent use
15	Lignocaine	Betablockers Anti-arrhythmic Drugs	Exagerrated cardiac depression – Avoid concurrent use

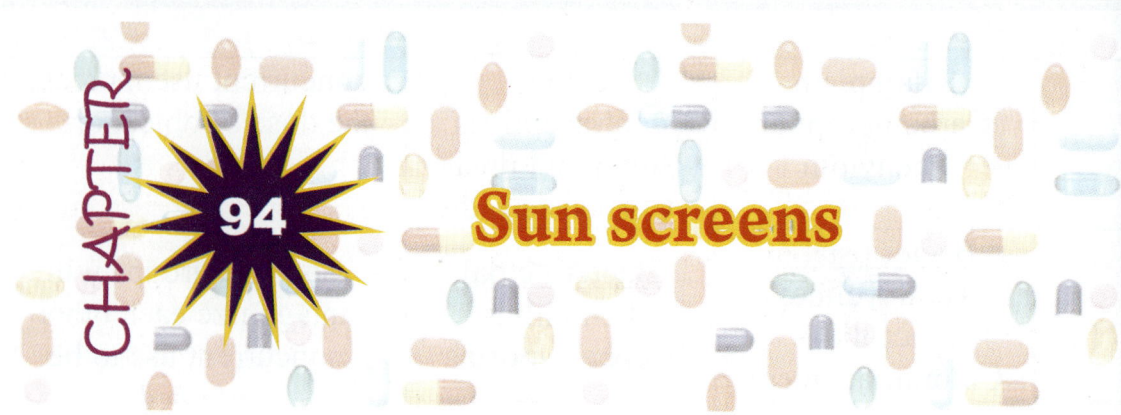

SUNSCREENS are substances that protect the skin from harmful effects of exposure to sunlight.

I.   Chemical sunscreen: They absorb and scatter the UV rays that are responsible for sun burn and phototoxicity, but allow longer wave length to penetrate, so that tanning occurs. The efficacy of the sun screens depends on the UVB radiation that produce minimal erythema on protected skin to that of unprotected skin

Para Amino Benzoic Acid(PABA) and its esters

They absorb UVB (290-320 nm)

They are used as 5% lotion or 10% cream

Other drugs: Benzophenones, Cinnamates

Uses: Chemical sun screens are used as adjunct in vitiligo therapy, in drug induced phototoxicity and facilitate tanning while preventing sun burn

2. To prevent premature ageing of skin

II. Physical sun screens: Heavy petroleum jelly, Titanium dioxide, Zinc oxide are opaque substances that stop and scatter not only UV but also visible light. They are also called as sun shade and have to be applied as a thick lotion . They withhold longer wave lengths also

Chloroquine is also effective in skin eruptions, but should be reserved in severe cases only

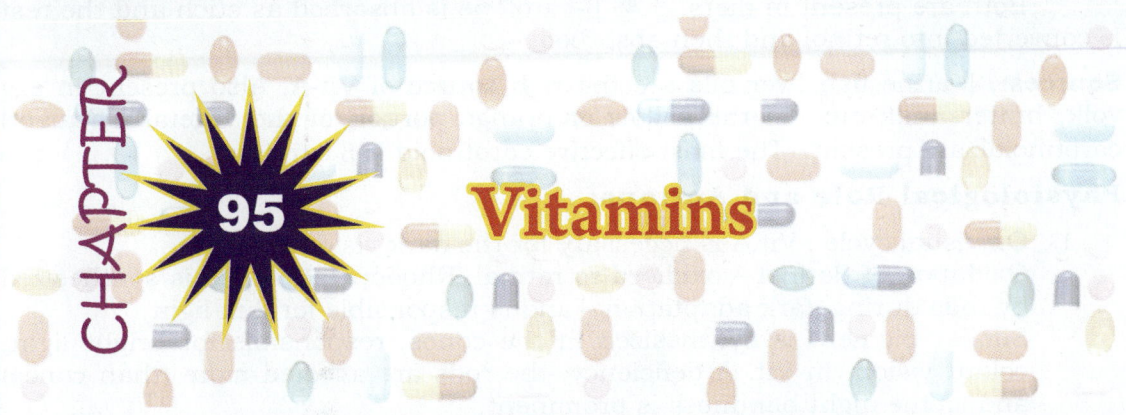

- Vitamins are nonenergy producing organic compounds, essential for normal human metabolism, that should be supplied in small quantity in the diet. This definition doesn't include the substances which are required large quantity for normal metabolism (ex: Essential Amino acids, minerals and fatty acids).
- The different chemical structure and other precursors of vitamins are called as 'vitamers' (analogy- isomer)
- The most important use of vitamins is in the treatment and prevention of deficiency states.
- The deficiency of vitamins is due to inadequate dietary intake, malabsorption (heavy alcohol intake), heavy bacterial growth in the gut(Vit B complex deficiency), increased excretion, increased metabolism, genetic variations, etc.
- Vitamins are over used,
- Vitamins are divided into two groups:

1. Fat soluble Vitamins (A,D,E,K)

Except Vit-K, other vitamins are stored in the body, and they are liable to produce cumulative toxicity, if consumed large quantity or used often.

2. Water soluble Vitamins (B complex and C)

Free radicals formed in our body destroy cells and inhibit DNA synthesis. The free radicals are removed from the body by antioxidants like Vit. E and Vit. C

FAT SOLUBLE VITAMINS:

VITAMIN- A

The naturally occurring vit. A is called 'retinol' (Vit. A_1) Vit A is in two forms. They are β-carotene (inactive form) converted into retinol (active form) β-carotene is called as provitamin-A.

Both are present in diets. 30% β-carotene is absorbed as such and the rest is converted into retinol and then absorbed.

Sources: Marine fish liver oils are the rich source of Vit-A. Also present in egg yolk, butter, milk etc., In the yellow or orange portion of the vegetable (carrot) carotinoids are present. The most effective carotinoid is β carotene

Physiological Role and Actions:

1. On visual cycle : Vit.A is necessary for the dark vision.
   Oxidation of Retinol – oxidised to retinal (Rhodopsin), which is synthesized by rods during dark adaptation – and is responsible for dim light.
   Similar pigment is synthesized in the cones, responsible for bright light, colour vision. In Vit. A deficiency, the rods are affected more (than cones) and so the night blindness is prominent.
2. On epithelial cells : Vit. A is necessary for differentiation and maintenance of healthy epithelial cells. It inhibits keratinisation and improves resistance to infection. It reduces the incidence of development of malignancies of epithelial structures.
3. On immunity: It is antiinfective. It increases proliferation of lymphocytes and killer cells function.
4. It is an antioxidant.
5. In reproduction : Retinol is necessary for spermatogenesis and foetal development.

Deficiency syndrome:

• EYE: It causes night blindness (nyctalopia), xerosis (dryness of cornea), bitot's spots (white spots on conjunctiva) and keratomalacia (necrosis of cornea). They are collectively called as 'xerophthalmia'
• On reproductive system : sterility in males and abortion, fetal abnormalities.
• On SKIN: It causes Hyperkeratinization, dry and rough skin
• On BONE: It causes faulty modelling of bone
• OTHERS: lung/skin malignancy

Clinical uses : 1. Prophylaxis of Vit. A deficiencies during infancy, pregnancy and lactation. (3000 – 5000 IU/day) of Retinol.

2. In treatment of Vit. A deficiency Retinol – (50,000 IU – 1,00,000 IU/day for 3 days)
3. Skin diseases like acne, psoriasis (Retinoic acid is preferred Ref : P.463)
4. As an antioxidant

Isotretinoin (Oral) used in acne vulgaris, prevention of cancer and psoriasis

Toxicity: Hypervitaminosis-A : dry and pruritic skin, hair loss, fissure of lips, tenderness of bone, brittle nail, oedema, reduce HDL level, fatigue

Treatment: Vit. E promotes the storage of Retinol into tissues and speeds recovery.

VITAMIN-E (TOCOFEROLS)

Alpha tocoferol is the most potent

It is a fat soluble vitamin

Dietary source: Wheat germ oil, vegetable seed oil, nuts, peas and egg yolk.

Physiological role:

- Antioxidant: It prevents the breakdown of polyunsaturated fatty acid, prevents cancer, coronary artery diseases (Atherosclerosis), Alzheimer's disease, cataract etc.

  It is an Antisterility factor

- Enhancement of use of Vit-A in the body.

Deficiency syndromes:

- Peripheral neuropathy,
- Sterility in males and recurrent abortions in females
- Muscular dystrophy and cardiomyopathy
- Haemolytic anaemia in premature infants (due to the deficiency of G6PDH enzyme)
- Altered gait, steatorroea

Clinical uses of VIT.E: 1. In Vit.E deficiency syndromes 2, In nocturnal muscle cramp 3. In fibrocystic breast diseases. 4, To increase the survival time of erythrocytes in G6PD deficiency (G6PD is essential to maintain the integrity of the cell membrane of the RBC) to prevent haemolysis. 5. As antioxidant to delay progressiveness of cataract, cardiovascular diseases and neurodegenerative disorders

VIT. K (ref: coagulants)

WATER SOLUBLE VITAMINS: (Vit. B complex & Vit. C)

Vit. B complex: Vit. B_{12} and Folic acid (ref: megaloblastic anaemia)

The vitamins belonging to this group tend to occur together in the food and hence the collective term 'Vit B complex'

The B vitamins are obtained from both meat and vegetables products except for Vit. B_{12}, which occurs only in meat, liver, fish, egg, milk and milk products (not vegetable source)

Vit. B_1 (Thiamine): Source : cereals, pulses, peanuts, green vegetables, egg and meat

Physiological role:

1. It acts as coenzyme in carbohydrate metabolism.
2. It also plays some role in neuromuscular transmission

Deficiency syndromes:

- Failure of carbohydrate metabolism, causing accumulation of pyruvic acid and lactic acid (Beri-Beri)
- Dry beri-beri affects CNS and peripheral nervous system causing peripheral neuropathy, numbness, cramps and muscular weakness,
- Wet beri-beri affects CVS causing palpitation, high out put cardiac failure
- In alcoholic poor diet → deficiency of Vit. B_1 → Werninicke Korsakoff syndrome (ophthalmoplegia, loss of memory, ataxia etc.,)

Clinical uses : 1. In Vit. B_1 deficiency

RIBOFLAVIN (VITAMIN B_2)

Source: As in Vit. B_1

Physiological role:

Acts as co-enzyme for flavoproteins involved in several oxidation-reduction reactions.

Deficiency syndromes: Glossitis, stomatitis, fissure on lips, cataract formation, local seborrheic dermatitis of trunk and extremities.

Clinical use: 1. In deficiency syndromes.

NIACIN (VITAMIN B_3) Ref: Antihyperlipidemic drugs

Deficiency syndromes: Pellagra (dermatitis, stomatitis, dementia, insomnia and depression)

Uses:

1. In deficiency syndromes (As prophylactic 25-50 mg/daily and treatment 250-500 mg/daily)

2. In hyperlipidemia

PANTOTHENIC ACID (VITAMIN B_5)

Physiological role: As that of Vit. B_1, Vit. B_2

Deficiency syndromes: leg cramp,flatulence, diarrhea.

Use: In deficiency syndromes

PYRIDOXINE (VITAMIN B_6)

Physiological role:

- Acts as coenzyme in the metabolism of carbohydrate, fat and protein
- Synthesis of GABA, Haem, amino acid (tryptophan- 5 HT precursor)
- Co-enzyme for INH metabolism

Deficiency syndromes: peripheral neuritis, anaemia, glossitis

Vomiting in pregnancy, anaemia, growth retardation in children

Clinical uses : 1. In deficiency syndromes 2. In vomiting due to pregnancy along with proper antiemetic drug 3. Along with INH in the treatment of tuberculosis, to minimise peripheral neuritis. 4. Convulsion in infants and children.

BIOTIN

Physiological role: same as other Vit. B complex

Deficiency syndromes: Nausea, vomiting, diarroea etc.

Use: As before

Toxicity: rare

VITAMIN B₁₂, FOLIC ACID (ref: megaloblastic anaemia)

NON B COMPLEX: VITAMIN- C (ASCORBIC ACID)

Dietary sources: citrus fruits, (lemon, orange, amla, tomato, potato, green chilli and cabbage).

Physiological role:

- It serves as cofactor in various oxidation-hyroxylation reactions .
- It plays a role in collagen synthesis, adrenal steroids, ADH, Oxytocin synthesis
- It stimulates the conversion of folic acid to folinic acid.
- To maintain Iron in ferrous state for its absorption.

Deficiency syndromes: Scurvy (defect in collagen synthesis, characterized by gingival bleeding, gingivitis, loosening of teeth and defect in tooth formation, failure of wound healing, capillaries rupture, anaemia, haematoma.

Use: 1. In deficiency syndromes. 2. To enhance healing in post-operatively 3. In iron deficiency anaemia with iron 4. To acidify urine in urinary tract infection and in basic drug poisoning.

VITAMIN D (Ref: Ca++ metabolism)

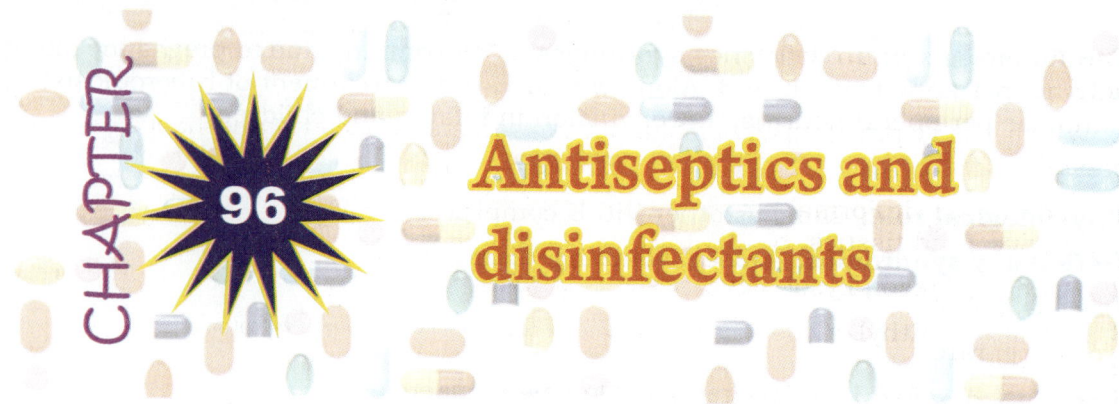

CHAPTER 96

Antiseptics and disinfectants

- Earlier, we discussed about those antimicrobials, which are used to treat systemic infections, since they are less toxic.
- Antiseptic-Disinfectants are also antimicrobial agents, but are toxic for systemic use. They are used only topically or locally.
- However, while providing medical care to the patients numerous instruments, glass wares and environmental surfaces get contaminated with patient's blood or pus, which are potential source of transmission of infection, particularly to the hospital staff.
- Hence, it is necessary to protect health care workers and also other patients from transmission of infection and its consequences. For that purpose the antimicrobial agents used are called as 'germicides' and used only externally.
- Germicides are divided into 1. ANTISEPTICS 2. DISINFECTANTS
- Antiseptics are chemical agents which destroy pathogenic bacteria (not spores) on animate (living) surfaces(skin, eye and mucous membranes)
- Disinfectants are chemical agents, which destroy or inhibit the growth of pathogenic bacteria on inanimate (non living) surfaces, such as glass wares, surgical instruments etc
- Sterilization is the ultimate goal of any infection control protocol. It is a process that kills all the living microorganisms (including spores),viruses, fungi. Usually sterilization is carried out by autoclaving at 15 lb pressure of steam at 120°C for atleast half an hour. But other methods such as infra-red, ultraviolet or gamma radiation are also used.
- Antimicrobial preservatives are used in sterile preparations such as eye drops and multi dose injections to maintain sterility during use. They are also used in oral liquids, food, ointments, creams to prevent microbial spoilage.
- The commonly used preservatives are benzyl alcohol, benzoic acid, parabens, mercuric salts (for eye drops and IM injections) Concomitant use of citric acid along with antioxidants preservatives increases their efficacy.

The antiseptics and disinfectants are classified according to their mechanism of action.

I. Which act by precipitating (coagulating) proteins of bacteria and hence death of bacteria.

1. Aldehydes: i) Formaldehyde (30% formaldehyde is formalin, which is used for preserving dead tissues, but irritant)

2. Phenols: Cresol, Lysol, Chloroxylenol with alcohol= DETTOL)

3. Alcohols: Ethyl alcohol, Isopropyl alcohol (as skin antiseptic before IM, IV injections)

4. Triclosan- used in soaps, hand wash, mouth wash, tooth pastes, etc.,

II. Which act by oxidising the SH groups of bacterial enzyme and hence death of the bacteria.

i) Hydrogen peroxide (broad spectrum germicidal agent) Effective against bacteria, viruses, fungi and spores. The oxidising agents liberate nascent Oxygen, which kill microorganisms.

It is used to clean the wound, abscesses, to remove ear wax.In dentistry, it is used to clean septic sockets in root canal and mouth wash

ii) Iodinated/chlorinated compounds.

Povidone-Iodine is used in burn, boils and as disinfectant spray in trichomonal vaginitis, as 10% solution is used to disinfect surgical instruments and as 1% solution for mouth wash.

Chlorinated lime (bleaching powder) is useful to disinfect swimming pool, tanks, toilets, drains etc.,

iii) Potassium permanganate: It Liberates nascent Oxygen, which oxidises bacterial proteins and enzymes and kills them. It is also used for gargling, irrigating cavities.

III. Which alter the properties of cell membrane:

Detergent action → they lower surface tension of cell membrane of bacteria → damage to the cell membrane → alter the cell membrane permeability → nutrients will leak out → bacteria die.

Example : Chlorhexidine + Cetrimide (SAVLON), commonly used antiseptic and disinfectant for surgical instruments, hand wash, mouth wash etc

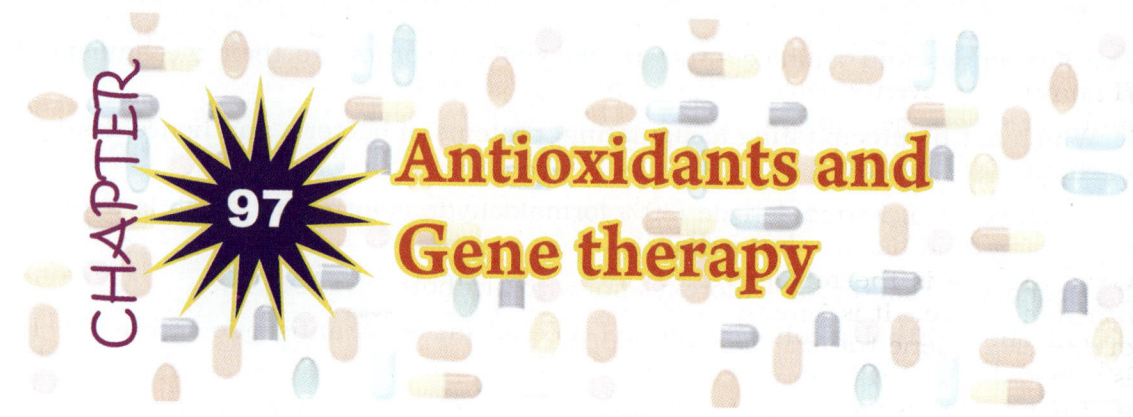

CHAPTER 97

Antioxidants and Gene therapy

ANTIOXIDANTS:

Due to the stimulation of some enzymes, free radicals (charged particles like nascent oxygen) are released, which are destructive to the various tissues in the body.

Antioxidants can intervene at any of the following levels between the process of free radicals generation to the causation of tissue injury.

1. Blockade of the generation of toxic free radicals.

2. Blockade of chain reactions set by free radicals.

3. Scavenging of free radicals

4. Blockade of secondary generation of toxic metabolite or mediators

5. Enhancing antioxidant capability

Endogenous antioxidants:

1. Super Oxidase Dismutase (SOD)

2. Glutathione reduced form (G-SH)

3. Carotenoid (Beta carotene)

4. Melatonin

5. Alpha tocoferol (Vit. E)

6. Ascorbic acid (Vit. C)

7. Adenosine

Agents augmenting the efficacy of endogenous antioxidants:

1. N-acetyl cysteine

2. Allopurinol, Selegiline, Selenium, Mn, Zn, Cu and Chromium

Antioxidants from plant sources: Garlic, Grapes, soya beans (isoflavones), turmeric, tomato, etc.,

Clinical uses of ANTIOXIDANTS: 1. It is of no use in any acute diseases. 2. However, it prevents some of the chronic conditions like atherosclerosis, cancer and tissue damage. They decrease the risk of atherosclerosis, MI, cancer, etc.,

GENE THERAPY

Gene therapy is the replacement of defective gene by the insertion of a normal, functional gene. It is genetic modification of cells for the prevention or treatment of diseases. Gene transfer may be done to replace defective genes. Gene therapy is aimed at genetically correcting the defect in the affected part of the body. Gene therapy can confer new functions in the cells.

Vector: Gene transfer requires the use of a vector (a suitable medium) to deliver the DNA material. An ideal vector should be safe and effective in inserting the therapeutic gene into the target cells. Biological vector (viral vector) is most commonly used. These viruses are not infectious and invade cells and use the metabolic processes of these host cells for replication. This property of viruses help to deliver the gene. Adenoviruses and retroviruses are used for this purpose.

Therapeutic applications of Gene therapy:

Though originally it was seen as a remedy for inherited single gene defects, Gene therapy has now been found to be useful in several acquired disorders.

1. Useful in thalassemia, cystic fibrosis, cancer, atherosclerosis, alzheimer's disease and many infectious diseases.
2. In familial hypercholesterolemia- LDL receptor gene is introduced into liver cells, which takes up cholesterol from blood to liver and reduces blood cholesterol level
3. In cancer-introducing the gene which makes the malignant cells sensitive to drugs. It inactivates the expression of oncogens. It introduces gene that attaches to the cancer cells and makes them susceptible to host defence cells. It also introduces genes to healthy cells to protect them from cytotoxic drugs.
4. In diabetes mellitus: It introduces the Insulin gene into pancreas which can produce Insulin
5. Coronary atherosclerosis- prevention of restenosis and ischaemia in coronary vessels by genes which inhibit the growth of vascular endothelial cells.

CHAPTER 98 — Critical evaluation (rationale combination of drugs) and advantages of the combinations

1. Adrenaline+ Lignocaine in infiltration anaesthesia;

In infiltration anaesthesia, if lignocaine is given alone, it produces vasodilatation.So, the drug will escape from the site of administration to the systemic action and produces the systemic toxicity.

secondly, the LA will escape through vasodilatation and the duration of action will be reduced

If it is combined with Adrenaline(a vasoconstrictor), prolong the duration of action of LA and reduces the systemic toxicity

Thirdly, bleeding will be reduced surrounding the field of surgery, since Adrenaline produces vasoconstriction.

For these reasons, it is better to combine Adrenaline with Lignocaine

Questions: i) What is infiltration anaesthesia? What are the USES of infiltration anaesthesia?

2. Estrogen +Progesteron as oral contraceptives (which are used to prevent pregnancy)

FSH and LH are very important for ovulation. Estrogen and Progesterone inhibit FSH and LH through negative feed back mechanism. So, ovulation is inhibited and hence pregnancy. If Estrogen or Progesterone is given alone, there is chance of missing ovulation and pregnancy may occur

so, for complete inhibition of ovulation, both drugs should be combined

Secondly, there is also synergistic action. Progesterone, apart from inhibition of ovulation, it produces thick cervical mucus and it is very difficult for the sperm to penetrate.

Thirdly, there are some health benefit of this combination i)Lower the risk of developing endometrial and ovarian carcinoma ii) if the menstruation is irregular become regular

Questions: i) What is emergency pill? What are the drugs and how they are administered? What is their Mechanism of action iii) What are the causes of contraceptive failure?

3 Neostigmine+ Atropine in myasthenia gravis.

Myasthenia gravis is an autoimmune disorder, in which there is a progressive loss of skeletal muscle tone, characterized by ptosis, difficulty in swallowing, difficulty in moving limbs etc. Nicotinic receptors are destroyed by antibodies, so ACh could not produce stimulation of skeletal muscles.

The treatment should be 1. Increase the concentration of ACh in the body 2.Prevent antibody production

Here, Neostimine increased the concentration of ACh in the body, by inhibiting the enzyme cholieesterase.That ACh produces both muscaranic and nicotinic actions. In myasthenia gravis, only the nocotinic action(stimulation of skeletal muscles) is wanted.   The muscaranic actions are not wanted. So,Atropine (muscaranic blocker)is given along with Neostigmine to block the unwanted muscaranic actions only without affecting the wanted nicotinic action

4. Cyclophophamide + Mesna In cancer treatment

Cyclophosphamide is converted by an enzyme to a toxic metabolite, Acroein, which produces haemorragic cystitis. Mesna inhibits that enzyme and prevent the conversion of cyclophophamide into toxic metabolite

5. Imipenem + Cilastatin in bacterial infection

Imipenem is a beta lactam antibiotic, and is used in g+ and g- infection. Imipenem is rapidly inactivated by the enzyme, dehydropeptidase. So, the efficacy of Imipenem is reduced.Cilastatin, inhibits the enzyme dehydropeptidase and prevents the inactivation of Imipenem and increases the efficacy of Imipenem.

6. Ampicillin+Clavulanic acid:

Ampicillin is a Beta lactam antibiotic. It is destroyed by the enzyme beta lactamase produced by some bacteria, which were previously sensitive to Ampicillin. In order to treat against beta lactamase producing bacteria, Ampicillin is combined with Clavulanic acid, a beta lactamase inhibitor.

7. L-Dopa + Carbidopa in Parkinsonism

Parkinsonism is due to the deficiency of Dopamine in the Basal ganglia.Dopamine doesn't cross blood brain barrier. But L-Dopa (inactive Prodrug)will cross BBB and is converted into Dopamine by the enyme Dopa Decarboxylase present in the BG. But most of L-Dopa is converted to Dopamine in the periphery before reaching BG by the peripheral dopa decarboxylase enzyme. If L-dopa alone given, the bioavailability in BG is very minimum. In order to block the peripheral conversion of L-dopa, a peripheral dopa decarboxylase inhibitor, Carbidopa is given with L-dopa. Now there will be maximum bioavailability of L-dopa at BG for action

Sulfamethaxazole + Trimathoprim (Ref : MOA of cotrimoxazole)

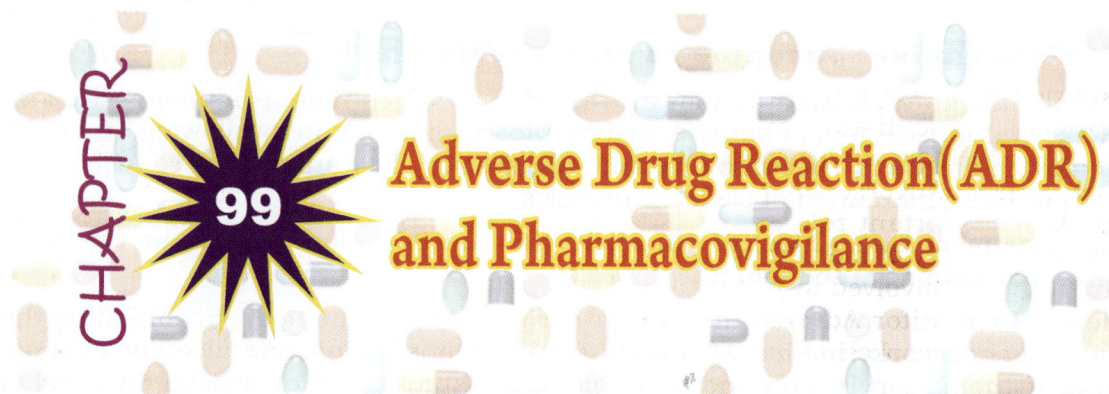

CHAPTER 99

Adverse Drug Reaction(ADR) and Pharmacovigilance

Adverse Drug Reactions: For the purpose of detecting and quantifying only those rare noxious effects of some import and occurs in ordinary therapeutic dose is termed as Adverse Drug Reaction, which requires treatment or decrease in dose or indicates caution in the future use of the drug This definition excludes trivial or expected side effects and poisoning or over dose.

Severity of adverse drug reaction has been grouped as:

Minor: No therapy, antidote or prolongation of hospitalization is required.

Moderate: requires change in drug therapy, specific treatment or prolonged hospital stay.

Severe: causes permanent organ damage, which is life threatening requires intensive medical treatment

Lethal: contributes to the death of the patient

Greek : Pharmakon = drug

Vigilare = To be observant

Pharmacovigilance is continuous monitoring for unwanted effects of marketed drugs. It is the science related to (DAUP) Detection Assessment, Understanding and prevention of adverse effects or any other drugs related problems.

Not all hazards can be known before a drug is marketed and used widely by the general population. Many facts about the drugs, i.e., their usefulness and harmfulness are only identified after the drug is widely used by a large community of the people (mainly through private practitioner) That stage is referred as clinical trial IV (post marketing surveillance)

Prior to drug approval:

It is very difficult to uncover every aspect of health of the approved drug. For example, the teratogenicity of thalidomide and recently of isotretinoin have been found out only after wide use of (Observational method) the drugs in pregnant women. The teratogenicity of the drugs (Experimental method) cannot be identified before approval of the drugs.

During the post marketing surveillance phase, the toxicity of fenfluramine and phentermine (appetite suppressants) the pulmonary hypertension and valvular heart disease have been revealed.

During the new drug status period of 4 years, the manufacturer is expected to report any new information about the drug like a rare side effects, a new clinical use, If any every six months for 2 years.

The information generated by pharmacovigilance is useful in educating doctor about Adverse Drug Reaction and in the official regulation of drug use. It has been important role in rational use of medicines, as it provides the basis for assessing safety of medicines.

The activities involved in pharmacovigilance are:

1. To monitor Adverse drug reaction: It is monitored the data received from post marketing surveillance, from voluntary report from doctor, prescription event, computerized medical report linkage as well as anecdotal case reports doctors. Even rare reaction can be detected by this method.

2. Bring awareness of Adverse Drug Reaction data through "drug alert", "medical letter", advisories sent to doctors by pharmaceuticals and regulatory agencies to take further necessary actions.

3. Instruction is to be given to the pharmaceutical companies to change in labeling of medicines indicating restriction in use or statuary warning, precautions or even withdrawal of drug.

So, WHO advised that every country should maintain a pharmaco-vigilance centre on 'safety monitoring of Medicinal products'.

Set up of pharmacovigilance centres in india:

In India, the pharmacovigilance centre is set up (in AIIMS, New- delhi) by drugs controller general of India under central drugs standard control organization (CDSCO).

National Pharmacovigilance centre
↓
Zonal Center → Two zonal centres
↑ ↓
Regional centre ← Four regional centers
↑ ↓
← Twenty eight pharmacovigilance centers
↓

Information fed to any of the peripheral centre (The data)

- The national pharmacovigilance centre will analyse the data, and how to manage those adverse effects or recommend to withdraw the drug from the market or recommend the new clinical use of the drug.
- The data base will be forwarded to global centre (WHO, Uppsala monitoring centre, Sweden), under the safety data exchange agreements.
- The signal or the data on the uses and risks of the new or old drug can be generated further by pharmacoepidemiological studies (Study of the effects of the drug when used in general population).

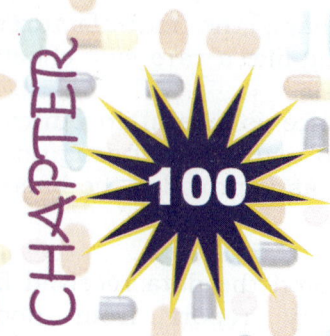

Geriatric and pediatric pharmacology

CHAPTER 100

GERIATRIC PHARMACOLOGY

In the elderly all the systems and organs progressively decline in function and structure. Especially renal function progressively declines due to loss of nephron and hence the drug dose have to be reduced. There is also a decline in the hepatic microsomal drug metabolizing activity even the blood flow to the liver and intestine is normal. This will have impact on the drug metabolism, drug absorption and hence the oral bioavailability. There is also lower plasma protein binding due to decreased plasma albumin.

The volume of distribution is increased or decreased due to hydrophilic or lipophilic nature of the drugs. The responsiveness and sensitivity to particular drugs is altered. For example: Due to prostatic enlargement, anticholinergic drugs should be used cautiously as it will lead to urinary retention.

The main concern in the drug therapy of elderly is renal clearance of drugs. The common formula used to calculate the creatinine clearance is Cockcroft -Gault Equation.

Creatinine clearance (male) (140 – Age) x weight in kg / Serum creatinine x 72 kg

Sex = male (1), Female (0.85)

clearance of drugs primarily excreted unchanged e.g. aminoglycosides are reduced parallel to decrease in creatinine clearance. A rough guideline is given below :

Correct dose = Normal adult dose x (patient's creatinine clearance / normal creatinine clearance) i.e. 100 ml/min

Creatinine clearance (Cr)	Dose rate
50 ml/min	50% of the adult dose
30 ml/min	30% of the adult dose
10 ml/min	10% of the adult dose
5 ml/min	5% of the adult dose

Poly pharmacy is very common in the elderly due to intake of multiple drugs such as antihypertensives, antiischemic drugs and antidiabetics which may lead to adverse drug interactions. The prescribing physician must limit the number of drugs in the elderly and prevent drug interactions. The drug interactions are proportional to the number of drugs prescribed.

Altered drug response in elderly

Geriatric patients are more sensitive to many drugs due to altered pharmacodynamic interactions with their receptors and diminished homeostatic response.

In elderly patients, the homeostatic response like damped baroreceptor reflex is seen. Hence, the reflex tachycardia is often blunted in the elderly after vasodilators therapy. In adult there is reflux tachycardia for hypotension.

Another common disorder seen in elderly persons are alzheimer's disease, due to the age-related deficiency of cholinergic transmission in CNS of the elderly.

Temperature regulation is also impaired in the elderly.

There is reduced response of β_2 agonists in the elderly. High dose of β_2 agonists is needed in elderly asthamatic patients.

Adverse reactions of the drugs are also high in elderly when compare to young adult.

Chronic use of some drugs in elderly will lead to vitamins deficiency, which are to be supplemented.

Age is an important physiological factor in the consideration of drug reactions and drug interactions. Studies indicate that there is an increased incidence of adverse drug reactions in geriatric patients. It is suggested that the risk of drug interactions in the patients of 60-70 years old is almost double to that in adults of 30-40 years old.

PEDIATRIC PHARMACOLOGY

The safety of drug usage in children is of paramount importance. The children may develop adverse drug reactions physiologically or iatrogenically. The pediatric population includes new born infants, infants, children and adolescents. Substantial physiological changes in body proportions and composition with growth and development occurs in pediatric population.The body fat, protein and extracellular water also change during childhood. The major organs like liver, kidney also change during growth, development and proportionately their functions.

Gastrointestinal tract and oral absorption of drugs are different from the adult. Gastric secretion is less, gastric emptying time is prolonged, excessive gastro-oesophageal reflux are seen in paediatrics. Distribution of medicine is altered due to high extracellular volume. Hepatic and renal function and elimination process is altered in the neonates and children. Hepatic drug metabolizing systems are inadequate in new borns e.g. Chloramphenicol can cause gray baby syndrome.

Blood brain barrier is more permeable to bilirubin and drugs which displace bilirubin can cause kernicterus e.g. Sulfonamides.

The elimination capacity of many drugs may even increase than the adults which makes administration of higher dose. Information about pharmacodynamic changes is limited still medicine targets such as receptors, transporters and channels are subject to developmental process.

The dose of a drug for children is calculated by following formulae :

Young's formula : Child's dose = Age/Age+12 x Adult dose

Dilling's formula: Child's dose = Age/20 X adult dose

On the basis of body weight.

Child's dose = (Weight of the child (lb) x Adult dose) / 150

More accurate dose is calculated on Body Surface Area (BSA)

Dubois formula BSA (m^2) = BW (kg)$^{0.425}$ x Height (cm)$^{0.725}$ x 0.007184

Some drugs are contraindicated/avoided in Children only. Example hydroxyl-chloroquine and Ethambutol cause optic nerve damage which lead to colour blindness, when they are used for long term. If it is found out earlier, the drug can be withdrawn to reverse that side effects, before going to severe condition (blindness). But children cannot reveal the defect in time and later on the condition becomes worse. So it is contraindicated in children below six years.

Some drugs are to be avoided in children. For example, Ethambutol is a antitubercular drug. Long term use of this drug causes night blindness (impairing visual acuity and red-green colour discrimination). This adverse effect is reversible after discontinuation of the drug. In adults, the defect can be found out earlier and the drug will be withdrawn. But in the case children (below 5 years) where it is difficult to assess the defect and later on it will lead to blindness. So, it is better to avoid ethambutol and hydroxyl chloroquine in children.
Tetracyclines in children are to be avoided because it leads to complexes with Ca++ in teeth and bones. They cause bone and teeth deformities in children.

However, the dose recommendations based on BSA are used only for anticancer and immunosuppressive drugs.

Children are growing and are susceptible to special adverse effects e.g suppression of growth with corticosteroids. Androgens may cause early fusion of epiphysis and short stature. Therefore it is mandatory to exercise caution in prescribing drugs to paediatric population and follow the dosage calculations to prevent unwanted drug effects.

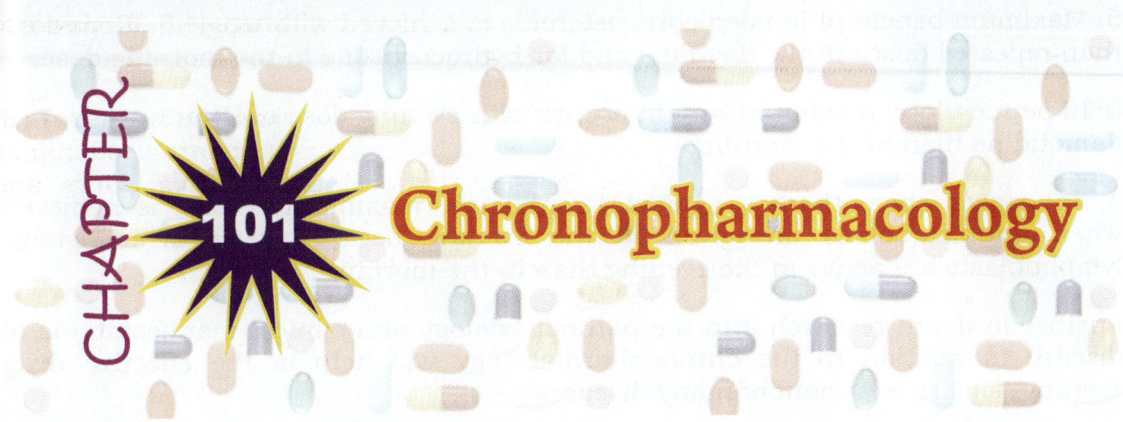

101 Chronopharmacology

Chronopharmacology is a science concerned with the effects of drugs upon the timing of biological processes and rhythms. It links the effects of drugs on biological clock to obtain dynamic activity. Chronopharmocokinetics is branch of chronopharmacology which deals with the changes in the pharmacokinetic parameters of the drugs with time.

There is synchrony between day and night cycles and the biological activities in the body. The pathophysiology of many diseases like bronchial asthma, Cardiovascular diseases, peptic ulcer etc results in exacerbation of symptoms in relation to time. Many drugs are given without considering the time of the day. To increase the therapeutic effect and to reduce the adverse effects of drugs it is important to administer drugs at most appropriate time of the day. The influence of circadian rhythms on pharmacological effects of drugs have become a big challenge for drug discovery and drug delivery.

Examples of disease conditions where chronopharmacology is currently applied are in cardiovascular diseases e.g. Hypertension, Ischemic heart diseases. Bronchial asthma, Peptic ulcer, Cancer chemotherapy etc.

1. Maximum B.P. reduction occurs with morning dose of ACE inhibitor like Enalapril.

2. Maximum vasodilatation occurs with morning dose of nitrates.

3. Maximum lipid lowering effect occurs for HMG COA reductase inhibitors e.g. Atorvastatin with night dose, because the enzyme is more active in the night time and cholesterol synthesis is also more in the night time.

4. Maximum brochodilatation occurs with evening 3 pm timed release theophylline, thereby achieving maximum bronchodilatation in the night and less side effects during day time.

5. Maximum benefit of inhaled corticosteroids is achieved with single 5.30pm dose than repeated doses in the day time and for hydrocortisone in the morning dose.

6. In peptic ulcer, maximum benefit occurs with evening dose of H_2 antagonist e.g. Famotidine than in the morning.

7. In cancer chemotherapy against lymphomas, maximum benefit is achieved when antimetabolites are given in the evening because residual malignant lymphoblasts are active in the evening than in the morning.

Further in depth research into the pathophysiology and clinical manifestations of disease in relation to the chronopharmacology will help in the effective drug therapy for the treatment of many diseases.

References :

1. Principles of Pharmacology, 2nd edition, By : HL. Sharma and KK. Sharma
2. Essentials of medical pharmacology, 6th edition, By : KD. Tripathi.

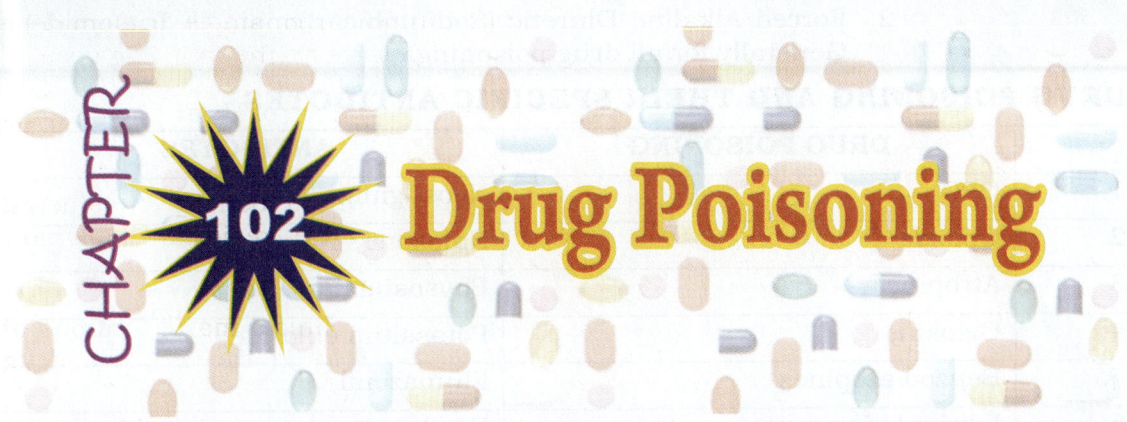

CHAPTER **102** **Drug Poisoning**

Poisoning means, which results from large dose of drugs endangering life by severely affecting one or more vital functions. Drugs, insecticides and other industrial products are also capable of producing poison in large dose. The type of poisoning can be detected by observing the signs and symptoms or by asking the relatives the possible type of poison the patient consumed. Once the poison is confirmed, the specific antidote is given, if available.

Whether the antidote is available or not, the following measures to be taken immediately

I. General measures
 1. Maintain the patent airway (Artificial respiration)
 2. Maintain B.P. and electrolytes balance

II. Termination of exposure:
 1. if the patient consumes volatile substance, the skin is washed thoroughly to remove the poison in order to prevent its absorption from the skin
 2. Gastric lavage: The gastric lavage is selected either to neutralize or to remove the unabsorbed poison, if it is consumed orally (Examples. Potassium permanganate, Activated charcoal (1 G/Kg). But many organic substances are not neutralized. Charcoal should not be tried in paralytic ileus.

III: Hastening elimination: (Fig:16.`C)
 1. By alkalinisation: In Phenobarbitone poisoining, its concentrasion is excess in the blood and so it is filtered as such (in the active form) without undergoing metabolism. Being an acidic drug, Phenobarbitone in normal acidic urine gets unionized, lipid soluble and reabsorbed and increase the blood level of Phenobarbitone and aggravate the poison. So, if the urine is made alkaline by IV Sodium bicarbonate, the active Phenobarbitone gets ionized, not reabsorbed from the urinary tract and excreted in the urine. In the same way the urine is made more acidic by Ammonium chloride/Ascorbic acid in case of poision due to basic drugs like Pethidine

2. Forced Alkaline Diuretic (Sodiumbicarbonate + frusemide) : Generally for all drug poisoning.

DRUG POISONING AND THEIR SPECIFIC ANTIDOTES

	DRUG POISONING	ANTIDOTES
1.	OPC	Neostigmine +Atropine
2.	Opioids	Naloxone/ Naltrexone
3.	Atropine	Physostigmine
4.	Digoxine	Potassium chloride
5.	Benzodiazepines	Flumazenil
6.	Fibrinolytic agents	Epsilon Amino caproic acid
7.	Heparin	Protamine sulphate
8.	Insulin	IV Glucose
9.	Warfarin sodium	Vit.K
10.	Heavy metals	Chelating agents++

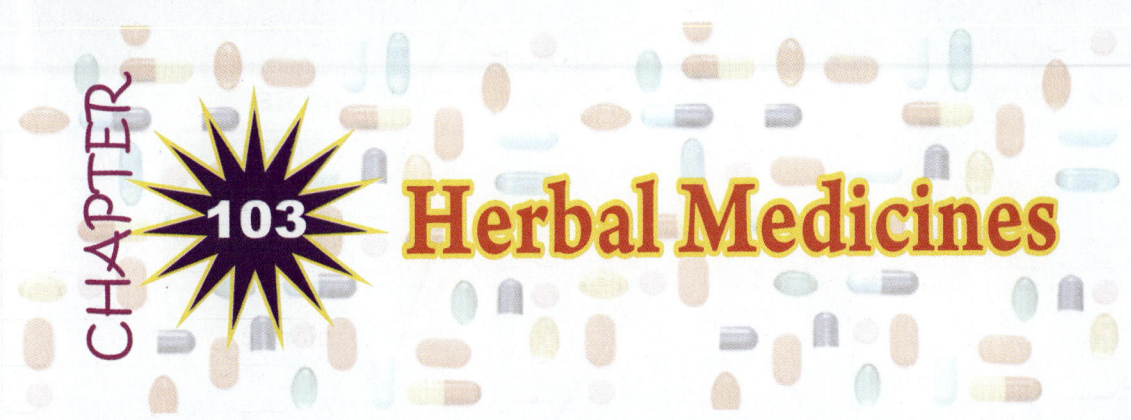

CHAPTER 103 Herbal Medicines

It is very clear that name for a drug is given from "drough" (French word, means herb). Most of the drugs used earlier are derived from herbs . Even though many drugs have been synthesized, the herbal medicines still occupy the important place in the treatment chronic diseases, since there is no side effects noticed even after a long period.. But they are slow acting and may not be suitable for immediate effect.. But they are cheap. They are also useful in some diseases which are not cured by modern medicines.

Some examples of successful herbal medicines and some are in research process.

1.	Bambusa arundinacea	Antiinflammatory and antiulcer (no allopaathy medicine is having both actions together)
2.	Ginger	prevents vomiting due to pregnancy
3.	Liv-52	effective liver tonic
4.	Artemesia annua	Artemisinine derivatives (Antimalarial)
5.	Aloe vera	Many uses (antiseptic, dandruff etc.)
6.	Neem	Antiseptic
7.	Manjal (haldi)	Antidiabetic, antiseptic
8.	Bitter gourd	Antidiabetic
9.	Drumstick	Aphrodisiac
10.	ALkALOIDS	Atropine, chloroquine, Ephedrine, Vincristine etc.
11.	Digitalis purpurea	Digoxin

-and many more herbals are in research progress

Homeopathy, Ayurveda, Siddha doctors prescribe herbal medicines

INDEX